2010
YEAR BOOK OF
**CRITICAL CARE
MEDICINE**®

The 2010 Year Book Series

Year Book of Anesthesiology and Pain Management™: Drs Chestnut, Abram, Black, Gravlee, Lee, Mathru, and Roizen

Year Book of Cardiology®: Drs Gersh, Cheitlin, Elliott, Graham, Sundt, and Waldo

Year Book of Critical Care Medicine®: Drs Dellinger, Parrillo, Balk, Dorman, Dries, and Zanotti-Cavazzoni

Year Book of Dermatology and Dermatologic Surgery™: Drs Thiers and Lang

Year Book of Diagnostic Radiology®: Drs Osborn, Abbara, Birdwell, Elster, Levy, Manaster, Oestreich, Offiah, Rosado de Christenson, and Walker

Year Book of Emergency Medicine®: Drs Hamilton, Bruno, Handly, Mullin, Quintana, and Ramoska

Year Book of Endocrinology®: Drs Schott, Apovian, Clarke, Eugster, Ludlam, Meikle, Ovalle, Schinner, Schteingart, and Toth

Year Book of Gastroenterology™: Drs Talley, Dempsey, Harnois, Lange, Pearson, Picco, Rombeau, and Scolapio

Year Book of Hand and Upper Limb Surgery®: Drs Yao and Steinmann

Year Book of Medicine®: Drs Barker, Berney, Garrick, Gersh, Khardori, LeRoith, Talley, and Thigpen

Year Book of Neonatal and Perinatal Medicine®: Drs Fanaroff, Benitz, Neu, and Papile

Year Book of Neurology and Neurosurgery®: Drs Klimo and Rabinstein

Year Book of Obstetrics, Gynecology, and Women's Health®: Drs Dungan and Shulman

Year Book of Oncology®: Drs Thigpen, Arceci, Bauer, Byhardt, Gordon, and Lawton

Year Book of Ophthalmology®: Drs Rapuano, Cohen, Eagle, Flanders, Hammersmith, Myers, Nelson, Penne, Sergott, Shields, Tipperman, and Vander

Year Book of Orthopedics®: Drs Morrey, Beauchamp, Huddleston, Swiontkowski, and Trigg

Year Book of Otolaryngology-Head and Neck Surgery®: Drs Sindwani, Balough, Franco, Gapany, and Mitchell

Year Book of Pathology and Laboratory Medicine®: Drs Raab, Parwani, Bejarano, and Bissell

Year Book of Pediatrics®: Dr Stockman

Year Book of Plastic and Aesthetic Surgery™: Drs Miller, Gosain, Gurtner, Gutowski, Ruberg, Salisbury, and Smith

Year Book of Psychiatry and Applied Mental Health®: Drs Talbott, Ballenger, Buckley, Frances, Krupnick, and Mack

Year Book of Pulmonary Disease®: Drs Barker, Jones, Maurer, Raza, Tanoue, and Willsie

Year Book of Sports Medicine®: Drs Shephard, Cantu, Feldman, Jankowski, Khan, Nieman, Pierrynowski, and Rowland

Year Book of Surgery®: Drs Copeland, Bland, Daly, Eberlein, Fahey, Jones, Mozingo, Pruett, and Seeger

Year Book of Urology®: Drs Andriole and Coplen

Year Book of Vascular Surgery®: Drs Moneta, Gillespie, Starnes, and Watkins

2010

The Year Book of CRITICAL CARE MEDICINE®

Editors-in-Chief:

R. Phillip Dellinger, MD
Professor of Medicine, Robert Wood Johnson Medical School, University of Medicine and Dentistry of New Jersey; Head, Division of Critical Care Medicine; Director, Medical/Surgical Intensive Care Unit, Cooper University Hospital, Camden, New Jersey

Joseph E. Parrillo, MD
Professor of Medicine, Robert Wood Johnson Medical School, University of Medicine and Dentistry of New Jersey; Chief, Department of Medicine, Edward D. Viner MD Chair, Department of Medicine; Director, Cooper Heart Institute, Cooper University Hospital, Camden, New Jersey

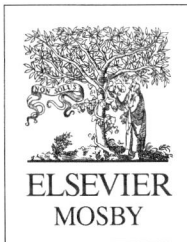

ELSEVIER
MOSBY

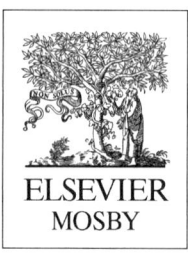

ELSEVIER
MOSBY

Vice President, Continuity: John A. Schrefer
Associate Developmental Editor: Yonah Korngold
Production Supervisor, Electronic Year Books: Donna M. Skelton
Electronic Article Manager: Jennifer C. Pitts
Illustrations and Permissions Coordinator: Dawn Vohsen

2010 EDITION

Printed in the United States of America
Composition by TNQ Books and Journals Pvt Ltd, India
Printing/binding by Sheridan Books, Inc.

Editorial Office:
Elsevier
Suite 1800
1600 John F. Kennedy Blvd.
Philadelphia, PA 19103-2899

International Standard Serial Number: 0734-3299
International Standard Book Number: 978-0-323-06826-0

Associate Editors

Robert A. Balk, MD
J. Bailey Carter, MD, Professor of Medicine, Rush Medical College; Director, Division of Pulmonary and Critical Care Medicine, Rush University Medical Center, Chicago, Illinois

Todd Dorman, MD
Associate Dean and Director of Continuing Medical Education; Professor and Vice-Chair for Critical Care Services; Departments of Anesthesiology/Critical Care Medicine, Internal Medicine, Surgery, and the School of Nursing, The Johns Hopkins University, Baltimore, Maryland

David J. Dries, MSE, MD
John F. Perry, Jr. Professor, Department of Surgery, University of Minnesota; Assistant Medical Director for Surgical Care, HealthPartners Medical Group, Minneapolis, Minnesota; Director of Critical Care Services and Director of Academic Programs, Regions Hospital, St. Paul, Minnesota

Sergio L. Zanotti-Cavazzoni, MD
Assistant Professor of Medicine, Robert Wood Johnson Medical School, University of Medicine and Dentistry of New Jersey; Program Director, Critical Care Fellowship, Division of Critical Care Medicine, Cooper University Hospital, Camden, New Jersey

Guest Editors

Guest Editor for Gastroenterology
Christopher W. Deitch, MD
*Assistant Professor of Medicine, Robert Wood Johnson Medical School,
University of Medicine and Dentistry of New Jersey; Division of
Gastroenterology, Cooper University Hospital, Camden, New Jersey*

Guest Editor for Transfusion in the Critically Ill
David R. Gerber, DO
*Associate Professor of Medicine, Robert Wood Johnson Medical School,
University of Medicine and Dentistry of New Jersey; Associate Director, Medical/
Surgical Intensive Care Unit, Cooper University Hospital, Camden, New Jersey*

Guest Editor for Infection
Anand Kumar, MD
*Associate Professor of Medicine, Robert Wood Johnson Medical College,
University of Medicine and Dentistry of New Jersey, Camden, New Jersey;
Division of Critical Care Medicine and Division of Infectious Diseases, Cooper
University Hospital, Camden, New Jersey; Associate Professor of Medicine,
Sections of Critical Care Medicine and Infectious Disease, University of
Manitoba, Winnipeg, Canada*

Guest Editor for Burns
Barbara A. Latenser, MD
*Clara L. Smith Professor of Burn Treatment, Department of Surgery, University
of Iowa; Director, Burn Treatment Center, University of Iowa Healthcare, Iowa
City, Iowa*

Guest Editor for Neurologic Care
Kiwon Lee, MD
*Assistant Professor, Neurology and Neurological Surgery, Columbia University
College of Physicians and Surgeons; Faculty Attending Staff, Neurological
Intensive Care Unit, New York Presbyterian Hospital, Columbia University
Medical Center, New York, New York*

Guest Editor for Postoperative Critical Care
Elizabeth A. Martinez, MD, MHS
*Associate Professor of Anesthesia/Critical Care Medicine and Surgery; Medical
Director, Adult Post Anesthesia Care Units, Johns Hopkins University School of
Medicine, Johns Hopkins Medical Institutions, Baltimore, Maryland*

Guest Editor for Ethics
Vijay K. Rajput, MD
*Assistant Professor of Medicine, Robert Wood Johnson Medical School,
University of Medicine and Dentistry of New Jersey; Program Director,*

Internal Medicine Residency, Cooper University Hospital, Camden, New Jersey; Associate Fellow, Center for Bioethics, University of Pennsylvania, Philadelphia, Pennsylvania

Guest Editor for Critical Care Performance Improvement and ICU Administration
Christa A. Schorr, RN, BSN
Assistant Professor of Medicine, University of Medicine and Dentistry of New Jersey; Director of Databases for Quality Improvement and Research, Program Director of Clinical Industry Trials in Critical Care, Cooper University Hospital, Camden, New Jersey

Guest Editor for Emergency Medicine
Stephen Trzeciak, MD, MPH
Assistant Professor of Medicine and Emergency Medicine, Robert Wood Johnson Medical School, University of Medicine and Dentistry of New Jersey; Department of Emergency Medicine and Division of Critical Care Medicine, Cooper University Hospital, Camden, New Jersey

Guest Editor for Nephrology and Poisoning/Overdose
Lawrence S. Weisberg, MD
Professor of Medicine, Robert Wood Johnson Medical School, University of Medicine and Dentistry of New Jersey; Head, Division of Nephrology, Cooper University Hospital, Camden, New Jersey

Guest Editor for Cardiology
Steven W. Werns, MD
Professor of Medicine, Robert Wood Johnson Medical School, University of Medicine and Dentistry of New Jersey; Director, Invasive Cardiovascular Services, Cooper University Hospital, Camden, New Jersey

Contributing Editors

Sharon M. Dostmann, JD
Deputy General Counsel, Legal Affairs, Cooper University Hospital, Camden, New Jersey

Duane Funk, MD, FRCP(C)
Assistant Professor of Anesthesia, University of Manitoba; Department of Anesthesia and Section of Critical Care Medicine, Winnipeg Health Sciences Center, Winnipeg, Manitoba, Canada

Zoulficar A. Kobeissi, MD
Department of Internal Medicine, Division of Critical Care, Methodist Hospital, Houston, Texas

Salimah H. Meghani, PhD, MBE, CRNP
Assistant Professor of Nursing, Associate Fellow of Bioethics, Biobehavioral and Health Sciences Division, University of Pennsylvania, Philadelphia, Pennsylvania

Sundip N. Patel, MD
Assistant Professor of Emergency Medicine, Robert Wood Johnson Medical School, University of Medicine and Dentistry of New Jersey; Clerkship Director of Medical Student Program, Department of Emergency Medicine, Cooper University Hospital, Camden, New Jersey

Collaborative Reviewers

Dhvani Doshi, BA
Medical Student, Robert Wood Johnson Medical School, University of Medicine and Dentistry of New Jersey, Piscataway, New Jersey

Shravan Kethireddy, MD
Postdoctoral Fellow, Department of Medicine, Section of Critical Care, University of Manitoba, Winnipeg, Canada

Munira Mehta, MD
Resident, Department of Medicine, Division of Internal Medicine, Cooper University Hospital, Camden, New Jersey

Ami A. Naik, BS
Medical Student, Robert Wood Johnson Medical School, University of Medicine and Dentistry of New Jersey, Camden, New Jersey

Raj Parekh, BA, BS
Medical Student, Robert Wood Johnson Medical School, University of Medicine and Dentistry of New Jersey, Piscataway, New Jersey

Utkal Patel, MD
Chief Resident, Department of Medicine, Division of Internal Medicine, Cooper University Hospital, Camden, New Jersey

Vivek Punjabi, MD
Resident, Department of Medicine, Division of Internal Medicine, Cooper University Hospital, Camden, New Jersey

Jean-Sebastien Rachoin, MD
Postdoctoral Fellow, Department of Medicine, Division of Critical Care Medicine, Cooper University Hospital, Camden, New Jersey

Kristin Robinson, BS
Medical Student, Robert Wood Johnson Medical School, University of Medicine and Dentistry of New Jersey, Camden, New Jersey

Nathan Samras, BSE, MPH
Medical Student, Robert Wood Johnson Medical School, University of Medicine and Dentistry of New Jersey, Camden, New Jersey

Imran Shariff, MD
Resident, Department of Medicine, Division of Internal Medicine, Cooper University Hospital, Camden, New Jersey

Hiren Shingala, MD
Postdoctoral Fellow, Department of Medicine, Division of Pulmonary/Critical Care Medicine, Cooper University Hospital, Camden, New Jersey

Table of Contents

Journals Represented

Journals represented in this YEAR BOOK are listed below.

Academic Emergency Medicine
Acta Anaesthesiologica Scandinavica
AJR American Journal of Roentgenology
American Heart Journal
American Journal of Emergency Medicine
American Journal of Gastroenterology
American Journal of Infection Control
American Journal of Neuroradiology
American Journal of Respiratory and Critical Care Medicine
American Journal of Surgery
American Surgeon
Anaesthesia
Anaesthesia and Intensive Care
Anesthesia & Analgesia
Anesthesiology
Annals of Internal Medicine
Annals of Neurology
Annals of Surgery
Annals of Thoracic Surgery
Archives of Neurology
Archives of Surgery
Brain Research
British Journal of Anaesthesia
British Journal of Radiology
British Journal of Surgery
Burns
Canadian Journal of Anaesthesia
Chest
Circulation
Clinical Infectious Diseases
Clinical Nuclear Medicine
Critical Care Medicine
European Journal of Internal Medicine
European Journal of Vascular and Endovascular Surgery
European Heart Journal
European Respiratory Journal
Gastrointestinal Endoscopy
Injury
Intensive Care Medicine
International Journal of Cardiology
Journal of Applied Physiology
Journal of Burn Care & Research
Journal of Cardiothoracic and Vascular Anesthesia
Journal of Clinical Neuroscience
Journal of Computer Assisted Tomography
Journal of Critical Care
Journal of Cutaneous Pathology

Journal of Emergency Medicine
Journal of Neurology Neurosurgery and Psychiatry
Journal of Neurosurgery
Journal of Pain and Symptom Management
Journal of Stroke and Cerebrovascular Diseases
Journal of Surgical Research
Journal of Vascular and Interventional Radiology
Journal of the American College of Cardiology
Journal of the American College of Surgeons
Journal of the American Medical Association
Journal of the Neurological Sciences
Journal of Trauma
Kidney International
Lancet
Mayo Clinic Proceedings
Neurosurgery
New England Journal of Medicine
Radiology
Seizure
Stroke
Surgery
Thorax
Thrombosis Research
Transfusion
Translational Research
Transplantation Proceedings
World Journal of Surgery

STANDARD ABBREVIATIONS

The following terms are abbreviated in this edition: acquired immunodeficiency syndrome (AIDS), cardiopulmonary resuscitation (CPR), central nervous system (CNS), cerebrospinal fluid (CSF), computed tomography (CT), deoxyribonucleic acid (DNA), electrocardiography (ECG), health maintenance organization (HMO), human immunodeficiency virus (HIV), intensive care unit (ICU), intramuscular (IM), intravenous (IV), magnetic resonance (MR) imaging (MRI), and ribonucleic acid (RNA).

NOTE

The YEAR BOOK OF CRITICAL CARE MEDICINE® is a literature survey service providing abstracts of articles published in the professional literature. Every effort is made to assure the accuracy of the information presented in these pages. Neither the editors nor the publisher of the YEAR BOOK OF CRITICAL CARE MEDICINE® can be responsible for errors in the original materials. The editors' comments are their own opinions. Mention of specific products within this publication does not constitute endorsement.

To facilitate the use of the YEAR BOOK OF CRITICAL CARE MEDICINE® as a reference tool, all illustrations and tables included in this publication are now identified as they appear in the original article. This change is meant to help the reader recognize that any illustration or table appearing in the YEAR BOOK OF CRITICAL CARE MEDICINE® may be only one of many in the original article. For this reason, figure and table numbers will often appear to be out of sequence within the YEAR BOOK OF CRITICAL CARE MEDICINE®.

1 Airways/Lungs

Acute Lung Injury/Acute Respiratory Distress Syndrome

The impact of the PAI-1 4G/5G polymorphism on the outcome of patients with ALI/ARDS

Tsangaris I, Tsantes A, Bonovas S, et al (Univ of Athens, Greece; Ctr for Diseases Control & Prevention, Athens, Greece)
Thromb Res 123:832-836, 2009

Introduction.—Increased levels of plasminogen activator inhibitor-1 (PAI-1) have been associated with worse outcome in ALI/ARDS. A single guanosine insertion/deletion (4G/5G) polymorphism in the promoter region of the PAI-1 gene, may play an important role in the regulation of PAI-1 expression. The objective of the study was to evaluate the effect of this polymorphism on the outcome of critically ill patients with ALI/ARDS.

Materials and Methods.—52 consecutive ventilated patients with ALI/ARDS were studied. Bronchoalveolar lavage was performed within 48 hours from diagnosis. Measurement of plasma and BALF PAI-1 activity and D-dimers levels, and 4G/5G genotyping of PAI-1 were carried out. The primary outcome was 28-day mortality, and secondary outcomes included organ dysfunction and ventilator-free days.

Results.—17 patients were homozygotes for the 4G allele. Severity scores were not different between subgroups upon study enrollment. 28-day mortality was 70.6% and 42.9% for the 4G-4G and the non-4G-4G patients, respectively (p = 0.06). PAI-1 activity levels and D-dimer in plasma and BALF were not significantly different between the 4G-4G and the non-4G-4G subgroups. In the multivariate analysis, genotype 4G/4G was the only variable independently associated with 28-day mortality (Odds Ratio = 9.95, 95% CI: 1.79-55.28, p = 0.009). Furthermore, genotype 4G/4G and plasma PAI-1 activity levels were independently negatively associated with ventilator free days (p = 0.033 and p = 0.008, respectively).

Conclusions.—ALI/ARDS patients, homozygous for the 4G allele of the PAI-1 gene, experienced higher 28-day mortality. This genotype was associated with a reduction in the number of days of unassisted ventilation and

TABLE 1.—Patients' Characteristics

	4G/4G (n = 17)	4G/5G and 5G/5G (n = 35)	P-value
Sex (male)	47.1%	68.6%	0.14
Age	63.2 ± 15.7	66.1 ± 16.9	0.43
Direct/Indirect	8/9	15/20	0.78
APACHE score	18.1 ± 6.1	20.2 ± 6.1	0.08
SOFA score	7.7 ± 3.7	8.6 ± 3.2	0.43
Lung injury score	2.5 ± 0.6	2.4 ± 0.6	0.81
PAI-1 activity in plasma (U/ml)	5.6 ± 1.6	5.4 ± 2.0	0.85
PAI-1 activity in alveolar fluid (U/ml)	0.22 ± 0.31	0.23 ± 0.48	0.91
D-dimer levels in plasma (ng/ml)	528.8 ± 468.2	624.3 ± 638.3	0.77
D-dimer levels in alveolar fluid (ng/ml)	310.1 ± 167.2	224.9 ± 198.2	0.10
28-day mortality	70.6%	42.9%	0.06
Days of unassisted ventilation	2.6 ± 5.2	7.1 ± 9.5	0.09
Days without organ failure besides lung	5.5 ± 8.9	10.5 ± 11.0	0.09

Data are presented as means ± SD, or percentages, when appropriate.

was inversely associated with the number of days without organ failure (Table 1).

▶ There has been consensus acknowledgement that sepsis, the systemic inflammatory response syndrome (SIRS), and sequelae such as acute lung injury (ALI), acute respiratory distress syndrome (ARDS), and multiple organ dysfunction syndrome (MODS) involve an interaction of the inflammatory pathways as well as the coagulation cascade. This interesting observation evaluated changes in plasminogen activator inhibitor function as a consequence of genetic polymorphism and found a potential marker to identify patients with a high risk of mortality. Although this represents only a small number of observations, the finding suggests the potential to uncover a true predictive marker for increased mortality and possibly a clue into the mechanism(s) of more severe disease. At this time, this exciting observation needs to be confirmed in a larger number of patients with well defined ALI and ARDS. If the observation continues to hold true, then perhaps some defined intervention may be used to improve outcome in these high-risk patients.

R. A. Balk, MD

A comparison of methods to identify open-lung PEEP
Caramez MP, Kacmarek RM, Helmy M, et al (Massachusetts General Hosp, Boston; et al)
Intensive Care Med 35:740-747, 2009

Purpose.—Many methods exist in the literature for identifying PEEP to set in ARDS patients following a lung recruitment maneuver (RM). We compared ten published parameters for setting PEEP following a RM.

Methods.—Lung injury was induced by bilateral lung lavage in 14 female Dorset sheep, yielding a PaO_2 100–150 mmHg at F_IO_2 1.0 and PEEP 5 cmH_2O. A quasi-static P–V curve was then performed using the supersyringe method; PEEP was set to 20 cmH_2O and a RM performed with pressure control ventilation (inspiratory pressure set to 40–50 cmH_2O), until $PaO_2 + PaCO_2 > 400$ mmHg. Following the RM, a decremental PEEP trial was performed. The PEEP was decreased in 1 cmH_2O steps every 5 min until 15 cmH_2O was reached. Parameters measured during the decremental PEEP trial were compared with parameters obtained from the P–V curve.

Results.—For setting PEEP, maximum dynamic tidal respiratory compliance, maximum PaO_2, maximum $PaO_2 + PaCO_2$, and minimum shunt calculated during the decremental PEEP trial, and the lower Pflex and point of maximal compliance increase on the inflation limb of the P–V curve (Pmci,i) were statistically indistinguishable. The PEEP value obtained using the deflation upper Pflex and the point of maximal compliance decrease on the deflation limb were significantly higher, and the true inflection point on the inflation limb and minimum $PaCO_2$ were significantly lower than the other variables.

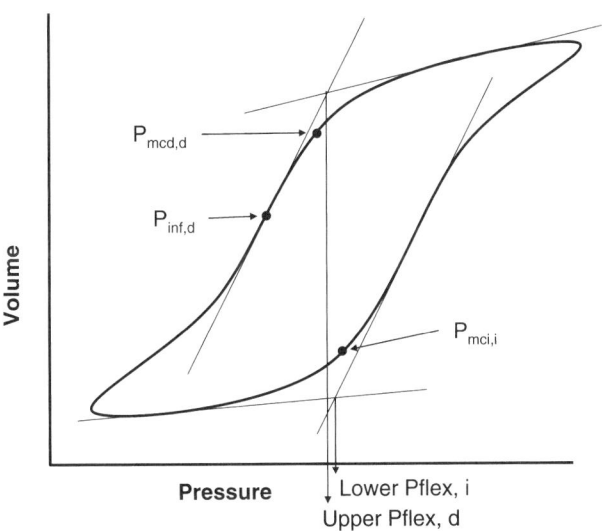

FIGURE 1.—Examples of different points on the P–V curve that have been proposed for setting PEEP. The lower inflection point of the inflation limb (lower Pflex,i) is identified by the intersection of two lines, one drawn through a region of low compliance at the beginning of inflation and one through the region of highest compliance. A similar method is done for the upper inflection point of the deflation limb (upper Pflex,d). The point of maximum compliance increase on the inflation limb (Pmci,i), point of maximum compliance decrease on the deflation limb (Pmcd,d) and true inflection point of the deflation limb (Pinf,d) are calculated from the curve-fitting parameters of the equation $V = a + b/(1 + e^{-(P - c)/d})$ [28, 29]. Editor's Note: Please refer to original journal article for full references. (Reprinted from Caramez MP, Kacmarek RM, Helmy M, et al. A comparison of methods to identify open-lung PEEP. *Intensive Care Med.* 2009;35:740-747, with permission from Springer-Verlag.)

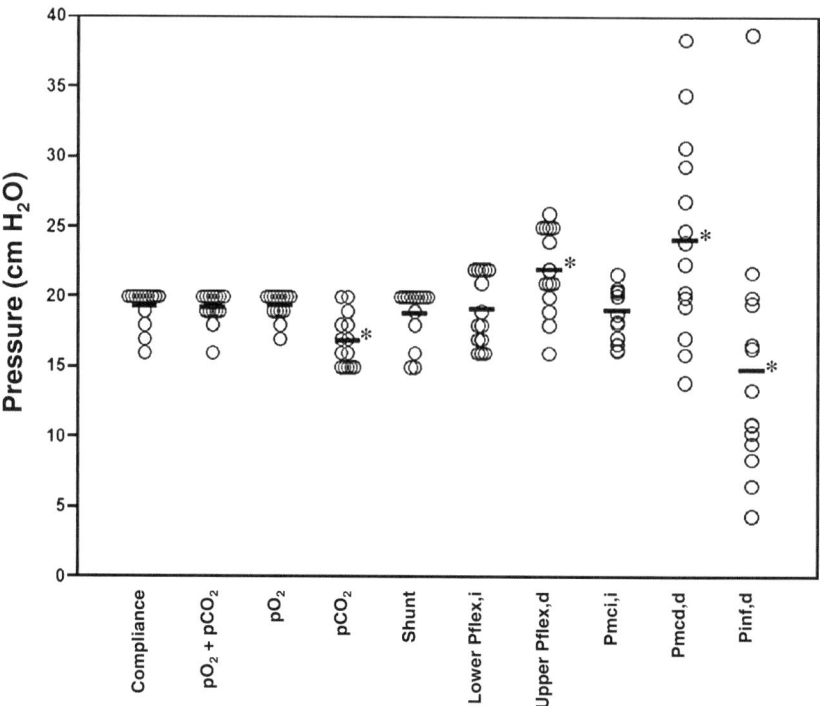

FIGURE 3.—Open-lung PEEP identified by ten different methods: Compliance, $PaO_2 + PaCO_2$, PaO_2, $PaCO_2$, shunt, inflation lower Pflex (Lower Pflex,i), deflation upper Pflex (Upper Pflex,d), point of maximum compliance increase on inflation (Pmci,i), point of maximum compliance decrease on deflation (Pmcd,d), and true inflection point of the deflation limb (Pinf,d). The *bars* represents mean values, the *open circles* are actual values for each animal. *$P < 0.05$ compared to all other variables. (Reprinted from Caramez MP, Kacmarek RM, Helmy M, et al. A comparison of methods to identify open-lung PEEP. *Intensive Care Med.* 2009;35:740-747, with permission from Springer-Verlag.)

Conclusion.—In this animal model of ARDS, dynamic tidal respiratory compliance, maximum PaO_2, maximum $PaO_2 + PaCO_2$, minimum shunt, inflation lower Pflex and Pmci,i yield similar values for PEEP following a recruitment maneuver (Figs 1 and 3).

▶ The best PEEP to use in the management of a patient with acute lung injury (ALI) or the acute respiratory distress syndrome (ARDS) has been a topic of debate almost since the initial description of ARDS in the late 1960s. While this study is an animal model of ARDS and may not be purely applicable to the human ALI/ARDS, it nonetheless, presents a good review of many of the techniques and end points that have been used to determine the best level of PEEP to use. The current recommendation for PEEP dosing in managing patients with ALI/ARDS is to use the ARDS network nomogram for PEEP and F_IO_2 titration.[1] However, a recent trial has suggested that using an esophageal pressure to guide PEEP dosing in ALI will result in improved outcome.[2]

In my opinion, at this time the ARDS network strategy has been shown to improve outcome in patient with ALI and ARDS and this strategy for ventilatory management, including PEEP dosing, should be the one we use as the standard of care until another large, prospective, multicenter trial leads us to a different conclusion.

R. A. Balk, MD

References

1. Ventilation with lower tidal volumes as compared with traditional tidal volumes for acute lung injury and the acute respiratory distress syndrome. The Acute Respiratory Distress Syndrome Network. *N Engl J Med.* 2000;342:1301-1308.
2. Talmor D, Sarge T, Malhotra A, et al. Mechanical ventilation guided by esophageal pressure in acute lung injury. *N Engl J Med.* 2008;359:2095-2104.

A 6-year review of total parenteral nutrition use and association with late-onset acute respiratory distress syndrome among ventilated trauma victims
Plurad D, Green D, Inaba K, et al (Univ of Southern California and Los Angeles County Hosp)
Injury 40:511-515, 2009

Aim.—To establish whether total parenteral nutrition (TPN) for ventilated trauma victims is associated with late-onset acute respiratory distress syndrome (ARDS) independent of ventilation and transfusion parameters.

Method.—Intensive care unit data over 6 years from a level I centre regarding all trauma victims ≥16 years old who underwent mechanical ventilation within the first 48 h of admission were examined. Patients were prospectively followed for late ARDS. Variables were examined for significant changes over time and independent associations with late ARDS were determined.

Results.—Of 2346 eligible patients among whom 404 (17.2%) were exposed to TPN, 192 (8.2%) met criteria for late ARDS. The incidence of late ARDS among those exposed to TPN was 28.7% (116/404) compared with 3.9% (76/1942) among those not so exposed. Adjustments for potential confounding associated risk factors were made.

Conclusions.—TPN administration is independently associated with late ARDS, and its use among critically ill trauma victims should be carefully scrutinised.

▶ Despite the inherent feeling by the critical care specialist that nutrients are necessary to sustain life during periods of critical illness, data on providing these nutrients by the parenteral route to improve survival is lacking. Although considerable literature exists that supports enteral feedings (and early enteral feeding), in the critically ill patient similar data for total parenteral nutrition (TPN) is lacking. The body has multiple amazing and complex methods for keeping the human engine going without external provision of fuels over an extended period of time. Interventions that were common place in the trauma and postoperative patient population in years past such as red blood cell transfusion and TPN now appear to be reserved for special cases and are not designated for general use. However, a decision for early enteral feeding appears to be in the patient's best interest.

R. P. Dellinger, MD

Exogenous Natural Surfactant for Treatment of Acute Lung Injury and the Acute Respiratory Distress Syndrome
Kesecioglu J, Beale R, Stewart TE, et al (Univ Med Ctr Utrecht, the Netherlands; Guy's and St Thomas' NHS Foundation Trust, London, UK; Univ of Toronto, Canada; et al)
Am J Respir Crit Care Med 180:989-994, 2009

Rationale.—Compositional changes in surfactant and/or decreased surfactant content of the lungs are common features in patients with acute respiratory failure. Instillation of exogenous surfactant into the lungs of neonates with respiratory distress syndrome or pediatric patients with acute respiratory distress syndrome (ARDS) has resulted in improved survival.

Objectives.—We conducted this trial to determine whether the instillation of exogenous surfactant would improve the Day 28 outcome of adult patients with acute lung injury (ALI) or ARDS.

Methods.—A total of 418 patients with ALI and ARDS were included in an international, multicenter, stratified, randomized, controlled, open, parallel-group study. We randomly assigned 418 patients to receive usual care either with or without instillation of exogenous natural porcine surfactant HL 10 as large boluses.

Measurements and Main Results.—The primary endpoint was death rate before or on Day 28. Secondary endpoints were adverse event and death rate on day 180. The 28-day death rate in the usual care group was 24.5% compared with 28.8% in the HL 10 group. The estimated odds ratio for death at Day 28 in the usual care group versus the HL10 group was 0.75 (95% CI, 0.48–1.18; $P = 0.22$). The most common adverse events related to HL 10 administration were temporary hypoxemia defined as oxygen saturation less than 88% (51.9% in HL 10 group vs. 25.2% in usual care) and hypotension defined as mean arterial blood pressure less than 60 mm Hg (34.1% in HL 10 group vs. 17.1% in usual care).

Conclusions.—In this study, instillation of a large bolus of exogenous natural porcine surfactant HL 10 into patients with acute lung injury and ARDS did not improve outcome and showed a trend toward increased mortality and adverse effects. Clinical trial registered with www. clinicaltrials.gov (NCT 00742482).

▶ The chalkboard logic for surfactant therapy of acute respiratory distress syndrome (ARDS) has always been appealing. Disruption of surfactant is one of the more reliable laboratory methods for producing ARDS. Natural surfactant has also been demonstrated to have anti-inflammatory effects in addition to capability to maintain open alveoli. Initial attempts with surfactant therapy in clinical trials failed to show benefit, but always with the question of whether it was delivered to the site of action. These initial trials were synthetic surfactants. This clinical trial used exogenous natural surfactant and again fails to show benefit with some suggestion that the therapy might even be harmful. Despite all the failures there continues to be discussion about the effect of surfactant on inflammation and whether different delivery techniques might still produce benefit.

R. P. Dellinger, MD

Diagnosing acute lung injury in the critically ill: a national survey among critical care physicians
Vlaar APJ, Honselaar WB, Binnekade JM, et al (Academic Med Ctr, Amsterdam, The Netherlands; et al)
Acta Anaesthesiol Scand 53:1293-1299, 2009

Background.—Incidence reports on acute lung injury (ALI) vary widely. An insight into the diagnostic preferences of critical care physicians when diagnosing ALI may improve identification of the ALI patient population.

Methods.—Critical care physicians in the Netherlands were surveyed using vignettes involving hypothetical patients and a questionnaire. The vignettes varied in seven diagnostic determinants based on the North American European Consensus Conference and the lung injury score. Preferences were analyzed using a mixed-effects logistic regression model and presented as an odds ratio (OR) with a 95% confidence interval.

Results.—From 243 surveys sent to 30 hospitals, 101 were returned (42%). ORs were as follows: chest X-ray consistent with ALI: OR 1.7 (1.3–2.3), high positive end-expiratory pressure (PEEP) (15 cmH$_2$O): OR 5.0 (3.9–6.6), low pulmonary artery occlusion pressures (PAOP) (<18 mmHg): OR 4.7 (3.6–6.1), low compliance (30 ml/cmH$_2$O): OR 0.7 (0.5–0.9), low PaO$_2$/FiO$_2$ (<250 mmHg): OR 9.2 (6.9–12.3), absence of heart failure: OR 1.2 (0.9–1.5), presence of a risk factor for ALI (sepsis): OR 1.0 (0.8–1.3). The questionnaire revealed that critical care physicians with an anesthesiology background differed from physicians with an internal medicine background with regard to hemodynamic variables when considering an ALI diagnosis ($P < 0.05$).

Conclusions.—Dutch critical care physicians consider the PEEP level, but not the presence of a risk factor for ALI, as an important factor to diagnose ALI. Background specialty of critical care physicians influences diagnostic preferences and may account for variance in the reported incidence of ALI.

▶ This study of critical care physicians in the Netherlands is revealing in quantifying how critical care physicians prioritize patient variables as to the likelihood of acute respiratory distress syndrome (ARDS). The value of greatest importance is a low PaO_2/FiO_2 ratio, followed by significant PEEP application, followed by low left heart filling pressures. Not having a history of heart failure or an admission diagnosis of sepsis did not play a key role. It is likely that since sepsis is a very common diagnosis, the presence of sepsis itself is not considered a major link to infiltrates being acute lung injury. Intensivists also likely relied more on current variables and less on history for their diagnostic suspicions.

R. P. Dellinger, MD

A multicenter, randomized, double-blind, placebo-controlled, dose-escalation trial assessing safety and efficacy of active site inactivated recombinant factor VIIa in subjects with acute lung injury or acute respiratory distress syndrome
Vincent J-L, Artigas A, Petersen LC, et al (Université libre de Bruxelles, Belgium; CIBER Enfermedades Respiratorias Autonomous Univ of Barcelona, Spain; Novo Nordisk, Bagsvaerd, Denmark)
Crit Care Med 37:1874-1880, 2009

Objective.—To evaluate the safety and efficacy of active site inactivated recombinant factor VIIa (FFR-rFVIIa) in patients with acute respiratory distress syndrome.

Design.—Phase II, randomized, double-blind, placebo-controlled, dose-escalation trial.

Setting.—Forty-six intensive care units (ICU) in ten countries.

Patients.—All adult ($\geq$18 years), mechanically ventilated patients with acute onset (within 48 hour) of acute lung injury/acute respiratory distress syndrome were included.

Interventions.—Four sequential (in ascending order) treatment groups (cohorts) in single and multiple dosing strategies. Subjects were randomized in a 2:1 ratio to either FFR-rFVIIa or placebo within each cohort.

Measurements and Results.—Data were collected daily for 7 days and on days 14 and 28 for efficacy variables including hematology and coagulation parameters, plasma D-dimer levels, plasma interleukin-6 levels, vital signs, ventilator parameters, lung injury score, and Sequential Organ Failure Assessment score. The study was discontinued prematurely by the Safety Committee based on statistical analysis of the mortality in cohort 3 (4×400 µg/kg), which suggested that, after adjusting for prognostic covariates, 28-day mortality was significantly higher in this cohort than in the placebo group and time to death was significantly shorter. A total of 214 patients (147 male) were included in the trial, mean age 59 years (range, 24–85 years). Overall, there were no significant differences in mortality rates in treated and placebo patients (36/144 deaths FFR-rFVIIa, 15/70 placebo). There was no treatment effect of FFR-rFVIIa on vital signs, blood chemistry parameters, hematology parameters, or amount of transfusion products required. There was a trend to increased bleeding with increasing FFR-rFVIIa dose.

Conclusion.—In this randomized double-blind, placebo-controlled, dose-escalation trial, FFR-rFVIIa had no beneficial effects on morbidity or outcome overall. The cohort of patients receiving 4×400 µg/kg of FFR-rFVIIa had increased mortality rates compared with placebo-treated patients, and there was a trend to increased risk of serious bleeding with increasing doses.

▶ There has been considerable interest in tissue factor (TF) as a trigger for the procoagulant pathway of sepsis and acute lung injury. This is particularly true in light of the integration of procoagulation activation with proinflammatory state and vice versa. TF pathway inhibition has been studied in patients with severe sepsis without evidence of clinical benefit. Another molecule that counters the procoagulant state of severe sepsis, rhAPC, was shown in one large clinical trial to provide benefit. Other anticoagulant compounds continue to be in development – such as soluble thrombomodulin. It is known that patients with acute lung injury have both proinflammatory and procoagulant states. Factor VIIa is most familiar to critical care physicians as the last resort for severe life-threatening hemorrhage. The compound studied in this trail was FFR-rFVIIa, a modified recombinant FVIIa. It is targeted to be an inactive recombinant FVIIa that retains TF binding capacity. This phase 1A study would be classified as failing to support additional development of this compound because there was no trend in better clinical outcome, but more importantly FFR-rFVIIa treatment did not decrease D-dimer or IL-6 levels.

R. P. Dellinger, MD

Recent trends in acute lung injury mortality: 1996–2005
Erickson SE, Martin GS, Davis JL, et al (Emory Univ, Atlanta, GA; Univ of California, San Francisco)
Crit Care Med 37:1574-1579, 2009

Objective.—Studies from single centers have suggested that mortality from acute lung injury (ALI) has declined over time. However, recent trends in ALI mortality from centers across the United States are unknown. We sought to determine whether recent advances in the treatment of ALI and related critical illnesses have resulted in decreased mortality from ALI.

Design.—Retrospective cohort study of patients enrolled in the Acute Respiratory Distress Syndrome (ARDS) Network randomized controlled trials.

Setting.—Adult intensive care units participating in the ARDS Network trials.

Patients.—2,451 mechanically ventilated patients with ALI enrolled in the ARDS Network randomized controlled trials between 1996 and 2005.

Measurements and Main Results.—Crude mortality was 35% in 1996–1997 and declined during each subsequent time period to a low of 26% in 2004–2005 (test for trend $p < 0.0005$). After adjusting for demographic and clinical covariates, including receipt of lower tidal volume ventilation and severity of illness, the temporal trend persisted (test for trend $p = 0.002$). When analyzed by individual causes of lung injury, there were not any statistically significant temporal trends in 60-day mortality for the most common causes of lung injury (pneumonia, sepsis, aspiration, and trauma).

Conclusions.—Over the past decade, there seems to be a clear temporal improvement in survival among patients with ALI treated at ARDS Network centers. Our findings strongly suggest that other advancements in critical care, aside from lower tidal volume ventilation, accounted for this improvement in mortality.

▶ Not only is the acute respiratory distress syndrome (ARDS) Network a valuable entity because it carries out government funded clinical trials to ascertain best therapy for ARDS, but it also gives us an opportunity to look at change in mortality over time in ARDS patients. Since most of the ARDS net studies enroll patients with common definition entry criteria, this is a very homogenous population over time. The significant reduction in mortality between 1996-2005 is also highlighted by data analysis support for this being driven more by nonARDS management factors. Another 4 years have gone by since 2005, and with the author's intimation that improvement in sepsis management may be a reason this changes over time, the role of the Surviving Sepsis Campaign performance improvement program that began in 2005 may intimate that mortality has continued to decrease.

R. P. Dellinger, MD

Cost-effectiveness of Implementing Low-Tidal Volume Ventilation in Patients With Acute Lung Injury
Cooke CR, Kahn JM, Watkins TR, et al (Univ of Washington, Seattle; Univ of Pennsylvania, Philadelphia; et al)
Chest 136:79-88, 2009

Background.—Despite widespread guidelines recommending the use of lung-protective ventilation (LPV) in patients with acute lung injury (ALI), many patients do not receive this lifesaving therapy. We sought to estimate the incremental clinical and economic outcomes associated with LPV and determined the maximum cost of a hypothetical intervention to improve adherence with LPV that remained cost-effective.

Methods.—Adopting a societal perspective, we developed a theoretical decision model to determine the cost-effectiveness of LPV compared to non-LPV care. Model inputs were derived from the literature and a large population-based cohort of patients with ALI. Cost-effectiveness was determined as the cost per life saved and the cost per quality-adjusted life-years (QALYs) gained.

Results.—Application of LPV resulted in an increase in QALYs gained by 15% (4.21 years for non-LPV vs 4.83 years for LPV), and an increase in lifetime costs of $7,233 per patient with ALI ($99,588 for non-LPV vs $106,821 for LPV). The incremental cost-effectiveness ratios for LPV were $22,566 per life saved at hospital discharge and $11,690 per QALY gained. The maximum, cost-effective, per patient investment in a hypothetical program to improve LPV adherence from 50 to 90% was $9,482. Results were robust to a wide range of economic and patient parameter assumptions.

Conclusions.—Even a costly intervention to improve adherence with low-tidal volume ventilation in patients with ALI reduces death and is cost-effective by current societal standards.

▶ It is approaching 10 years since the first landmark ARDSnet trial compared ventilation with lower tidal volumes versus traditional tidal volumes for acute lung injury and acute respiratory distress syndrome. This has changed and continues to change the way we mechanically ventilate patients with acute lung injury with regard to size of tidal volume. It is generally accepted that an initial target tidal volume of 6 mL/kg predicted body weight followed by additional lowering of tidal volume if necessary to achieve an inspiratory plateau pressure of 30 cm H_2O is best practice. However, this best practice is not necessarily followed on a day-to-day basis, especially with some physicians and in some institutions. As we discuss national health policy with a fervor not seen in our lifetime, we should pay attention to studies such as this one demonstrating that paying up to approximately $10 000 per patient to increase low tidal volume compliance from 50% to 90% is cost effective. The take-home message here is that the costs of assuring that this strategy is followed is not $10 000; it is minimal. Therefore, this is low-hanging fruit for cost-effective medicine.

R. P. Dellinger, MD

Surviving critical illness: Acute respiratory distress syndrome as experienced by patients and their caregivers
Cox CE, Docherty SL, Brandon DH, et al (Duke Univ, Durham, NC; Duke Univ School of Nursing, Durham, NC; et al)
Crit Care Med 37:2702-2708, 2009

Objective.—To characterize the effects of critical illness in the daily lives and functioning of acute respiratory distress syndrome survivors. Survivors of acute respiratory distress syndrome, a systemic critical illness, often report poor quality of life based on responses to standardized questionnaires. However, the experiences of acute respiratory distress syndrome survivors have not been reported.

Design.—We conducted semistructured interviews with 23 acute respiratory distress syndrome survivors and 24 caregivers 3 to 9 mos after intensive care unit admission, stopping enrollment after thematic saturation was reached. Transcripts were analyzed, using Colaizzi's qualitative methodology, to identify significant ways in which survivors' critical illness experience impacted their lives.

Setting.—Medical and surgical intensive care units of an academic medical center and a community hospital.

Patients.—We recruited consecutively 31 acute respiratory distress syndrome survivors and their informal caregivers. Eight patients died before completing interviews.

Interventions.—None.

Measurements and Main Results.—Participants related five key elements of experience as survivors of acute respiratory distress syndrome: 1) pervasive memories of critical care; 2) day-to-day impact of new disability; 3) critical illness defining the sense of self; 4) relationship strain and change; and 5) ability to cope with disability. Survivors described remarkable disability that persisted for months. Caregivers' interviews revealed substantial strain from caregiving responsibilities as well as frequent symptom minimization by patients.

Conclusions.—The diverse and unique experiences of acute respiratory distress syndrome survivors reflect the global impact of severe critical illness. We have identified symptom domains important to acute respiratory distress syndrome patients who are not well represented in existing health outcomes measures. These insights may aid the development of targeted interventions to enhance recovery and return of function after acute respiratory distress syndrome.

▶ There is a high prevalence and persistence of cognitive deficits among acute respiratory distress syndrome (ARDS) survivors that has been previously described.[1,2] The key addition to the literature from this paper is the underappreciation of this occurrence with long-term follow-up by physicians and the dismissal of this possibility by the physician once the patient reports these findings. Much work needs to be done with interventions targeting ICU-acquired weakness in ARDS patients as well as aggressive rehabilitation

programs targeting not only motor but also cognitive defect. It might be postulated that a long-term follow-up meeting with patients, intensivists, and chronic
caregivers would be important to fix intervention plans.

R. P. Dellinger, MD

References

1. Larson MJ, Weaver LK, Hopkins RO. Cognitive sequelae in acute respiratory
distress syndrome patients with and without recall of the intensive care unit.
J Int Neuropsychol Soc. 2007;13:595-605.
2. Hopkins RO, Weaver LK, Collingridge D, et al. Two-year cognitive, emotional
and quality-of-life outcomes in acute respiratory distress syndrome. *Am J Respir
Crit Care Med.* 2005;171:340-347.

**Traumatic memories, post-traumatic stress disorder and serum cortisol
levels in long-term survivors of the acute respiratory distress syndrome**
Hauer D, Weis F, Krauseneck T, et al (Ludwig-Maximilians-Univ, Munich,
Germany; et al)
Brain Res 1293:114-120, 2009

Survivors of the acute respiratory distress syndrome (ARDS) often
report traumatic memories from the intensive care unit (ICU) and display
a high incidence of post-traumatic stress disorder (PTSD). As it is known
that subjects with PTSD often show sustained reductions in circulating
cortisol concentrations, we examined the relationship between serum
cortisol, traumatic memories and PTSD in patients after ARDS. We
evaluated 33 long-term survivors of ARDS (7.5 ± 2.9 years after discharge
from the ICU) for pre-defined categories of traumatic memory from the
ICU, hypothalamic–pituitary–adrenocortical axis reactivity to cortico-
tropin and PTSD (by psychiatric interview). During evaluation, patients
with multiple traumatic memories had significantly lower basal serum
cortisol levels when compared to patients with no or only 1 category of
traumatic memory, with no differences in peak cortisol levels after cortico-
tropin stimulation between both subgroups. There was a significant
negative correlation between basal cortisol levels and the number of
traumatic memories present. PTSD symptom scores correlated with the
number of traumatic memories but not with cortisol levels. These findings
indicate that lower baseline cortisol levels in long-term survivors of ARDS
are associated with an increased incidence of traumatic memories from the
ICU, and that more traumatic memories are related to a higher incidence
and intensity of PTSD symptoms.

▶ This is a must-read article for those who provide chronic care for patients
having experienced acute respiratory distress syndrome (ARDS). ARDS
patients have significant long-term sequelae to include minimal but measurable
pulmonary dysfunction, neurocognitive defects, posttraumatic stress disorder,
and traumatic memories. This article, although retrospective in nature, offers

strong support for the posttraumatic stress disorder and traumatic memories being linked to low cortisol levels. This becomes even more fascinating when looking at literature that reveals prolonged administration of glucocorticoids during septic shock or cardiac surgery results in reduced posttraumatic stress disorder and chronic stress symptoms in long-term survivors.[1] Low-dose hydrocortisone has also been shown in small studies to improve symptomatology.[2]

R. P. Dellinger, MD

References

1. Schelling G, Briegel J, Roozendaal B, Stoll C, Rothenhäusler HB, Kapfhammer HP. The effect of stress doses of hydrocortisone during septic shock on posttraumatic stress disorder in Survivors. *Biol Psychiatry.* 2001;50:978-985.
2. Schelling G, Kilger E, Roozendaal B, et al. Stress doses of hydrocortisone, traumatic memories and post-traumatic stress disorder in patients after cardiac surgery: a randomized study. *Biol Psychiatry.* 2004;55:627-633.

ECMO in ARDS: a long-term follow-up study regarding pulmonary morphology and function and health-related quality of life
Lindén VB, Lidegran MK, Frisén G, et al (Karolinska Univ Hosp, Stockholm, Sweden)
Acta Anaesthesiol Scand 53:489-495, 2009

Background.—A high survival rate can be achieved in patients with severe acute respiratory distress syndrome (ARDS) using extracorporeal membrane oxygenation (ECMO). The technique and the costs are, however, debated and follow-up studies in survivors are few. The aim of this study was to evaluate long-term pulmonary health after ECMO and severe ARDS.

Methods.—Twenty-one long-term survivors of severe ARDS and ECMO were studied in a follow-up program including high-resolution computed tomography (HRCT) of the lungs, extensive pulmonary function tests, pulmonary scintigraphy and the pulmonary disease-specific St George's Respiratory Questionnaire (SGRQ).

Results.—The majority of patients had residual lung parenchymal changes on HRCT suggestive of fibrosis, but the extension of morphologic abnormalities was limited and without the typical anterior localization presumed to indicate ventilator-associated lung injury. Pulmonary function tests revealed good restitution with mean values in the lower normal range, while $T_{\frac{1}{2}}$ for outwash of inhaled isotope was abnormal in all patients consistent with subclinical obstructivity. Most patients had reduced health-related quality of life (HRQoL), according to the SGRQ, but were stating less respiratory symptoms than conventionally treated ARDS patients in previous studies. The majority were integrated in normal work.

Conclusion.—The majority of ECMO-treated ARDS patients have good physical and social functioning. However, lung parenchymal changes on HRCT suggestive of fibrosis and minor pulmonary function abnormalities remain common and can be detected more than 1 year after ECMO. Furthermore, most patients experience a reduction in HRQoL due to the pulmonary sequelae.

▶ Although integrating intermediate and longer term follow-up of critical care patients is part of the critical care training program, it is difficult to offer first-hand accounts of health-related quality of life late after ICU care. The publication of literature such as this which can be presented to trainees and established intensivists as well and remind us of long-term impact of critical illness despite in those patients being perceived a "save" at the time of discharge from the ICU and hospital. It has long been known that pulmonary parenchymal changes as detected by high-resolution CT persist and are suggestive of minor pulmonary function abnormalities. These are likely less debilitating than quality of life issues that influence family and job capabilities.

R. P. Dellinger, MD

Hypercapnia in late-phase ALI/ARDS: providing spontaneous breathing using pumpless extracorporeal lung assist
Weber-Carstens S, Bercker S, Hommel M, et al (Universitätsmedizin Berlin, Germany; Univ of Leipzig, Germany)
Intensive Care Med 35:1100-1105, 2009

Objective.—The fibroproliferative phase of late ALI/ARDS as described by Hudson and Hough is associated with pronounced reductions in pulmonary compliance and an accompanying hypercapnia complicating low tidal volume mechanical ventilation. We report the effects of extracorporeal CO_2 removal by means of a novel pumpless extracorporeal lung assist (p-ECLA) on tidal volumes, airway pressures, breathing patterns and sedation management in pneumonia patients during late-phase ARDS.

Design.—Retrospective analysis.

Setting.—Fourteen-bed university hospital ICU.

Patients.—Ten consecutive late-phase ALI/ARDS patients with low pulmonary compliance, and severe hypercapnia.

Intervention.—Gas exchange, tidal volumes, airway pressures, breathing patterns and sedation requirements before (baseline) and after (2–4 days) initiation of treatment with p-ECLA were analysed. Patients were ventilated in a pressure-controlled mode with PEEP adjusted to pre-defined oxygenation goals.

Measurements and Main Results.—Median reduction in pCO_2 was 50% following institution of p-ECLA. Extracorporeal CO_2 removal enabled significant reduction in tidal volumes (to below 4 mL/kg predicted body weight) and inspiratory plateau pressures [30 (28.5/32.3) cmH_2O, median 25, 75% percentiles]. Normalization of pCO_2 levels permitted significant reduction in the dosages of analgesics and sedatives. The proportion of assisted spontaneous breathing increased within 24 h of instituting p-ECLA.

Conclusion.—Elimination of CO_2 by p-ECLA therapy allowed reduction of ventilator-induced shear stress through ventilation with tidal volumes below 4 mL/kg predicted body weight in pneumonia patients with severely impaired pulmonary compliance during late-phase ARDS. p-ECLA treatment supported control of breathing pattern while sedation requirements were reduced and facilitated the implementation of assisted spontaneous breathing.

▶ From a conceptual standpoint, extracorporeal membrane oxygenation and extracorporeal CO_2 elimination are very appealing in acute respiratory distress syndrome (ARDS) patients with severe refractory hypoxemia and high airway pressures, despite maximization of current ARDSnet strategy. Despite this conceptual potential, all randomized trials of these technologies have failed to show improvement in clinical outcome. In this novel experiment, pumpless extracorporeal lung assist was used to facilitate elimination of CO_2 with the hypothesis that this would allow tidal volumes of 4 mL/kg predicted body weight to be used and tolerated with assisted ventilation. I have witnessed intolerance of low tidal volume ventilations on many occasions, but never considered whether the patient's drive was related to CO_2 or primary dislike of the low tidal air movement. The results of this study would support that CO_2 is at least a major factor in tolerance, and with this technique low tidal volumes with less sedation can be used.

R. P. Dellinger, MD

Airway

Tracheostomy in the Intensive Care Unit: A Nationwide Survey
Kluge S, Baumann HJ, Maier C, et al (Univ Med Ctr, Hamburg-Eppendorf, Germany)
Anesth Analg 107:1639-1643, 2008

Background.—The indication, timing and technique of tracheostomy have changed over the last several years. We performed a survey to assess the current practice of tracheostomy in German intensive care units (ICUs).

Methods.—A postal questionnaire was sent to the head physicians of 513 German ICUs, excluding pediatric ICUs.

Results.—We obtained responses from 455 of the 513 ICUs (89%). In 90% of the ICUs, tracheostomies were performed during the first 14 d of mechanical ventilation. Eighty-six percent of the ICUs routinely performed percutaneous dilatational tracheostomy; the modified Ciaglia technique was the most popular percutaneous technique (69%). The majority (98%) of the percutaneous procedures were performed under bronchoscopic control. Surgical tracheostomy is usually performed in the operating room (72%) by a surgeon (61%), whereas percutaneous dilatational tracheostomies are usually performed at the patient's bedside in the ICU (98%) by an intensivist (93%). Tracheostomized patients were followed up routinely in 26% of the ICUs, and in 45% of the ICUs there were guidelines regarding the indication, the timing and the technique of tracheostomy.

Conclusion.—Percutaneous dilatational tracheostomy is the procedure of choice for tracheostomy in critically ill patients in Germany. The modified Ciaglia technique is the preferred percutaneous technique, and nearly all physicians routinely use bronchoscopic guidance. Most tracheostomies are done during the second week of mechanical ventilation.

▶ The performance of bedside percutaneous dilational tracheostomy appears to be the predominant procedure for prolonged airway management in most of the European ICUs and particularly in the United Kingdom and Germany. From this survey study, it appears that most use bronchoscopic guidance, and the procedure is typically performed within the first 2 weeks of ventilatory support. I would expect this practice to continue to gain in popularity, and it will be interesting to see what happens to the timing of the procedure as changes occur in ventilatory management and reimbursement overtime.

R. A. Balk, MD

Etomidate versus ketamine for rapid sequence intubation in acutely ill patients: a multicentre randomised controlled trial

Jabre P, on behalf of the KETASED Collaborative Study Group (Université Paris 13, Bobigny, France; et al)
Lancet 374:293-300, 2009

Background.—Critically ill patients often require emergency intubation. The use of etomidate as the sedative agent in this context has been challenged because it might cause a reversible adrenal insufficiency, potentially associated with increased in-hospital morbidity. We compared early and 28-day morbidity after a single dose of etomidate or ketamine used for emergency endotracheal intubation of critically ill patients.

Methods.—In this randomised, controlled, single-blind trial, 655 patients who needed sedation for emergency intubation were prospectively enrolled from 12 emergency medical services or emergency departments and 65 intensive care units in France. Patients were randomly assigned by a computerised random-number generator list to receive 0·3 mg/kg of etomidate (n = 328) or 2 mg/kg of ketamine (n = 327) for intubation. Only the emergency physician enrolling patients was aware of group assignment. The primary endpoint was the maximum score of the sequential organ failure assessment during the first 3 days in the intensive care unit. We excluded from the analysis patients who died before reaching

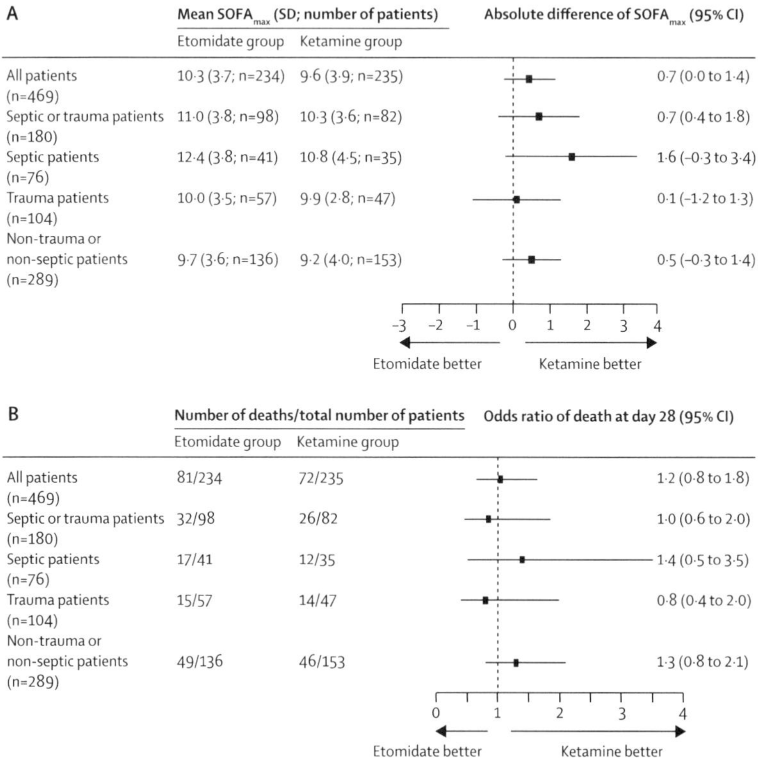

A

	Mean SOFA$_{max}$ (SD; number of patients)		Absolute difference of SOFA$_{max}$ (95% CI)
	Etomidate group	Ketamine group	
All patients (n=469)	10·3 (3·7; n=234)	9·6 (3·9; n=235)	0·7 (0·0 to 1·4)
Septic or trauma patients (n=180)	11·0 (3·8; n=98)	10·3 (3·6; n=82)	0·7 (0·4 to 1·8)
Septic patients (n=76)	12·4 (3·8; n=41)	10·8 (4·5; n=35)	1·6 (−0·3 to 3·4)
Trauma patients (n=104)	10·0 (3·5; n=57)	9·9 (2·8; n=47)	0·1 (−1·2 to 1·3)
Non-trauma or non-septic patients (n=289)	9·7 (3·6; n=136)	9·2 (4·0; n=153)	0·5 (−0·3 to 1·4)

−3 −2 −1 0 1 2 3 4

← Etomidate better   Ketamine better →

B

	Number of deaths/total number of patients		Odds ratio of death at day 28 (95% CI)
	Etomidate group	Ketamine group	
All patients (n=469)	81/234	72/235	1·2 (0·8 to 1·8)
Septic or trauma patients (n=180)	32/98	26/82	1·0 (0·6 to 2·0)
Septic patients (n=76)	17/41	12/35	1·4 (0·5 to 3·5)
Trauma patients (n=104)	15/57	14/47	0·8 (0·4 to 2·0)
Non-trauma or non-septic patients (n=289)	49/136	46/153	1·3 (0·8 to 2·1)

0 1 2 3 4

← Etomidate better   Ketamine better →

FIGURE 3.—Outcomes of patients receiving etomidate or ketamine for emergency intubation according to subgroups (A) Absolute difference in maximum score on the sequential organ failure assessment (SOFA$_{max}$). (B) Death within 28 days. (Reprinted from Jabre P, on behalf of the KETASED Collaborative Study Group. Etomidate versus ketamine for rapid sequence intubation in acutely ill patients: a multicentre randomised controlled trial. *Lancet*. 2009;374:293-300, with permission from Elsevier.)

the hospital or those discharged from the intensive care unit before 3 days (modified intention to treat). This trial is registered with ClinicalTrials.gov, number NCT00440102.

Findings.—234 patients were analysed in the etomidate group and 235 in the ketamine group. The mean maximum SOFA score between the two groups did not differ significantly (10·3 [SD 3·7] for etomidate *vs* 9·6 [3·9] for ketamine; mean difference 0·7 [95% CI 0·0–1·4], p = 0·056). Intubation conditions did not differ significantly between the two groups (median intubation difficulty score 1 [IQR 0–3] in both groups; p = 0·70). The percentage of patients with adrenal insufficiency was significantly higher in the etomidate group than in the ketamine group (OR 6·7, 3·5–12·7). We recorded no serious adverse events with either study drug.

TABLE 3.—Adrenal Function Assessment in Study Patients†

	Etomidate (n = 116)	Ketamine (n = 116)	p value
Cortisol (nmol/L; median [IQR])			
Baseline	441 (304–717)	690 (469–938)	<0·0001
30 min after ACTH test	497 (331–800)	911 (690–1131)	<0·0001
60 min after ACTH test	524 (386–828)	1048 (776–1324)	<0·0001
Non-responder in ACTH test (n [%, 95% CI])*	93 (81%, 76–86)	49 (42%, 36–48)	<0·0001
Adrenal insufficiency (n [%, 95% CI])	100 (86%, 82–90)	56 (48%, 42–54)	<0·0001

ACTH = adrenocorticotropin hormone.
*Patient was a non-responder if maximum change was less than 250 nmol/L.
†Patient had adrenal insufficiency if baseline cortisol was less than 276 nmol/L or the maximum change (peak cortisol minus baseline cortisol) was less than 250 nmol/L, or both.

Interpretation.—Our results show that ketamine is a safe and valuable alternative to etomidate for endotracheal intubation in critically ill patients, and should be considered in those with sepsis.

▶ Emergency control of the airway requires procedural skill and knowledge into the pharmacology and pharmacodynamics of induction agents. Such knowledge allows the practitioner to choose the best agent in each circumstance. The 2 most common induction agents, barbiturates, and propofol are typically not used in hemodynamically unstable patients as these can contribute to further instability. Thus, the debate usually comes down to etomidate versus ketamine. Previously, it was known that etomidate administration by infusion was associated with adrenal insufficiency and in the recent few years a growing body of data has supported the notion that even a single dose can lead to such an event thus possibly tipping the scale to the use of ketamine. Ketamine, however, directly inhibits myocardial contractility and provides hemodynamic stability through an indirect release of catecholamines; so many have thought that if the patient was already experiencing maximum catecholamine release that ketamine might also worsen instability. These authors have performed a randomized comparison of these 2 agents and have seemingly demonstrated that there was no difference in maximum sequential organ failure assessment (SOFA) score or mortality (Fig 3) and that the only identifiable difference was in a higher rate of adrenal insufficiency (Table 3). Unfortunately, only slightly more than 10% of patients in both groups were in shock at the time of enrollment, and thus the questions as to whether ketamine is better or equivalent in patients already in shock remains unanswered.

T. Dorman, MD

Effect of manual in-line stabilization of the cervical spine in adults on the rate of difficult orotracheal intubation by direct laryngoscopy: a randomized controlled trial

Thiboutot F, Nicole PC, Trépanier CA, et al (Univ of Ottawa, Ontario, Canada; Université Laval, Quebec City, Canada)
Can J Anesth 56:412-418, 2009

Purpose.—Although manual in-line stabilization (MILS) is commonly used during endotracheal intubation in patients with either known or suspected cervical spine instability, the effect of MILS on orotracheal intubation is poorly documented. This study evaluated the rate of failed tracheal intubation in a fixed time interval with MILS.

Methods.—Two hundred elective surgical patients were randomized into two groups. In the MILS group, the patient's head was stabilized in a neutral position by grasping the patient's mastoid processes to minimize any head movement during tracheal intubation. In the control group, the patient's head rested in an optimal position for tracheal intubation. A 30-sec period was allowed to complete tracheal intubation with a #3 Macintosh laryngoscope blade. The primary endpoint was the rate of failed tracheal intubation at 30 sec. Secondary endpoints included tracheal intubation time and the Cormack & Lehane grade of laryngoscopy.

Results.—Patient characteristics were similar with respect to demographic data and risk factors for difficult tracheal intubation. The rate of failed tracheal intubation at 30 sec was 50% (47/94) in the MILS group compared to 5.7% (6/105) in the control group (P < 0.0001). Laryngoscopic grades 3 and 4 were more frequently observed in the MILS group. Mean times for successful tracheal intubation were 15.8 ± 8.5 sec and 8.7 ± 4.6 sec for the MILS and control groups, respectively (mean difference 7.1, $CI_{95\%}$ 5.0–9.3, P < 0.0001). All patients who failed tracheal intubation in the MILS group were successfully intubated when MILS was removed.

Conclusion.—In patients with otherwise normal airways, MILS increases the tracheal intubation failure rate at 30 sec and worsens laryngeal visualization during direct laryngoscopy.

▶ This study intended to evaluate manual in-line stabilization in over 500 patients for elective intubation being performed by experienced anesthesiologists. The same individual performed all of the stabilization maneuvers. Only 200 patients were enrolled because the investigators thought that an interim analysis was required because they believed it would show a marked difference in the primary outcome. When that interim analysis indeed showed a difference, the study was stopped. It should be noted that early stopping of a study can impact the findings in very perverse manners that are not always predictable. As can be seen in Fig 1, all patients were ultimately intubated easily once in-line stabilization was removed. It should be noted, however, that all intubations were done with a single blade type and size, and no adjuncts such as cricoid pressure or intubating stylets was permitted. These restrictions may have

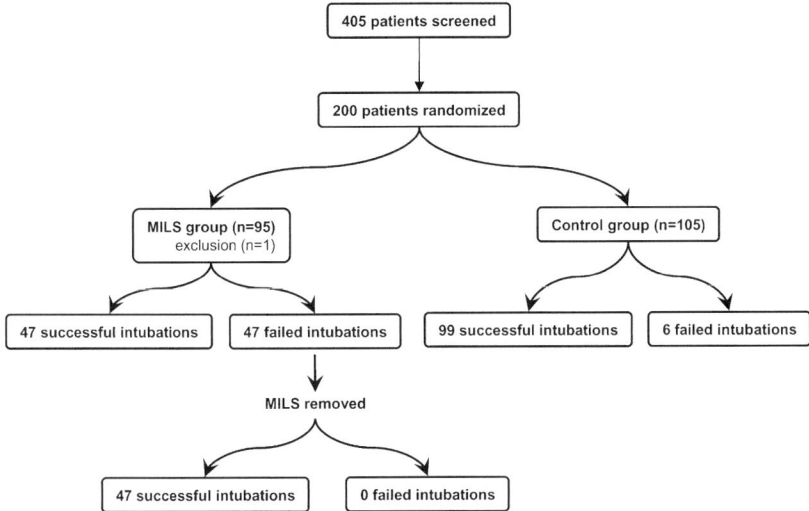

FIGURE 1.—Flow diagram of the experimental protocol. Patients of the MILS group who could not be successfully intubated within the first 30-sec attempt had MILS removed for the second tracheal intubation attempt. *MILS* manual in-line stabilization. (Reprinted from Thiboutot F, Nicole PC, Trépanier CA, et al. Effect of manual in-line stabilization of the cervical spine in adults on the rate of difficult orotracheal intubation by direct laryngoscopy: a randomized controlled trial. *Can J Anesth.* 2009;56:412-418.)

TABLE 2.—Tracheal Intubation Data

	MILS Group ($n = 94$)	Control Group ($n = 105$)	P
Failed tracheal intubation, no. (%)			
1st attempt[a]	47 (50.0)	6 (5.7)	<0.0001
2nd attempt[b]	0 (0.0)	–	
Intubation time (sec)[c]			
1st attempt[a]	15.8 ± 8.5	8.7 ± 4.6	<0.0001
Mean difference (CI$_{95\%}$)	7.1 (5.0–9.3)		
2nd attempt[b]	9.4 ± 4.2	–	
Cormack and Lehane grades[d]			
I	7 (7.4)	77 (73.3)	<0.0001
II	32 (34.0)	23 (21.9)	
III	44 (46.8)	5 (4.8)	
IV	11 (11.7)	0	

Data are presented as number and percentage or mean ± SD.

[a]1st attempt = number of failed tracheal intubations within the first 30-sec attempt.

[b]2nd attempt = number of failed tracheal intubations within the second 30-sec attempt with MILS removed, in the patients who could not be intubated at the first attempt with MILS.

[c]Intubation time = time from the insertion of the laryngoscope blade to inflation of the orotracheal tube cuff during the first or the second 30-sec attempt.

[d]Cormack and Lehane scale of glottic exposure = grade I, complete visualization of the vocal cords; grade II, visualization of the posterior portion of the glottis; grade III, visualization of the epiglottis only; grade IV, inability to visualize the epiglottis.

significantly impacted the finding as these sorts of tools are not routinely restricted in clinical practice. In spite of these restrictions though, the important findings here are that in-line stabilization was associated with a worse laryngo-scopic view and a lower rate of rapid intubation (less than 30 seconds). These findings, as listed in Table 2, support the long-held belief that appropriate posi-tion when it is clinically possible is associated with easier airway control. The optimal approach in patients in whom we are concerned about cervical spine stability remains unclear.

T. Dorman, MD

Mechanical Ventilation/Weaning

Early physical and occupational therapy in mechanically ventilated, critically ill patients: a randomised controlled trial
Schweickert WD, Pohlman MC, Pohlman AS, et al (Univ of Pennsylvania, Philadelphia; Univ of Chicago, IL; et al)
Lancet 373:1874-1882, 2009

Background.—Long-term complications of critical illness include inten-sive care unit (ICU)-acquired weakness and neuropsychiatric disease. Immobilisation secondary to sedation might potentiate these problems. We assessed the efficacy of combining daily interruption of sedation with physical and occupational therapy on functional outcomes in patients receiving mechanical ventilation in intensive care.

Methods.—Sedated adults (≥18 years of age) in the ICU who had been on mechanical ventilation for less than 72 h, were expected to continue for at least 24 h, and who met criteria for baseline functional independence were eligible for enrolment in this randomised controlled trial at two university hospitals. We randomly assigned 104 patients by computer-generated, permuted block randomisation to early exercise and mobilisation (physical and occupational therapy) during periods of daily interruption of sedation (intervention; n=49) or to daily interruption of sedation with therapy as ordered by the primary care team (control; n=55). The primary endpoint—the number of patients returning to inde-pendent functional status at hospital discharge—was defined as the ability to perform six activities of daily living and the ability to walk indepen-dently. Therapists who undertook patient assessments were blinded to treatment assignment. Secondary endpoints included duration of delirium and ventilator-free days during the first 28 days of hospital stay. Analysis was by intention to treat. This trial is registered with ClinicalTrials.gov, number NCT00322010.

Findings.—All 104 patients were included in the analysis. Return to independent functional status at hospital discharge occurred in 29 (59%) patients in the intervention group compared with 19 (35%) patients in the control group (p=0·02; odds ratio 2·7 [95% CI 1·2–6·1]). Patients in the intervention group had shorter duration of delirium (median 2·0 days, IQR 0·0–6·0 *vs* 4·0 days, 2·0–8·0; p=0·02), and more

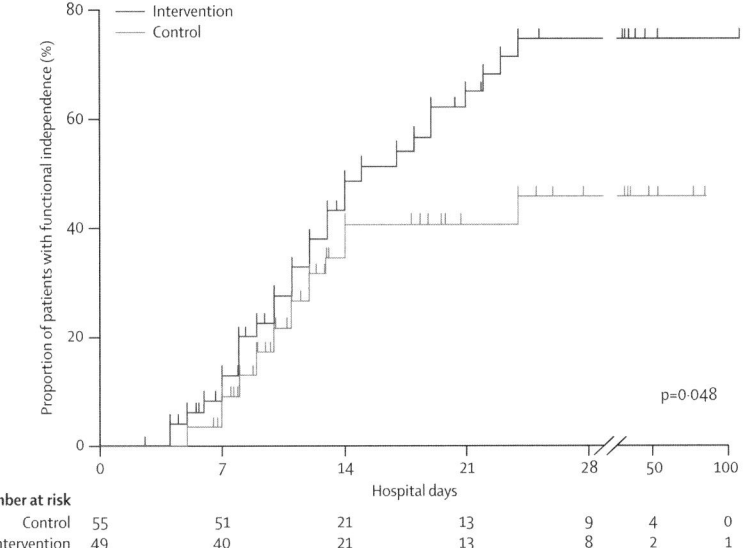

FIGURE 2.—Probability of return to independent functional status in intervention and control groups. (Reprinted from Schweickert WD, Pohlman MC, Pohlman AS, et al. Early physical and occupational therapy in mechanically ventilated, critically ill patients: a randomised controlled trial. *Lancet.* 2009;373:1874-1882, with permission from Elsevier.)

TABLE 3.—Main Outcomes According to Study Group

	Intervention (n=49)	Control (n=55)	p Value
Return to independent functional status at hospital discharge	29 (59%)	19 (35%)	0·02
ICU delirium (days)	2·0 (0·0–6·0)	4·0 (2·0–7·0)	0·03
Time in ICU with delirium (%)	33% (0–58)	57% (33–69)	0·02
Hospital delirium (days)	2·0 (0·0–6·0)	4·0 (2·0–8·0)	0·02
Hospital days with delirium (%)	28% (26)	41% (27)	0·01
Barthel Index score at hospital discharge	75 (7·5–95)	55 (0–85)	0·05
ICU-acquired paresis at hospital discharge	15 (31%)	27 (49%)	0·09
Ventilator-free days*	23·5 (7·4–25·6)	21·1 (0·0–23·8)	0·05
Duration of mechanical ventilation (days)	3·4 (2·3–7·3)	6·1 (4·0–9·6)	0·02
Duration of mechanical ventilation, survivors (days)	3·7 (2·3–7·7)	5·6 (3·4–8·4)	0·19
Duration of mechanical ventilation, non-survivors (days)	2·5 (2·4–5·5)	9·5 (5·9–14·1)	0·04
Length of stay in ICU (days)	5·9 (4·5–13·2)	7·9 (6·1–12·9)	0·08
Length of stay in hospital (days)	13·5 (8·0–23·1)	12·9 (8·9–19·8)	0·93
Hospital mortality	9 (18%)	14 (25%)	0·53

Data are n (%), median (IQR), or mean (SD). ICU=intensive care unit.
Barthel Index scale 0–100, APACHE II scale 0–71.
*Ventilator-free days from study day 1 to day 28.

ventilator-free days (23·5 days, 7·4–25·6 vs 21·1 days, 0·0–23·8; p=0·05) during the 28-day follow-up period than did controls. There was one serious adverse event in 498 therapy sessions (desaturation less than 80%). Discontinuation of therapy as a result of patient instability occurred in 19 (4%) of all sessions, most commonly for perceived patient-ventilator asynchrony.

Interpretation.—A strategy for whole-body rehabilitation—consisting of interruption of sedation and physical and occupational therapy in the earliest days of critical illness—was safe and well tolerated, and resulted in better functional outcomes at hospital discharge, a shorter duration of delirium, and more ventilator-free days compared with standard care (Fig 2 and Table 3).

▶ The aftermath of critical illness is often overshadowed by the fact that the patient made a significant enough improvement to be discharged from the ICU to a floor or rehab facility. While we are all aware that critical illness neuro-myopathy often leads to prolonged weaning and resumption of usual physical activities, most of us did not realize how long it may take for a patient recovering from a critical illness to regain their ability to walk independently and accomplish 6 basic activities of daily living, which were used as the primary endpoints in this trial. While the cost in effort, personnel, and time to provide the physical and occupational therapy for these critically ill ventilator managed patients is likely huge for most of us, the improved outcome is impressive. Even with all of this effort, only 59% of the patients were able to return to independent function at hospital discharge. However, the control group had only 35% of patients able to independently function at hospital discharge. The overall benefit of the improved function at discharge needs to be put into context of the total cost savings for our health care system. The ability of these survivors to return to work and avoid the need for prolonged rehabilitation and other support services post hospital discharge may be well worth the additional costs and resource use during the ICU stay. We will await further studies and an economic analysis to help direct our adoption of this whole-body rehabilitation model for the critically ill ventilator managed patient.

R. A. Balk, MD

Nonthyroidal Illness Syndrome and Prolonged Mechanical Ventilation in Patients Admitted to the ICU
Bello G, Pennisi MA, Montini L, et al (Policlinico Universitario A. Gemelli, Università Cattolica del Sacro Cuore, Rome, Italy)
Chest 135:1448-1454, 2009

Background.—The effect of the nonthyroidal illness syndrome (NTIS) on the duration of mechanical ventilation (MV) has not been extensively investigated. This study aims to determine whether the NTIS is associated with the duration of MV in patients admitted to the ICU.

TABLE 1.—Characteristics of Study Population and Main Outcomes*

Variables	Normal-Hormone Group (n = 56)	Low-fT3 Group (n = 208)	p Value
Age, yr	70 (58–76)	71 (60–77)	0.959
Male sex	30 (54)	105 (50)	0.681
Underlying disease			
COPD	11 (20)	50 (24)	0.489
Neurologic	13 (23)	57 (27)	0.528
ARF of various etiologies	32 (57)	101 (49)	0.254
Pneumonia			
Overall	32 (57)	134 (64)	0.317
VAP	21 (38)	102 (49)	0.124
CAP	11 (20)	32 (15)	0.444
SAPS II	38 (31–45)	43 (35–53)	< 0.001
Duration of MV, d	10 (4–14)	13 (7–21)	< 0.001
ICU LOS, d	19 (11–27)	22 (15–33)	0.008
ICU deaths	3 (5.4)	78 (37.5)	< 0.001
Thyroid hormones†			
fT3, pg/mL	2.5 (2.4–2.7)	1.6 (1.1–1.9)	< 0.001
fT4, pg/mL	11.9 (10.9–13.7)	10.0 (8.1–12.3)	< 0.001
TSH, mIU/mL	1.70 (0.93–2.17)	1.06 (0.69–1.70)	< 0.001

*Data are expressed as median (25th to 75th percentile) or No. (%), unless otherwise indicated. CAP = community-acquired pneumonia; VAP = ventilator-associated pneumonia.
†Serum levels at the first dosage.

Methods.—We evaluated all patients admitted over a 6-year period to our ICU who underwent invasive MV and had measurement of serum free triiodothyronine (fT3), free thyroxine (fT4), and thyroid-stimulating hormone (TSH) performed in the first 4 days after ICU admission and, subsequently, at least every 8 days during the time they received MV. The primary outcome measure was prolonged MV (PMV), which was defined as dependence on MV for > 13 days.

Results.—Two hundred sixty-four patients were included. Fifty-six patients (normal-hormone group) had normal thyroid function test results, whereas 208 patients (low-fT3 group) had, at least in one hormone dosage, low levels of fT3 with normal (n = 145)/low (n = 63) levels of fT4 and normal (n = 189)/low (n = 19) levels of TSH. Patients in the low-fT3 group showed significantly higher mortality and simplified acute physiology score II, and significantly longer duration of MV and ICU length of stay compared with the normal-hormone group. Two of the variables studied were associated with PMV, as follows: the NTIS (odds ratio [OR], 2.25; 95% confidence interval [CI], 1.18 to 4.29; p = 0.01); and the presence of pneumonia (OR, 1.17; 95% CI, 1.06 to 3.01; p = 0.03).

Conclusion.—The NTIS represents a risk factor for PMV in mechanically ventilated, critically ill patients (Table 1).

▶ Endocrine abnormalities, such as adrenal insufficiency, hypo or hyperthyroidism may present additional challenges to the management of critically ill patients; the impact of sick euthyroid syndrome or nonthyroidal illness syndrome is still uncertain. Whether this thyroid function test abnormality represents a true illness or a biochemical phenomenon remains to be answered. Another question is the clinical value of treating the nonthyroidal ill syndrome with some specific (yet to be determined) agent. For now this finding of increased likelihood of prolonged mechanical ventilation associated with the presence of nonthyroidal illness syndrome should give rise to further studies designed to better understand the specific role of the abnormal hormone values in this disorder.

R. A. Balk, MD

The impact of delirium on clinical outcomes in mechanically ventilated surgical and trauma patients
Lat I, McMillian W, Taylor S, et al (The Univ of Chicago Hosps, IL; Fletcher Allen Health Care, Burlington, VT; Via Christi Regional Med Ctr, Wichita, KS; et al)
Crit Care Med 37:1898-1905, 2009

Objective.—Previously, delirium has been identified as an independent risk factor for mortality in critically ill medical patients. We undertook this study to examine the relationships among medication usage, delirium, and clinical outcomes in a critically ill surgical/trauma population.

Design.—Prospective, multicentered, observational study.

Setting.—Two surgical intensive care units in level 1 trauma centers.

Patients.—One hundred thirty-four consecutive surgical adult patients requiring mechanical ventilation (MV) for greater than 24 hours.

Interventions.—Daily delirium assessment with the Confusion Assessment Method-Intensive Care Unit tool, outcomes assessment, and prospective data collection.

Measurement and Main Results.—Of the 134 patients who met inclusion criteria, 84 patients (63%) developed delirium at some point during their intensive care unit (ICU) stay. Delirium was associated with more MV days (9.1 vs. 4.9 days, $p < 0.01$), longer ICU stay (12.2 vs. 7.4 days, $p < 0.01$), longer hospital stay (20.6 vs. 14.7 days, $p < 0.01$). Additionally, greater cumulative lorazepam dose ($p = 0.012$), and higher cumulative fentanyl dose ($p = 0.035$) were administered in the delirium group.

Conclusions.—Delirium in the surgical/trauma ICU cohort is independently associated with more days requiring MV, longer ICU length of stay, and longer hospital length of stay. Additionally, greater amounts of lorazepam and fentanyl were administered to patients with delirium.

▶ The impact of delirium on outcome and clinical course of critically ill patients is now well established.[1,2] Because trauma typically involves younger individuals, we often assume that they would be less likely to develop delirium and ICU psychosis. This observational study from 2 different hospitals demonstrates the adverse impact of delirium in the mechanically ventilated postsurgical and posttrauma patients. It is now clear that strategies to accurately diagnose and treat delirium are important in the management of all critically ill patients. Perhaps, our efforts should now be focused on ways to prevent delirium, not just recognize and treat it in our critically ill patients.

R. A. Balk, MD

References

1. Ely EW, Inouye SK, Bernard GR, et al. Delirium in mechanically ventilated patients: Validity and reliability of the confusion assessment method for the intensive care unit (CAM-ICU). *JAMA.* 2001;286:2703-2710.
2. Ely EW, Shintani A, Truman B, et al. Delirium as a predictor of mortality in mechanically ventilated patiens in the intensive care unit. *JAMA.* 2004;291: 1753-1762.

Echocardiographic diagnosis of pulmonary artery occlusion pressure elevation during weaning from mechanical ventilation

Lamia B, Maizel J, Ochagavia A, et al (Université Paris Sud, Le Kremlin-Bicêtre, France; et al)
Crit Care Med 37:1696-1701, 2009

Objective.—Weaning-induced pulmonary edema is a cause of weaning failure in high-risk patients. The diagnosis may require pulmonary artery catheterization to demonstrate increased pulmonary artery occlusion pressure (PAOP) during weaning. Transthoracic echocardiography can

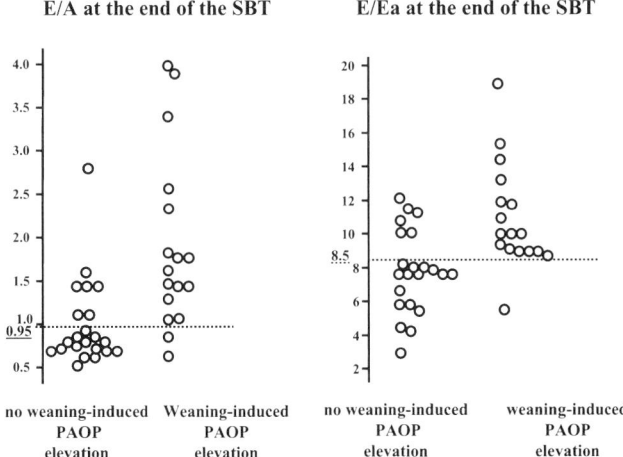

FIGURE 1.—Individual values of ratio of early (E) to late (A) peak diastolic velocities measured using Doppler transmitral flow (*E/A*) and ratio of early (E) diastolic velocity measured with Doppler transmitral flow to early (Ea) peak diastolic velocity of mitral annulus measured with tissue Doppler imaging (*E/Ea*) at the end of the spontaneous breathing trial (*SBT*) in patients with weaning-induced pulmonary artery occlusion pressure elevation and in patients with no weaning-induced pulmonary artery occlusion pressure elevation. (Courtesy of Lamia B, Maizel J, Ochagavia A, et al. Echocardiographic diagnosis of pulmonary artery occlusion pressure elevation during weaning from mechanical ventilation. *Crit Care Med.* 2009;37:1696-1701.)

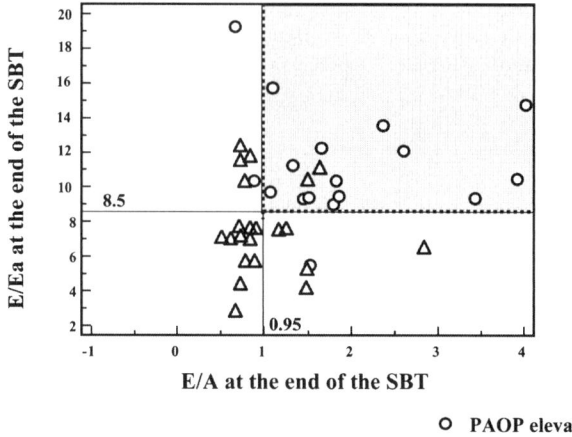

○ PAOP elevation

△ no PAOP elevation

FIGURE 2.—Individual plots of ratio of early (E) to late (A) peak diastolic velocities measured using Doppler transmitral flow (*E/A*) and ratio of early (E) diastolic velocity measured with Doppler transmitral flow to early (Ea) peak diastolic velocity of mitral annulus measured with tissue Doppler imaging (*E/Ea*) at the end of the spontaneous breathing trial (*SBT*) in patients with weaning-induced pulmonary artery occlusion pressure (*PAOP*) elevation (*circles*) and in patients with no weaning-induced PAOP elevation (*triangles*). The *gray upper right quadrant* includes weaning-induced patients with PAOP well diagnosed by transthoracic echocardiography: they all had an E/A >0.95 and an E/Ea >8.5 at the end of the SBT. The three remaining *white quadrants* include patients without weaning-induced PAOP elevation well diagnosed by transthoracic echocardiography. (Courtesy of Lamia B, Maizel J, Ochagavia A, et al. Echocardiographic diagnosis of pulmonary artery occlusion pressure elevation during weaning from mechanical ventilation. *Crit Care Med.* 2009;37:1696-1701.)

estimate left ventricular filling pressures using early (E) and late (A) peak diastolic velocities measured with Doppler transmitral flow, and tissue Doppler imaging of mitral annulus velocities including early (Ea) peak diastolic velocity. We tested the hypothesis that E/A and E/Ea could be used to detect weaning-induced PAOP elevation defined by a PAOP ≥ 18 mm Hg during a spontaneous breathing trial (SBT).

Measurements and Main Results.—We included 39 patients who previously failed two consecutive SBTs. A third SBT was performed over a maximum 1-hour period using a T-piece. The PAOP, E/A, and E/Ea were measured before and during this SBT. Receiver operating characteristic curves were constructed to determine the optimal sensitivity and specificity values of E/A and E/Ea obtained at the end of the SBT for predicting a weaning-induced PAOP elevation. Weaning-induced PAOP elevation occurred in 17 patients. A value of E/A > 0.95 at the end of the SBT predicted weaning-induced PAOP elevation with a sensitivity of 88% and a specificity of 68%. A value of E/Ea > 8.5 at the end of the SBT predicted weaning-induced PAOP elevation with a sensitivity of 94% and a specificity of 73%. The combination of E/A > 0.95 and E/Ea > 8.5 predicted a weaning-induced PAOP elevation with a sensitivity of 82% and a specificity of 91%.

Conclusion.—At the end of an SBT, the combination of E/A > 0.95 and E/Ea > 8.5 measured with transthoracic echocardiography allowed an accurate noninvasive detection of weaning-induced PAOP elevation (Figs 1 and 2).

▶ Cardiac factors, whether from ischemia, arrhythmias, or over decompensation, and heart failure are well-known causes of weaning failure.[1] Unfortunately, this clinical situation is not always easy to diagnose before a spontaneous breathing trial until there is overt failure. Diagnosing cardiac decompensation from an elevated pulmonary artery occlusion pressure has typically required the insertion of a pulmonary artery catheter. As we all know, there has been a progressive movement away from using these catheters for a variety of reasons, so it is important to note that echocardiography can identify those patients with an elevated pulmonary artery occlusion pressure during the weaning process in a noninvasive and reliable fashion. The combination of the elevated early (E)/late (A) and E/Ea ratios yielded a reasonably high sensitivity and specificity as well as a good positive and negative predictive index. As the intensivist learns and becomes more familiar with ultrasound techniques, including echocardiography, we will see this technology become a standardized part of our daily evaluation process, particularly in complex critically ill patients.

R. A. Balk, MD

Reference

1. Balk RA. *Weaning from Mechanical Ventilation: What Strategies do Randomized Controlled Trials Recommend? Mechanical Ventilation: Trends in Adult and Pediatric Practice.* Mount Prospect, IL: Society of Critical Care Medicine; 2009; 141-155.

Effects of staff training on the care of mechanically ventilated patients: a prospective cohort study
Bloos F, Müller S, Harz A, et al (Univ Hosp Jena, Germany; et al)
Br J Anaesth 103:232-237, 2009

Background.—Adherence to guidelines to avoid complications associated with mechanical ventilation is often incomplete. The goal of this study was to assess whether staff training in pre-defined interventions (bundle) improves the quality of care in mechanically ventilated patients.

Methods.—This study was performed on a 50-bed intensive care unit of a tertiary care university hospital. Application of a ventilator bundle consisting of semirecumbent positioning, lung protective ventilation in patients with acute lung injury (ALI), ulcer prophylaxis, and deep vein thrombosis prophylaxis (DVTP) was assessed before and after staff training in postsurgical patients requiring mechanical ventilation for at least 24 h.

Results.—A total of 133 patients before and 141 patients after staff training were included. Overall bundle adherence increased from 15 to

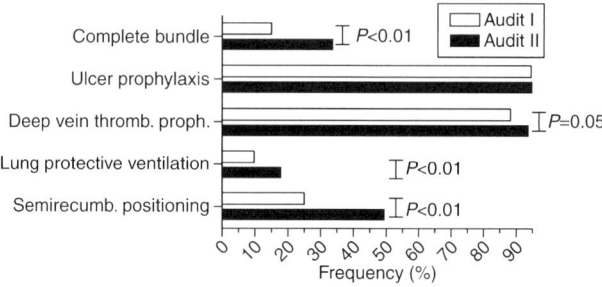

FIGURE 1.—Frequency of successful implementation of treatment bundles before and after staff training. Data are given in percentage of patient days. Lung protective ventilation applies to patients with ALI only. (Reprinted from Bloos F, Müller S, Harz A, et al. Effects of staff training on the care of mechanically ventilated patients: a prospective cohort study. *Br J Anaesth*. 2009;103:232-237, by permission of The Board of Management and Trustees of the British Journal of Anaesthesia, Oxford University Press.)

TABLE 4.—Outcome in all Patients, and in Patients with Ventilator-associated Pneumonia. Data are Expressed as Median and Interquartile Range

	Audit I	Audit II	P-value
All patients			
	$n = 133$	$n = 141$	
Duration of mechanical ventilation (days)	6.0 (2.0–15.0)	4.0 (2.0–9.0)	0.02
ICU mortality	27.8%	25.5%	0.68
ICU length of stay (days)	12.0 (5.0–21.5)	13.0 (6.0–21.0)	0.71
Frequency of VAP	33.1%	32.4%	0.68
Patients with ventilator-associated pneumonia (subgroup analysis)			
	$n = 44$	$n = 45$	
Duration of mechanical ventilation (days)	18 (13–26)	10 (6–17)	<0.01
ICU mortality	43.2%	35.6%	0.52
ICU length of stay (days)	30.0 (17.3–45)	21 (11.5–35)	0.04
Duration until onset of VAP (days)	5.3 (3.5–8.9)	6.4 (4.1–11.0)	0.18

33.8% (*P*<0.001). Semirecumbent position was achieved in 24.9% of patient days before and 46.9% of patient days after staff training (*P*<0.001). Administration of DVTP increased from 89.5 to 91.5% (*P*=0.048). Ulcer prophylaxis of >90% was achieved in both groups. Median tidal volume in patients with ALI remained unaltered. Days on mechanical ventilation were reduced from 6 (interquartile range 2.0–15.0) to 4 (2.0–9.0) (*P*=0.017). Rate of ventilator-associated pneumonia (VAP), ICU length of stay, and ICU mortality remained unaffected. In patients with VAP, the median ICU length of stay was reduced by 9 days (*P*=0.04).

Conclusions.—Staff training by an ICU change team improved compliance to a pre-defined ventilator bundle. This led to a reduction in the days spent on mechanical ventilation, despite incomplete bundle implementation (Table 4).

▶ In an effort to improve clinical outcomes and reduce complications, almost all intensive care units have adopted the use of specialized care protocols to ensure the provision of best practice management and provide some degree of uniformity in patient care. To assist with implementation and ensure frequent use, most of us have turned to the use of simplified groups of care, so-called bundles. Bundles of care are now popular for the management of sepsis and have been used for ventilator management and to facilitate weaning from mechanical ventilatory support.[1,2] The components of the bundle come from evidenced-based data and reflect best practice. This study demonstrates the use of a ventilator bundle decreased the overall ventilatory support by 2 days. Unfortunately, developing and deploying the bundle for your ICU does not necessarily translate into universal acceptance and use for all applicable patients. The use of the ventilator management bundle in this study was preceded by an educational process and the actual use and outcomes were subsequently assessed in comparison with the preimplementation period. As shown in Fig 1, some aspects of care are used in almost everyone; however, surprisingly, some components are used in a very small percentage of patients, while some remained low even with the educational process.

The use of bundles to improve patient outcome and quality of care is a good idea, but is surprisingly hard to get complete buy in. Computer prompts and performance reviews will likely help increase use. However, it will probably require some type of outcome comparison report among different clinicians to fully drive this practice change. Physicians tend to be fairly competitive and type A in behavior, with no one wanting to be less effective than their peers at anything.

R. A. Balk, MD

References

1. Nguyen HB, Corbett SW, Steele R, et al. Implementation of a bundle of quality indicators for the early management of severe sepsis and septic shock is associated with decreased mortality. *Crit Care Med.* 2007;35:1105-1112.
2. Resar R, Pronovost P, Haraden C, Simmonds T, Rainey T, Nolan T. Using a bundle approach to improve ventilator care processes and reduceventilator-associated pneumonia. *Jt Comm J Qual Patient Saf.* 2005;31:243-248.

Age, Duration of Mechanical Ventilation, and Outcomes of Patients Who Are Critically Ill

Feng Y, Amoateng-Adjepong Y, Kaufman D, et al (Bridgeport Hosp, CT; et al)

Chest 136:759-764, 2009

Background.—Age and duration of mechanical ventilation (MV) are strongly associated with mortality and hospital discharge disposition.

Methods.—Electronic administrative records from a 425-bed community teaching hospital were obtained for 9,912 patients who were admitted to hospital ICUs between 2003 and 2008. Risk estimates of age and duration of MV for in-hospital mortality and discharge to home vs extended-care facilities (ECFs) also were obtained.

Results.—Of 9,912 patients, 37 were discharged to hospice care, and 668 were < 18 years of age. Of the remaining 9,207 patients, 4,238 received invasive MV. Mortality or hospital discharge to ECFs increased consistently for each decade of age > 65 years and as the duration of MV increased. Although only 11.7% of patients < 65 years age who received MV for 1 or 2 days died during hospitalization, the mortality rate increased to 72.1% for patients > 85 years of age who had received MV for > 7 days. For patients requiring MV for ≥ 7 days, < 10% of the ≥ 65 years of age and < 5% of patients ≥ 85 years of age survived to be discharged home from the hospital. Multivariate logistic regression analyses showed that age > 65 years and duration of MV remained significantly associated with outcomes, even after adjustment for hospital discharge diagnoses (Charlson scores).

Conclusions.—This study suggests that age and duration of MV are strongly associated with mortality and posthospital disposition. If confirmed, the simple combination of age and duration of MV provides prognostic information that could be used with trajectory of illness and in the context of patients' values to inform end-of-life discussions with patients or their surrogates during a trial of critical care.

▶ Elderly individuals typically do not fare as well as younger people with critical illness. This was well demonstrated by Ely et al and Hudson et al in acute lung injury and acute respiratory distress syndrome patients.[1,2] This study also nicely demonstrates the negative effect advanced age has on hospital survival. The authors pose a potential new tool (the age duration of mechanical ventilation index), which may have use in advising patients and/or families (decision makers) about the potential outcome of critically ill, ventilated elderly patients.

R. A. Balk, MD

References

1. Ely EW, Wheeler AP, Thompson BT, Ancukiewicz M, Steinberg KP, Bernard GR. Recovery rate and prognosis in older persons who develop acute lung injury and the acute respiratory distress syndrome. *Ann Intern Med.* 2002;136:25-36.
2. Milberg JA, Davis DR, Steinberg KP, Hudson LD. Improved survival of patients with acute respiratory distress syndrome (ARDS): 1983-1993. *JAMA.* 1995;273:306-309.

Role of the respiratory muscles in acute respiratory failure of COPD: lessons from weaning failure

Tobin MJ, Laghi F, Brochard L (Edward Hines Jr. Veterans Affairs Hosp and Loyola Univ of Chicago Stritch School of Medicine, Hines, IL; Albert Chenevier-Henri Mondor Teaching Hosp, Créteil, France)
J Appl Physiol 107:962-970, 2009

It is problematic to withhold therapy in a patient with chronic obstructive pulmonary disease (COPD) who presents with acute respiratory failure so that detailed physiological measurements can be obtained. Accordingly, most information on respiratory muscle activity in patients experiencing acute respiratory failure has been acquired by studying patients who fail a trial of weaning after a period of mechanical ventilation. Such patients experience marked increases in inspiratory muscle load consequent to increases in resistance, elastance, and intrinsic positive end-expiratory pressure. Inspiratory muscle strength is reduced secondary to hyperinflation and possibly direct muscle damage and the release of inflammatory mediators. Most patients recruit both their sternomastoid and expiratory muscles, even though airflow limitation prevents the expiratory muscles from lowering lung volume. Even when acute hypercapnia is present, patients do not exhibit respiratory center depression; indeed, voluntary activation of the diaphragm, in absolute terms, is greater in hypercapnic patients than in normocapnic patients. Instead, the major mechanism of acute hypercapnia is the development of rapid shallow breathing. Despite the marked increase in mechanical load and decreased force-generating capacity of the inspiratory muscles, patients do not develop long-lasting muscle fatigue, at least over the period of a failed weaning trial. Although the disease originates within the lung parenchyma, much of the distress faced by patients with COPD, especially during acute respiratory failure, is caused by the burdens imposed on the respiratory muscles.

▶ This is an excellent review of respiratory muscle function and its role in respiratory failure. The authors have extensive experience in the evaluation of respiratory mechanics and have drawn heavily on the response of the respiratory muscles to a weaning trial to piece together the important aspects of the response of the respiratory muscles to increased load and changes in respiratory mechanics during acute respiratory failure. Understanding the forces in action and the root of the problem can better delineate management approach. This article should be required reading for those who manage patients with obstructive lung disease.

R. A. Balk, MD

Predicting the risk of documented ventilator-associated pneumonia for benchmarking: Construction and validation of a score

Zahar J-R, Nguile-Makao M, Français A, et al (Necker Teaching Hosp, Paris France; Albert Bonniot Inst, Grenoble, France; et al)
Crit Care Med 37:2545-2551, 2009

Objectives.—To build and validate a ventilator-associated pneumonia risk score for benchmarking. The rate of ventilator-associated pneumonia varies widely with case-mix, a fact that has limited its use for measuring intensive care unit performance.

Methods.—We studied 1856 patients in the OUTCOMEREA database treated at intensive care unit admission by endotracheal intubation followed by mechanical ventilation for >48 hrs; they were allocated randomly to a training data set (n = 1233) or a validation data set (n = 623). Multivariate logistic regression was used. Calibration of the final model was assessed in both data sets, using the Hosmer-Lemeshow chi-square test and receiver operating characteristic curves.

Measurements and Main Results.—Independent risk factors for ventilator-associated pneumonia were male gender (odds ratio = 1.97, 95% confidence interval = 1.32–2.95); SOFA at intensive care unit admission (<3 [reference value], 3–4 [2.57, 1.39–4.77], 5–8 [7.37, 4.24 –12.81], >8 [5.81 (3.2–10.52)], no use within 48 hrs after intensive care unit admission of parenteral nutrition (2.29, 1.52–3.45), no broad-spectrum antimicrobials (2.11, 1.46–3.06); and mechanical ventilation duration (<5 days (1); 5–7 days (17.55, 4.01–76.85); 7–15 days (53.01, 12.74 –220.56); >15 days (225.6, 54.3–936.7). Tests in the training set showed good calibration and good discrimination (area under the curve-receiver operating characteristic curve = 0.881), and both criteria remained good in the validation set (area under the curve-receiver operating characteristic curve = 0.848) and good calibration (Hosmer-Lemeshow chi-square = 9.98, *p* = .5). Observed ventilator-associated pneumonia rates varied across intensive care units from 9.7 to 26.1 of 1000 mechanical ventilation days but the ratio of observed over theoretical ventilator-associated pneumonia rates was >1 in only two intensive care units.

Conclusions.—The ventilator-associated pneumonia rate may be useful for benchmarking provided the ratio of observed over theoretical rates is used. External validation of our prediction score is needed.

▶ One of the criticisms of using incidence of ventilator-acquired pneumonia (VAP) as a quality indicator in the ICU is the difficulty in being assured that the diagnosis is present. Despite this, VAP continues to be incredibly emphasized across the United States in quality programs. The ventilator bundles, although including some elements that would have no effect on VAP, nevertheless are instituted with the indicator being incidence of VAP. Attempts at better sensitivity and specificity for the diagnosis of VAP are encouraged as is demonstrated in this article. However, even this score has clear limitations, as pointed out by the authors, as to influence of the ratio of observed over theoretical rates. External validation of this score awaits.

R. P. Dellinger, MD

Epidemiology of Mechanical Ventilation: Analysis of the SAPS 3 Database
Metnitz PGH, on behalf of the SAPS 3 Investigators (Med Univ of Vienna, Austria; et al)
Intensive Care Med 35:816-825, 2009

Objective.—To evaluate current practice of mechanical ventilation in the ICU and the characteristics and outcomes of patients receiving it.

Design.—Pre-planned sub-study of a multicenter, multinational cohort study (SAPS 3).

Patients.—13,322 patients admitted to 299 intensive care units (ICUs) from 35 countries.

Interventions.—None.

TABLE 1.—Demographic and Clinical Data

	NoMV		NIV		invMV		
	n	%	n	%	n	%	p-value
Number of patients	6261		554		6507		
ICU LOS, days (median, Q1-Q3)	3.0 (1.0-4.9)		4.0 (1.7-8.3)		4.0 (1.8-10.3)		<0.001
Gender							<0.001
Female	2614	41.8	219	39.5	2460	37.8	
Male	3641	58.2	335	60.5	4042	62.1	
Missing	6	0.1			5	0.1	
Age, years (median, Q1-Q3)	63 (48-74)		69 (56-77)		64 (48-74)		<0.001
ICU admission status							<0.001
Planned	1036	16.5	74	13.4	1463	22.5	
Unplanned	5050	80.7	463	83.6	4874	74.9	
Missing	175	2.8	17	3.1	170	2.6	
Acute Infection at ICU admission							<0.001
No infection	4781	76.4	323	58.3	4608	70.8	
Clinically improbable/colonization	91	1.5	24	4.3	154	2.4	
Clinically probable/documented	940	15.0	156	28.2	1213	18.6	
Microbiologically documented	446	7.1	51	9.2	524	8.1	
Missing	3	0.0			8	0.1	
Surgical status							<0.001
No surgical procedure	3903	62.3	373	67.3	2748	42.2	
Scheduled surgery	1054	16.8	88	15.9	1530	23.5	
Emergency surgery	876	14.0	60	10.8	1896	29.1	
Missing	428	6.8	33	6.0	333	5.1	
SOFA score (median, Q1-Q3)	2 (1-4)		5 (3-6)		5 (3-8)		<0.001
SAPS 3 score (median, Q1-Q3)	45 (37-54)		58 (51-66)		58 (47-70)		<0.001
Outcome							
ICU mortality (%)		12.1		18.4		29.8	
Hospital mortality (%)		17.5		27.8		37.1	

NoMV, NIV and inv MV are explained in the Methods section. LOS: length of stay; Q1, Q3: first and third quartiles; The exact definition of all variables can be found in the ESM of the original SAPS 3 report [9]. Editor's Note: Please refer to original journal article for full references.

Main Measurements and Results.—Patients were divided into three groups: no mechanical ventilation (MV), noninvasive MV (NIV), and invasive MV. More than half of the patients (53% [CI: 52.2-53.9%]) were mechanically ventilated at ICU admission. FiO_2, V_T and PEEP used during invasive MV were on average 50% (40-80%), 8 mL/kg actual body weight (6.9-9.4 mL/kg) and 5 cmH$_2$O (3-6 cmH$_2$O), respectively. Several invMV patients (17.3% (CI:16.4-18.3%)) were ventilated with zero PEEP (ZEEP). These patients exhibited a significantly increased risk-adjusted hospital mortality, compared with patients ventilated with higher PEEP (O/E ratio 1.12 [1.05-1.18]). NIV was used in 4.2% (CI: 3.8-4.5%) of all patients and was associated with an improved risk-adjusted outcome (OR 0.79, [0.69-0.90]).

Conclusion.—Ventilation mode and parameter settings for MV varied significantly across ICUs. Our results provide evidence that some ventilatory modes and settings could still be used against current evidence and recommendations. This includes ventilation with tidal volumes >8mL/kg body weight in patients with a low PaO2/FiO2 ratio and ZEEP in invMV patients. Invasive mechanical ventilation with ZEEP was associated with a worse outcome, even after controlling for severity of disease. Since our study did not document indications for MV, the association between MV settings and outcome must be viewed with caution (Table 1).

▶ It is important to assess our practice patterns at regular intervals to know that we are actually doing what the evidence says we should and to know that what we think is happening is actually taking place. Nothing speaks louder than data when it comes to addressing these important questions. This study presents data from almost 300 intensive care units in 35 countries. The data set involves over 13 000 patients. There are several important conclusions that can be drawn from this information. First, as much as we discuss the increasing popularity of noninvasive ventilatory support, it is used in less than 5% of patients. The use of noninvasive ventilation was associated with a better outcome in comparison with invasive ventilatory support. Second, despite guidelines for use of tidal volume and positive end-expiratory pressure (PEEP) for patients with oxygenation abnormalities consistent with acute lung injury and/or acute respiratory distress syndrome (ARDS), those recommendations were not uniformly followed. In fact tidal volumes exceeded 8 mL/kg in most patients ventilated in this study.

I would again emphasize the importance of actually looking at what is being done in comparison with what you think is being done, to determine whether optimum practice patterns are being used.

R. A. Balk, MD

Acute respiratory failure in intensive care units. FINNALI: a prospective cohort study
Linko R, The FINNALI-study group (Helsinki Univ Hosp, Finland; et al)
Intensive Care Med 35:1352-1361, 2009

Objective.—To evaluate the incidence, treatment and mortality of acute respiratory failure (ARF) in Finnish intensive care units (ICUs).
Study Design.—Prospective multicentre cohort study.
Methods.—All adult patients in 25 ICUs were screened for use of invasive or non-invasive ventilatory support during an 8-week period. Patients needing ventilatory support for more than 6 h were included and defined as ARF patients. Risk factors for ARF and details of prior chronic health status were assessed. Ventilatory and concomitant treatments were

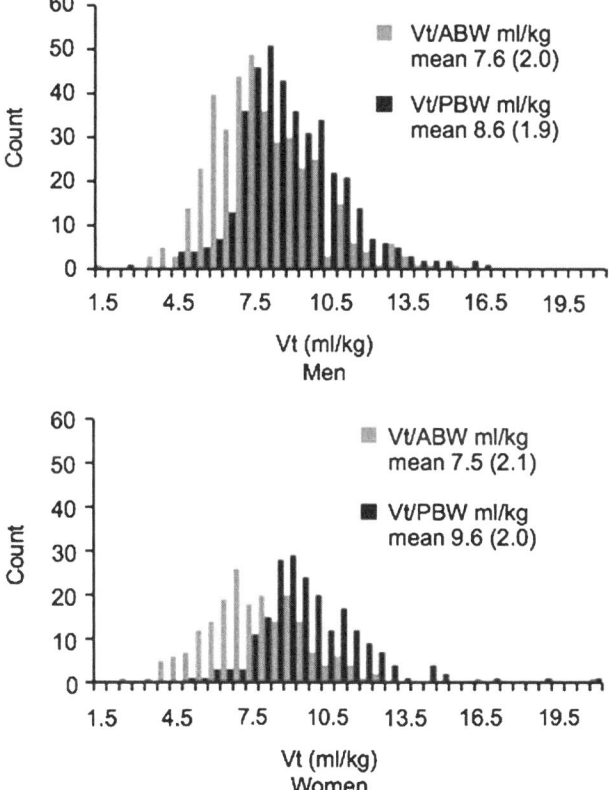

FIGURE 2.—Tidal volume distribution at baseline (at 6 h after treatment start). V_t Tidal volume (ml/kg), *ABW* actual body weight, *PBW* predicted body weight, values are mean ± SD, PBW men 0.91 × (height − 152.4) + 50, PBW women 0.91 × (height − 152.4) + 45.5 (height in cm). (Reprinted from Linko R, The FINNALI-study group. Acute respiratory failure in intensive care units. FINNALI: a prospective cohort study. *Intensive Care Med.* 2009;35:1352-1361, with permission from Springer-Verlag.)

evaluated and recorded daily throughout the ICU stay. ICU and 90-day mortalities were assessed.

Results.—A total of 958 (39%) from the 2,473 admitted patients were treated with ventilatory support for more than 6 h. Incidence of ARF, acute lung injury (ALI) and acute respiratory distress syndrome (ARDS) was 149.5, 10.6 and 5.0/100,000 per year, respectively. Ventilatory support was started with non-invasive interfaces in 183 of 958 (19%) patients. Ventilatory modes allowing triggering of spontaneous breaths were preferred (81%). Median tidal volume/predicted body weight was 8.7 (7.6–9.9) ml/kg and plateau pressure 19 (16–23) cmH$_2$O. The 90-day mortality of ARF was 31%.

Conclusions.—While the incidence of ARF requiring ventilatory support is higher, the incidence of ALI and ARDS seems to be lower in Finland than previously reported in other countries. Tidal volumes are higher than recommended in the concept of lung protective strategy. However, restriction of peak airway pressure was used in the majority of ARF patients (Fig 2).

▶ An important component of our efforts to improve the management and outcome of our critically ill patients is to determine and evaluate the care we are actually providing. All too often what we think and say we are doing, is far different from what we are doing. The only way to truly know is to carefully look and obtain data. I applaud the efforts of these Finnish investigators who undertook just such a project on the provision of mechanical ventilation to patients with acute respiratory failure. As we might expect, they found some interesting facts. While we all think we are using lower tidal volumes and providing lung protective ventilatory support strategies, we don't really know until we collect the data. I urge all of us to look at our own performance and actually collect and analyze the information to ensure that we are actually doing what we say and think we are doing.

R. A. Balk, MD

Screening for ocular surface disease in the intensive care unit
McHugh J, Alexander P, Kalhoro A, et al (St George's Hosp, London, UK; Moorfields Eye Hosp at St George's Hosp, London, UK)
Eye 22:1465-1468, 2008

Purpose.—Ventilated patients in the intensive care unit (ICU) often develop exposure keratopathy. This predisposes to the development of bacterial keratitis, which in ICU is often bilateral, with a high risk of perforation. As regular examinations of all ventilated patients by ophthalmologists would be impractical, the purpose of this study was to assess whether ICU staff can screen reliably for keratopathy.

Methods.—A prospective study was performed in a general adult ICU. Twice each week, two junior ICU doctors examined the lid position and ocular surface of all patients who had been continuously sedated for more than 24 h, using fluorescein and a pen torch with a blue filter. An ophthalmologist performed similar examinations using a portable slit lamp.

Results.—A total of 48 ocular examinations were performed in 18 patients. Exposure keratopathy was found by the ophthalmologist in 37.5% of examinations and by ICU doctors in 31.3% of examinations. ICU doctors had a sensitivity of 77.8% and a specificity of 96.7% in detecting keratopathy, when compared with the findings of the ophthalmologist. All cases missed by ICU doctors had punctate erosions of less than 5% of the corneal surface. Keratopathy was significantly commoner in patients with incomplete lid closure than in patients with closed lids (70.0 *vs* 28.9%; two-tailed Fisher's exact test $P = 0.027$).

Conclusions.—ICU staff can perform screening examinations for exposure keratopathy with reasonable sensitivity and specificity. Regular screening by ICU staff would facilitate appropriate treatment of exposure keratopathy and promote earlier identification of cases of keratitis.

▶ This study draws attention to eye injuries that can occur during periods of critical illness that require ventilatory assistance. It highlights the importance of incomplete eye closure as a risk factor for keratopathy and alerts the intensivist that common intensive care bacteria, such as *Pseudomonas*, may infect the ulcerations of the cornea. This finding suggests that intensive care management strategies should also adopt simple measures, such as eye closure, to prevent the development of keratopathy in sedated patients. A future study might also evaluate the development of keratopathy using a sedation protocol versus a nonprotocol provision of sedation.

R. A. Balk, MD

Bilevel vs ICU Ventilators Providing Noninvasive Ventilation: Effect of System Leaks: A COPD Lung Model Comparison

Ferreira JC, Chipman DW, Hill NS, et al (Univ of Sao Paulo, Brazil; Instituto do Coração, Sao Paulo, Brazil; et al)
Chest 136:448-456, 2009

Background.—Noninvasive positive-pressure ventilation (NPPV) modes are currently available on bilevel and ICU ventilators. However, little data comparing the performance of the NPPV modes on these ventilators are available.

Methods.—In an experimental bench study, the ability of nine ICU ventilators to function in the presence of leaks was compared with a bilevel ventilator using the IngMar ASL5000 lung simulator (IngMar Medical; Pittsburgh, PA) set at a compliance of 60 mL/cm H_2O, an inspiratory resistance of 10 cm $H_2O/L/s$, an expiratory resistance of 20 cm $H_2O/L/s$, and a respiratory rate of 15 breaths/min. All of the ventilators were set at

TABLE 1.—Ventilator Specifications

Ventilator	Leak Compensation	Trigger Type	Rise Time Type	IT Type	Timax	Bias Flow
e360	25 L/min	P or V' 0–5 cm H_2O	1–19	5–50%	No	3 L/min
e500	25 L/min	P or V' 0–5 cm H_2O	1–19	5–50%*	No	3 L/min
e500 auto	25 L/min	P or V' 0–5 cm H_2O	1–19	Auto	No	3 L/min
Esprit	20 L/min	V' 0.5–20 L/min	0.1–0.9 s	10–80%	No	5 L/min
Esprit Auto-Trak	60 L/min	Auto	0.1–0.9 s	Auto	No	Pt leak + 5 L/min
Evita XL	30 L/min	V' 0.3–15 L/min	0–2 s	Fixed 25%	Yes	None
IVent	65 L/min	P 0.5–20 cm H_2O, V' 1–20 L/min	Auto or 0.1–1.5 s	10–90%	Yes	2 L/min
PB840	None	V' 0.1–20 L/min	1.0–100%	1.0–80%	Yes	1.5 L/min
Raphael	No information	V' 1–10 L/min	50–200 ms	5–70%	Yes	0–10 L/min
Servo I	50 L/min	Auto	0–0.4 s	0–70%	Yes	7.5 L/min
Vela	No information	V' 1–20 L/min	No control	5–30%	Yes	10–20 L/min
Vision	Up to 60 L/min	Auto	0.05–0.4 s	Auto	No	No control

Pt = patient; IT type = approach and/or range of insiratory termination criteria (cycling); Timax = ability to set maximum inspiratory time; V' = flow; P = pressure.
*International version adjustment is automatic or manual and the range is 5 to 55%.

12 cm H_2O pressure support and 5 cm H_2O positive end-expiratory pressure. The data were collected at baseline and at three customized leaks.

Main Results.—At baseline, all of the ventilators were able to deliver adequate tidal volumes, to maintain airway pressure, and to synchronize with the simulator, without missed efforts or auto-triggering. As the leak was increased, all of the ventilators (except the Vision [Respironics; Murrysville, PA] and Servo I [Maquet; Solna, Sweden]) needed adjustment of sensitivity or cycling criteria to maintain adequate ventilation, and some transitioned to backup ventilation. Significant differences in triggering and cycling were observed between the Servo I and the Vision ventilators.

Conclusions.—The Vision and Servo I were the only ventilators that required no adjustments as they adapted to increasing leaks. There were differences in performance between these two ventilators, although the clinical significance of these differences is unclear. Clinicians should be aware that in the presence of leaks, most ICU ventilators require adjustments to maintain an adequate tidal volume (Table 1).

▶ Noninvasive ventilatory support is being used more frequently in the management of patients with acute respiratory failure, particularly associated with chronic obstructive pulmonary disease (COPD) and/or pulmonary edema. Most often noninvasive ventilatory support is initiated on a standard ventilator with a full-face mask. For the therapy to be effective, the clinician puts faith in the ventilatory to compensate for leaks and maintain synchrony with the patient. This study used a test lung to evaluate the capability of many popular ICU ventilators to compensate for leaks in the system and maintain synchrony with the respiratory effort of the simulated patient. All of the ventilators performed well at baseline (without leaks) and were able to maintain airway pressure, tidal volume, and avoid autocycling or missed respiratory efforts. However, as the leak in the system increased, as frequently happens in clinical management, only 2 ventilators were able to maintain airway pressure, tidal volume, and avoid ventilator dyssynchrony because they were able to auto adjust the triggering and cycling functions. All of the other ventilators would require recognition of the problem and a manual adjustment to correct the triggering and cycling functions. This information is important to know, because sometimes the failure of noninvasive ventilation may not be the technique, but failure to adjust for the leaks in the system.

R. A. Balk, MD

Iron lung versus mask ventilation in acute exacerbation of COPD: a randomised crossover study
Corrado A, Gorini M, Melej R, et al (Universitaria Careggi, Padiglione San Luca, Italy; Servizio di Fisiopatologia Respiratoria—UTIR, AOU Parma, Italy)
Intensive Care Med 35:648-655, 2009

Objective.—To compare iron lung (ILV) versus mask ventilation (NPPV) in the treatment of COPD patients with acute on chronic respiratory failure (ACRF).

Design.—Randomised multicentre study.

Setting.—Respiratory intermediate intensive care units very skilled in ILV.

Patients and Methods.—A total of 141 patients met the inclusion criteria and were assigned: 70 to ILV and 71 to NPPV. To establish the failure of the technique employed as first line major and minor criteria for endotracheal intubation (EI) were used. With major criteria EI was promptly established. With at least two minor criteria patients were shifted from one technique to the other.

Results.—On admission, PaO_2/FiO_2, 198 (70) and 187 (64), $PaCO_2$, 90.5 (14.1) and 88.7 (13.5) mmHg, and pH 7.25 (0.04) and 7.25 (0.05), were similar for ILV and NPPV groups. When used as first line, the success of ILV (87%) was significantly greater ($P = 0.01$) than NPPV (68%), due to the number of patients that met minor criteria for EI; after the shift of the techniques; however, the need of EI and hospital mortality was similar in both groups. The total rate of success using both techniques increased from 77.3 to 87.9% ($P = 0.028$).

Conclusions.—The sequential use of NPPV and ILV avoided EI in a large percentage of COPD patients with ACRF; ILV was more effective than NPPV on the basis of minor criteria for EI but after the crossover the need of EI on the basis of major criteria and mortality was similar in both groups of patients.

▶ The use of face mask noninvasive positive pressure ventilatory support in the setting of acute exacerbation of chronic obstructive pulmonary disease (COPD) or the management of pulmonary edema has become common place with expected good results and prevention of many of the complications associated with invasive ventilatory support. As Larry "Yogi" Berra would say, "It's deja vu, all over again,"[1] as this study has gone back to the use on iron lung negative pressure ventilators to compare with noninvasive ventilatory support for the management of acute on chronic respiratory failure. I think we are all surprised at how well the iron lung treatment actually did. I would not, however, expect to see a widespread resurgence of iron lung ventilators in the United States for treating acute respiratory failure. Previous experience with the use of negative pressure devices has emphasized the potential for upper airway obstruction and worsening of obstructive sleep apnea in some patients. In addition, the iron lung makes it difficult to examine and instrument our patients.

R. A. Balk, MD

Reference

1. Bera Y. *When you Come to a Fork in the Road, Take It!* New York; 2001.

Noninvasive ventilation for acute respiratory failure after lung resection: an observational study

Lefebvre A, Lorut C, Alifano M, et al (Université Paris 5, France)
Intensive Care Med 35:663-670, 2009

Background.—A single prospective randomized study found that, in selected patients with acute respiratory failure (ARF) following lung resection, noninvasive ventilation (NIV) decreases the need for endotracheal mechanical ventilation and improves clinical outcome.

Method.—We prospectively evaluated early NIV use for ARF after lung resection during a 4-year period in the setting of a medical and a surgical ICU of a university hospital. We documented demographics, initial clinical characteristics and clinical outcomes. NIV failure was defined as the need for tracheal intubation.

Results.—Among 690 patients at risk of severe complications following lung resection, 113 (16.3%) experienced ARF, which was initially supported by NIV in 89 (78.7%), including 59 with hypoxemic ARF (66.3%) and 30 with hypercapnic ARF (33.7%). The overall success rate of NIV was 85.3% (76/89). In-ICU mortality was 6.7% (6/89). The mortality rate following NIV failure was 46.1%. Predictive factors of NIV failure in univariate analysis were age ($P = 0.046$), previous cardiac comorbidities ($P = 0.0075$), postoperative pneumonia ($P = 0.0016$), admission in the surgical ICU ($P = 0.034$), no initial response to NIV ($P < 0.0001$) and occurrence of noninfectious complications ($P = 0.037$). Only two independent factors were significantly associated with NIV failure in multivariate analysis: cardiac comorbidities (odds ratio, 11.5;

TABLE 4.—Outcomes of the Two NIV Groups

Outcomes	Overall Population $n = 89$	Hypoxemic ARF Group $n = 59$	Hypercapnic ARF Group $n = 30$	P Value
NIV duration (days), mean ± SD	3.4 ± 1.9 (1–10)	3.4 ± 2	3.3 ± 1.7	0.79
ETMV, n (%)	13 (14.6)	11 (18.6)	2 (6.6)	0.1
ICU length of stay (days), mean ± SD	10.3 ± 11 (2–81)	11.1 ± 10.9	8.86 ± 13.7	0.4
ICU mortality, n (%)	6 (6.7)	6 (10.1)	0	0.07
Hospital mortality, n (%)	9 (10)	8 (13.5)	1 (3)	0.26
Hospital length of stay (days), mean ± SD	17.4 ± 12	18 ± 10	16.8 ± 13	0.7

ARF acute respiratory failure, *ETMV* endotracheal mechanical ventilation, *ICU* intensive care unit.

95% confidence interval, 1.9–68.3; $P = 0.007$) and no initial response to NIV (odds ratio, 117.6; 95% confidence interval, 10.6–1305.8; $P = 0.0001$).

Conclusion.—This prospective survey confirms the feasibility and efficacy of NIV in ARF following lung resection (Table 4).

▶ The use of noninvasive ventilation continues to grow, particularly when clinicians become comfortable with the technique and skilled in its use. Arguably, there are few clinicians more comfortable with the technique and skilled in its use than the French. This study evaluated the use of noninvasive ventilatory support in management of acute respiratory failure after lung resection. Whether the respiratory failure was hypoxemic or hypercapnic there were similar outcomes. The use of noninvasive ventilatory support can be expected to continue to increase in utilization, however, clinicians must also note when noninvasive support is not adequate and quickly move to invasive ventilatory support to avoid morbidity and mortality.

R. A. Balk, MD

Miscellaneous

Comparison of Lung Scintigraphy With Multi-Slice Spiral Computed Tomography in the Diagnosis of Pulmonary Embolism
Wang F, Fang W, Lv B, et al (Chinese Academy of Med Sciences and Peking Union Med College, Beijing, People's Republic of China)
Clin Nucl Med 34:424-427, 2009

Purpose.—To compare the diagnostic efficacy of lung perfusion scans combined with ventilation (V/Q) scans and/or chest radiography (CR) with contrast-enhanced multislice spiral CT pulmonary angiography (CTPA) in diagnosing pulmonary embolism (PE).

Materials and Methods.—Eighty-two consecutive patients with suspected PE underwent CTPA, lung perfusion scan, and CR. Of them, 28 patients underwent V/Q scans. The final diagnosis was made using a composite reference test.

Results.—The overall sensitivity and specificity were 89.2% and 92.1% for V/Q scan or perfusion scan combined with CR, and 97.3% and 97.4% for CTPA. For the 28 patients with V/Q scan, the sensitivity and specificity were 91.7% and 92.9% for V/Q scan, and 91.7% and 100.0% for CTPA. The segmental agreement rate between perfusion scan and CTPA was 69.5% (kappa = 0.30, $P < 0.05$). The perfusion scan revealed significantly more subsegmental abnormalities than CTPA (59 vs 10, χ^2 test, $P < 0.05$).

Conclusions.—V/Q scan, perfusion scan combined with CR and CTPA all show high efficacy in diagnosing PE. V/Q scan or perfusion scan combined with CR is as accurate as CTPA.

▶ After years of being pushed aside to a considerable degree by computed angiographic tomography, lung scintigraphy appears to be making a significant comeback. This is one of the several recent studies that support equivalent diagnostic capability of lung scintigraphy when compared with computed angiographic tomography in the diagnosis of pulmonary embolism. Lung scintigraphy, from my viewpoint, is most effective in patients without previous cardiopulmonary disease, and it is particularly effective when chest radiograph is without infiltrates. In that circumstance, there is neither chronic abnormality nor major acute primary ventilatory problems that would produce secondary perfusion changes. The primary value of lung scintigraphy over computed tomography is decreased radiation and no dye exposure. It is important to remember, however, that in patients who are intubated and mechanically ventilated and/or not capable of cooperating, the 8 views needed for optimum lung perfusion and ventilation imaging makes scintigraphy of limited use.

R. P. Dellinger, MD

Etomidate versus ketamine for rapid sequence intubation in acutely ill patients: a multicentre randomised controlled trial
Jabre P, Combes X, Lapostolle F, et al (Université Paris, Bobigny, France; Hôpital Henri Mondor, AP-HP, Créteil, France; et al)
Lancet 374:293-300, 2009

Background.—Critically ill patients often require emergency intubation. The use of etomidate as the sedative agent in this context has been challenged because it might cause a reversible adrenal insufficiency, potentially associated with increased in-hospital morbidity. We compared early and 28-day morbidity after a single dose of etomidate or ketamine used for emergency endotracheal intubation of critically ill patients.

Methods.—In this randomised, controlled, single-blind trial, 655 patients who needed sedation for emergency intubation were prospectively enrolled from 12 emergency medical services or emergency departments and 65 intensive care units in France. Patients were randomly assigned by a computerised random-number generator list to receive 0·3 mg/kg of etomidate (n=328) or 2 mg/kg of ketamine (n=327) for intubation. Only the emergency physician enrolling patients was aware of group assignment. The primary endpoint was the maximum score of the sequential organ failure assessment during the first 3 days in the intensive care unit. We excluded from the analysis patients who died before reaching the hospital or those discharged from the intensive care unit before 3 days (modified intention to treat). This trial is registered with ClinicalTrials.gov, number NCT00440102.

Findings.—234 patients were analysed in the etomidate group and 235 in the ketamine group. The mean maximum SOFA score between the two groups did not differ significantly (10·3 [SD 3·7] for etomidate *vs* 9·6 [3·9] for ketamine; mean difference 0·7 [95% CI 0·0–1·4], p=0·056). Intubation conditions did not differ significantly between the two groups (median intubation difficulty score 1 [IQR 0–3] in both groups; p=0·70). The percentage of patients with adrenal insufficiency was significantly higher in the etomidate group than in the ketamine group (OR 6·7, 3·5–12·7). We recorded no serious adverse events with either study drug.

Interpretation.—Our results show that ketamine is a safe and valuable alternative to etomidate for endotracheal intubation in critically ill patients, and should be considered in those with sepsis.

▶ Critically ill patients often require emergency orotracheal intubation for airway control. Rapid sequence intubation with administration of a sedative and a paralytic agent is commonly used in emergency departments. In patients who have hemodynamic instability, etomidate is the sedative drug that is most often used in rapid sequence intubation. However, over recent years, the use of etomidate has been brought to question because it can cause a reversible adrenal insufficiency. This adrenal insufficiency is secondary to a dose dependent inhibition of 11β-hydroxylase.[1] Multiple studies have reported an association between the use of etomidate and the development of adrenal insufficiency, and some studies suggest increased morbidity in critically ill patients, particularly in those with sepsis.[2] Development of adrenal insufficiency in a patient who is critically ill can increase the risk of death and has led some experts to advise against the use of etomidate (even as a single bolus).[3] Clinicians must balance the potential risks of causing adrenal insufficiency with the advantages of using etomidate in hemodynamically unstable patients who require emergent orotracheal intubation.

In this prospective randomized single-blinded study, Jabre et al compared early and 28-day morbidity after a single dose of etomidate or ketamine was used for emergency endotracheal intubation of critically ill patients. This study showed that 1 dose of 0.03 mg/kg of etomidate for emergency intubation can result in adrenal access dysfunction to a higher degree than when 2 mg/kg of ketamine is used. There was no difference between patients treated with eto-midate or ketamine when the primary endpoint of sequential organ failure assessment (SOFA) score during the first 3 days was compared. Both agents provided similar intubation conditions, and there were no differences in mortality or other complications. This well-conducted randomized trial provides useful information for clinicians. First, it seems to show that ketamine can be safety used in rapid sequence intubation and may constitute an alternative to etomidate. Second, this study confirms that etomidate is associated with an increased incidence of adrenal axis dysfunction as measured by cortisone levels and cosyntropin stimulation tests. What this study does not show is that the etomidate-induced adrenal insufficiency is associated with increased organ failure as measured by SOFA or increased mortality. One limitation of the study perhaps is the small number of patients with sepsis who were studied. In this group, no differences in morbidity or mortality were identified. However, the small number of patients with sepsis may have precluded a more definitive finding. So where does this leave the clinician at the bedside? It seems that there is a real risk of adrenal insufficiency with etomidate. This adrenal insuffi-ciency is transient. As of the results of this study, they do not indicate that there is an increased associated mortality. However, clinicians must weigh and balance the possible implications of adrenal insufficiency, especially in sepsis patients when deciding which agent to use. Finally, maybe the results of this study will encourage physicians to take a second look at ketamine as an alter-native for rapid sequence intubation in hemodynamically unstable patients.

S. L. Zanotti-Cavazzoni, MD

References

1. Malerba G, Romano-Girad F, Caravoisy A, et al. Risk factors of relative adren-cortical deficiency in intensive care patients needing mechanical ventilation. *Intensive Care Med.* 2005;31:388-392.
2. Lipiner-Friedman D, Sprung CL, Laterre PF, et al. Adrenal function in sepsis: the retrospective Corticus cohort study. *Crit Care Med.* 2007;35:1012-1018.
3. Annane D. ICU physicians should abandon the use of etomidate! *Intensive Care Med.* 2005;65:325-326.

Mechanical determinants of early acute ventilatory failure in COPD patients: a physiologic study

Purro A, Appendini L, Polillo C, et al (Gradenigo Hosp, Turin, Italy; Rehabilitation Inst of Veruno, Italy)
Intensive Care Med 35:639-647, 2009

Objective.—The purpose of this study is to investigate the respiratory mechanics, breathing pattern, and pressure-generating capacity of respira-tory muscles during the early phases of an acute exacerbation of COPD.

Design.—Prospective study.

Setting.—Division of Emergency Critical Care and Chronic Ventilator Unit.

Patients.—A total of 24 COPD patients: nine patients requiring ventilatory support because of acute respiratory acidosis due to COPD exacerbation (NPPV group, pH 7.28 ± 0.02); seven patients successfully managed with medical therapy only (SB group, pH 7.39 ± 0.04); eight clinically stable, long term mechanically ventilated, COPD patients (IPPV group).

Measurements.—Respiratory mechanics during a period of unsupported breathing.

Results.—A rapid shallow breathing, in the presence of a high drive to breath and a high diaphragmatic tension-time index (TT_{di}), was found in NPPV and IPPV groups compared to the SB group (f/V_T ratio: 118 ± 43 and 137 ± 65, respectively, versus 37 ± 12 breaths/min/l.; $P_{0.1}$: 5.0 ± 1.0 and 5.4 ± 1.4, respectively, versus 2.2 ± 0.2 cmH$_2$O, TT_{di}: 0.168 ± 0.035 and 0.161 ± 0.039, respectively, versus 0.057 ± 0.033); at variance, PEEPi$_{dyn}$ was greater in IPPV compared to the other two groups. A significant relationship was observed between TT_{di} ratio and f/V_T (Rho 0.756).

Conclusion.—During the early phases of an acute exacerbation, patients with COPD and acute respiratory failure had an imbalance between the decreased capacity of the respiratory muscles to generate pressure and the increased respiratory load. This imbalance was similar to that recorded in patients with COPD and chronic ventilatory failure. In both groups, the imbalance was associated with rapid shallow breathing. Among the

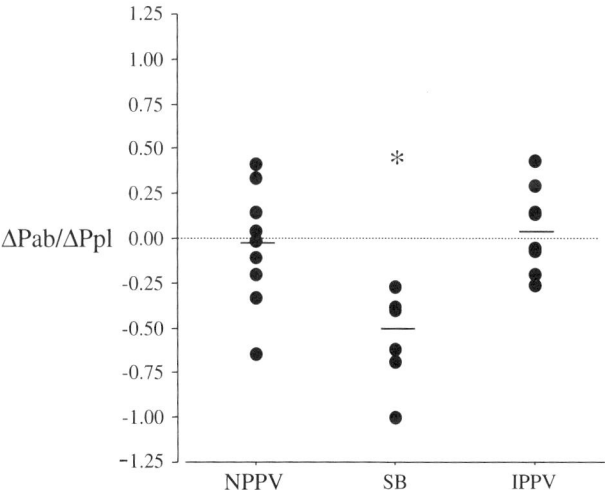

FIGURE 5.—Ventilatory muscle recruitment. $\Delta P_{ab}/\Delta P_{pl}$ ribcage and expiratory muscles recruitment index. *Horizontal bars* mean values. Both NPPV and IPPV showed a greater activation of ribcage and expiratory muscles in comparison to SB group (mean values −0.028 ± 0.353, 0.020 ± 0.061, and −0.550 ± 0.262, for NPPV, IPPV, and SB groups, respectively; *$P < 0.05$, SB versus both NPPV and IPPV groups). (Reprinted from Purro A, Appendini L, Polillo C, et al. Mechanical determinants of early acute ventilatory failure in COPD patients: a physiologic study. *Intensive Care Med.* 2009;35:639-647, with permission from Springer-Verlag.)

mechanical constraints to ventilation, only PEEPi,dyn was different between acute and chronic patients with ventilatory failure (Fig 5).

▶ This interesting, but small study attempted to better understand the reason for respiratory failure in a group of patients with chronic obstructive pulmonary disease (COPD) and admission for an acute exacerbation. Comparing patients treated with noninvasive ventilatory support to spontaneously breathing patients and patients on chronic invasive (through a tracheostomy) ventilatory support would allow evaluation of whether the acute respiratory failure resulted form problems with the respiratory control center, decreased respiratory muscle strength, or increased load on the respiratory muscles. In this small group of subjects, there were no problems with the respiratory controller function. There, however, was evidence of increased respiratory load and decreased respiratory muscle strength. Unfortunately, the study did not elucidate the contribution of various factors known to affect respiratory muscle function and/or load. The authors did note that the clinical manifestation of this imbalance of muscle function and respiratory load takes the form of rapid shallow breathing or an increased ratio of respiratory fate to tidal volume. Further studies and larger number of subjects will be needed to better guide our future management of these patients with treatments directed to improve the balance between respiratory muscle function and the stress they must overcome.

R. A. Balk, MD

Impact of a Monitored Program of Care on Incidence of Ventilator-Associated Pneumonia: Results of a Longterm Performance-Improvement Project

Weireter LJ Jr, Collins JN, Britt RC, et al (Eastern Virginia Med School, Norfolk)
J Am Coll Surg 208:700-705, 2009

Background.—Ventilator-associated pneumonia (VAP) remains a major source of morbidity, mortality, and expense in the ICU despite therapies directed against it.

Study Design.—A retrospective review of a prospectively developed performance-improvement project monitoring the incidence of VAP in two adjacent ICUs was conducted. In response to an excessive VAP rate, weekly multidisciplinary team meetings were instituted to review data, develop care protocols, and modify care routines. Protocol compliance was monitored daily and feedback provided weekly to the care teams. VAP rates were determined by the institutional Infection Control Committee and reviewed monthly with the ICU multidisciplinary team. Duration of the investigational period was 10 years.

Results.—A standardized ventilator-weaning protocol was instituted with confirmed 95% use. Additional modifications of care, such as patient positioning, use of specific endotracheal tubes to minimize aspiration of supraglottic secretions, an oral-care regimen, and aggressive antibiotic stewardship were standardized, with a compliance rate >90%. VAP rates dropped from 12.8 per 1,000 patient-days in 1998 to 1.1 in 2007 in the burn trauma ICU and from 21.2 to <1 in the neurotrauma ICU in the same time frame. Also, mean ventilator length of stay decreased from 6 days to 4.2 and from 5.8 days to 4.75 simultaneously in the respective ICUs. Such performance improvement has been sustained since implementation of the program.

Conclusion.—A systematic, monitored program of standardized care protocols can markedly reduce VAP rate in the ICU.

▶ Striving for excellence in decreasing events in the critically ill requires diligence and ongoing evaluation of performance and goal achievement. Although many processes and therapeutic interventions may be put in place, eliminating ventilator-associated pneumonia (VAP) completely is unlikely.[1]

This is a 10-year study that observed significant decreases in the VAP rates to near elimination in a burn trauma and the neurosurgical unit. There were several multidisciplinary processes put in place, including a directed antibiotic stewardship, directed bedside initiatives, and protocolization of ventilator weaning assessment and extubation. Audit and feedback was implemented with audit program for adherence to protocols. There were mechanisms put in place to reduce the time on mechanical ventilation, to modify the endotracheal tube, and to manage gastrointestinal feeding to minimize aspiration. Changes in the protocols and or algorithms were made based on the findings during the study period.

There were several processes put in place over the 10-year period. The investigators report taking a systems approach to decrease the VAP rate taking advantage of factors that were modifiable. The cumulative effect over time was outstanding, but there were periods when the VAP rate increased without any real identifiable cause. Yet, selecting 1 or even 2 interventions put in place to decrease VAP was not easily identifiable by the investigators. A study in Brazil found that decreasing VAP in an ICU setting requires a multifaceted approach and only when compliance exceeded 95% did the VAP rate drop to zero.[2] Weireter and colleagues report successful key elements in starting this project, including a break down of the data, developing new methods to deal with the problem, and testing the protocols. Rapid cycle testing was reported to be helpful in this 10-year period.

A model that includes physicians, nurses, and respiratory therapists within a team can help decrease VAP.[3] There are several important messages to take from this study. (1) Not only may the interventions be of significance, but also the culture change wanting to achieve a zero VAP rate was thought to contribute to the sustainability. (2) It is important to build on small successes and not overreact when there is a spike or several months with no VAP reported. (3) The improvements identified in this study found that the system needs a purpose and cooperation, and the system must be managed and led.

C. A. Schorr, RN, MSN

References

1. Palmer LB. Ventilator-associated infection. *Curr Opin Pulm Med*. 2009;15: 230-235.
2. Marra AR, Cal RG, Silva CV, et al. Successful prevention of ventilator-associated pneumonia in an intensive care setting. *Am J Infect Control*. 2009;37:619-625.
3. El-Khatib MF, Zeineldine S, Ayoub C, Husari A, Bou-Khalil PK. Clinicians' knowledge of evidence-based guidelines for preventing ventilator-associated pneumonia. *Am J Crit Care*. 2009 Aug 17 [Epub ahead of print].

2 Cardiovascular

Cardiopulmonary Resuscitation/Other

Epidemiologic Study of In-Hospital Cardiopulmonary Resuscitation in the Elderly

Ehlenbach WJ, Barnato AE, Curtis JR, et al (Univ of Washington, Seattle; Univ of Pittsburgh School of Medicine; et al)
N Engl J Med 361:22-31, 2009

Background.—It is unknown whether the rate of survival after in-hospital cardiopulmonary resuscitation (CPR) is improving and which characteristics of patients and hospitals predict survival.

Methods.—We examined fee-for-service Medicare data from 1992 through 2005 to identify beneficiaries 65 years of age or older who underwent CPR in U.S. hospitals. We examined temporal trends in the incidence of CPR and the rate of survival after CPR, as well as patient- and hospital-level predictors of survival to discharge.

Results.—We identified 433,985 patients who underwent in-hospital CPR; 18.3% of these patients (95% confidence interval [CI], 18.2 to 18.5) survived to discharge. The rate of survival did not change substantially during the period from 1992 through 2005. The overall incidence of CPR was 2.73 events per 1000 admissions; the incidence was higher among black and other nonwhite patients. The proportion of patients undergoing in-hospital CPR before death increased over time and was higher for nonwhite patients. The survival rate was lower among patients who were men, were older, had more coexisting illnesses, or were admitted from a skilled-nursing facility. The adjusted odds of survival for black patients were 23.6% lower than those for similar white patients (95% CI, 21.2 to 25.9). The association between race and survival was partially explained by hospital effects: black patients were more likely to undergo CPR in hospitals that have lower rates of post-CPR survival. Among patients surviving in-hospital CPR, the proportion of patients discharged home rather than to a health care facility decreased over time.

Conclusions.—Survival after in-hospital CPR did not improve from 1992 through 2005. The proportion of in-hospital deaths preceded by CPR increased, whereas the proportion of survivors discharged home after undergoing CPR decreased. Black race was associated with higher rates of CPR but lower rates of survival after CPR.

▶ Using a Medicare database from 1992 through 2005, the authors performed an analysis of trends in survival after in-hospital cardiopulmonary resuscitation (CPR). They found no improvement in survival after CPR over this time period. There are several possible explanations. First, many of the advances in delivering CPR are only pertinent to out-of-hospital cardiac arrest, such as the development of sophisticated emergency medical services (EMS) and training bystanders in CPR. Second, only recently has CPR quality become identified as a major determinant of outcome, and it is likely that CPR quality may have been similarly suboptimal throughout the entire study period. Lastly, postresuscitation therapeutic hypothermia has only recently been identified as a beneficial strategy for improving outcome, and hypothermia has also had very slow penetration into routine clinical practice. Therefore, this report is important for establishing a baseline for outcome in a Medicare population; however, the more important question is whether these new innovations will eventually be able to change a trajectory of this disease in a large population.

S. Trzeciak, MD, MPH

Epidemiologic Study of In-Hospital Cardiopulmonary Resuscitation in the Elderly
Ehlenbach WJ, Barnato AE, Curtis JR, et al (Univ of Washington, Seattle; Univ of Pittsburgh School of Medicine; et al)
N Engl J Med 361:22-31, 2009

Background.—It is unknown whether the rate of survival after in-hospital cardiopulmonary resuscitation (CPR) is improving and which characteristics of patients and hospitals predict survival.

Methods.—We examined fee-for-service Medicare data from 1992 through 2005 to identify beneficiaries 65 years of age or older who underwent CPR in U.S. hospitals. We examined temporal trends in the incidence of CPR and the rate of survival after CPR, as well as patient- and hospital-level predictors of survival to discharge.

Results.—We identified 433,985 patients who underwent in-hospital CPR; 18.3% of these patients (95% confidence interval [CI], 18.2 to 18.5) survived to discharge. The rate of survival did not change substantially during the period from 1992 through 2005. The overall incidence of CPR was 2.73 events per 1000 admissions; the incidence was higher among black and other nonwhite patients. The proportion of patients undergoing in-hospital CPR before death increased over time and was higher for nonwhite patients. The survival rate was lower among patients who were men, were older, had more coexisting illnesses, or were admitted from a skilled-nursing facility. The adjusted odds of survival for black patients were 23.6% lower than those for similar white patients (95% CI, 21.2 to

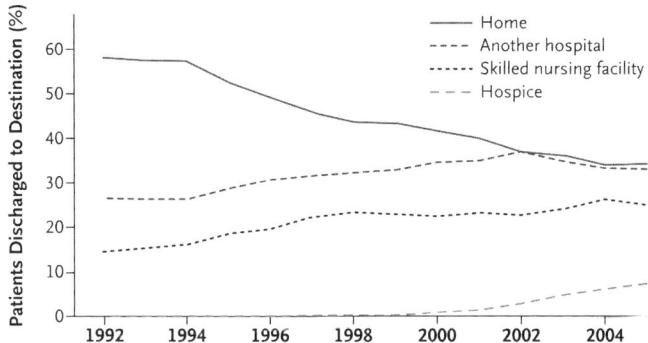

FIGURE 3.—Trends in the discharge destination of survivors of in-hospital CPR. Patients discharged home include both those with and those without home health or intravenous services. Patients discharged to a skilled nursing facility were covered by Medicare or Medicaid. Patients discharged to another hospital include those discharged to another acute care hospital, an intermediate care facility, a long-term care hospital, a non–acute care bed within the same hospital, or a rehabilitation hospital. Patients discharged to hospice include those discharged to hospice care either at home or at a medical facility; this category was used beginning in 1997. P for linear trend was less than 0.001 for all analyses. (Reprinted from Ehlenbach WJ, Barnato AE, Curtis JR, et al. Epidemiologic study of in-hospital cardiopulmonary resuscitation in the elderly. *N Engl J Med.* 2009;361:22-31. Copyright 2009 Massachusetts Medical Society. All rights reserved.)

25.9). The association between race and survival was partially explained by hospital effects: black patients were more likely to undergo CPR in hospitals that have lower rates of post-CPR survival. Among patients surviving in-hospital CPR, the proportion of patients discharged home rather than to a health care facility decreased over time.

Conclusions.—Survival after in-hospital CPR did not improve from 1992 through 2005. The proportion of in-hospital deaths preceded by CPR increased, whereas the proportion of survivors discharged home after undergoing CPR decreased. Black race was associated with higher rates of CPR but lower rates of survival after CPR (Table 1).

▶ The standard in the United States is that all hospitalized patients will undergo cardiopulmonary resuscitation (CPR) should they arrest unless specifically declined. This approach is in place despite the fact that CPR was originally crafted specifically for arrhythmic arrests, and it persists despite data that survival to discharge is fairly low and that survival to discharge rates are extremely poor when the patient has sepsis, renal failure, or metastatic cancer. This epidemiologic study adds some important information to the field especially during the present national debate on the future of health care. The data from this extremely large trial on over 400 000 admissions shows that survival to hospital discharge may be as low as 11% and as high as 22% (mean 18.3%). CPR is performed less often, and survival is less likely the higher the severity of illness (Deyo-Charlson score). Interestingly, CPR is performed more often as age increases from 65 to 79, but then less often from 80 and older, while the rate of survival declines steadily with advancing age. Fig 3 shows what is happening at discharge to the survivors, and fewer are heading

TABLE 1.—Percentage of Patients who Underwent In-Hospital Cardiopulmonary Resuscitation (CPR) and Survived to Hospital Discharge, According to Patient and Hospital Characteristics

Variable	In-Hospital CPR (N = 433,985) number (percent)	Survival to Hospital Discharge* percent (95% CI)
Patient characteristics		
Sex		
Male	219,377 (50.5)	17.5 (17.3–17.6)
Female	214,608 (49.5)	19.2 (19.1–19.4)
Age (yr)		
65–69	63,299 (14.6)	22.2 (21.9–22.6)
70–74	84,353 (19.4)	20.9 (20.6–21.1)
75–79	98,263 (22.6)	19.1 (18.9–19.3)
80–84	91,471 (21.1)	17.0 (16.8–17.3)
85–89	62,530 (14.4)	15.1 (14.8–15.4)
≥90	34,069 (7.9)	12.2 (11.9–12.6)
Race†		
White	352,173 (81.1)	19.2 (19.1–19.3)
Black	59,682 (13.8)	14.3 (14.0–14.6)
Other	22,130 (5.1)	15.9 (15.4–16.4)
Deyo–Charlson score‡		
0	77,349 (17.8)	18.7 (18.5–19.0)
1	145,627 (33.6)	19.1 (18.9–19.3)
2	116,401 (26.8)	18.9 (18.7–19.2)
≥3	94,608 (21.8)	16.1 (15.8–16.3)
Admitted from a skilled nursing facility		
Yes	10,924 (2.5)	11.5 (10.9–12.1)
No	423,061 (97.5)	18.5 (18.4–18.6)
ZIP Code median annual income		
<$15,000	10,626 (2.5)	13.3 (12.7–14.0)
$15,000–$29,999	87,164 (20.1)	17.9 (17.7–18.2)
$30,000–$44,999	178,536 (41.1)	19.1 (19.0–19.3)
$45,000–$59,999	70,429 (16.2)	18.4 (18.1–18.7)
$60,000–$74,999	22,083 (5.1)	18.3 (17.8–18.8)
≥$75,000	15,458 (3.6)	17.6 (17.0–18.2)
No data	49,489 (11.4)	17.4 (17.1–17.7)
Diagnosis§		
Myocardial infarction		
Yes	92,986 (21.4)	20.4 (20.1–20.7)
No	340,999 (78.6)	17.8 (17.7–17.9)
Congestive heart failure		
Yes	168,515 (38.8)	20.4 (20.2–20.6)
No	265,470 (61.2)	17.1 (16.9–17.2)
Stroke		
Yes	38,121 (8.8)	18.2 (17.8–18.5)
No	395,864 (91.2)	18.4 (18.2–18.5)
Diabetes mellitus		
Yes	78,840 (18.2)	17.3 (17.0–17.6)
No	355,145 (81.8)	18.6 (18.5–18.7)
Chronic obstructive pulmonary disease		
Yes	116,997 (27.0)	18.9 (18.6–19.1)
No	316,988 (73.0)	18.2 (18.0–18.3)
Hospital characteristics		
Location		
Metropolitan	345,808 (79.7)	18.0 (17.9–18.1)
Nonmetropolitan	73,397 (16.9)	21.1 (20.9–21.5)
Unknown	14,780 (3.4)	12.6 (12.0–13.1)
Teaching status		
Teaching hospital	144,385 (33.3)	17.4 (17.2–17.6)
Nonteaching hospital	288,774 (66.5)	18.8 (18.6–18.9)
Unknown	826 (0.2)	26.3 (23.3–29.3)
		(Continued)

TABLE 1. *(continued)*

Variable	In-Hospital CPR (N = 433,985) number (percent)	Survival to Hospital Discharge* percent (95% CI)
No. of beds		
<250	165,514 (38.1)	19.6 (19.4–19.8)
250–449	142,462 (32.8)	17.7 (17.5–17.9)
≥450	125,183 (28.9)	17.3 (17.1–17.5)
Unknown	826 (0.2)	26.3 (23.3–29.3)

*P<0.001 for all between-category differences except stroke, for which P = 0.32 (by the chi-square test).
†Information on race was obtained from Medicare data and is based on self-reporting by patients at the time of enrollment.
‡The Deyo–Charlson score ranges from 0 to 33, with higher scores indicating a higher burden of chronic illness.
§Diagnoses were for the hospitalization during which CPR was performed.

TABLE 2.—Multivariable Analyses for Factors Associated with Survival to Discharge

Predictor	Adjusted Odds Ratio (95% CI)	P Value
Analysis for patient and hospital factors*		
Age	0.97 (0.97–0.97)	<0.001
Male sex	0.84 (0.82–0.85)	<0.001
Race†		
White	Reference	
Black	0.70 (0.67–0.73)	<0.001
Other	0.85 (0.82–0.89)	<0.001
Deyo–Charlson score‡	0.93 (0.92–0.94)	<0.001
Admission from a skilled nursing facility	0.60 (0.54–0.67)	<0.001
Nonmetropolitan hospital	1.13 (1.08–1.18)	0.001
No. of hospital beds§	0.98 (0.96–0.98)	<0.001
Teaching hospital	1.00 (0.97–1.07)	0.38
Analysis with adjustment for hospital where CPR was performed¶		
Age	0.97 (0.97–0.97)	<0.001
Male sex	0.83 (0.82–0.84)	<0.001
Race†		
White	Reference	
Black	0.76 (0.74–0.79)	<0.001
Other	0.92 (0.88–0.96)	<0.001
Deyo–Charlson score‡	0.93 (0.92–0.94)	<0.001
Admission from a skilled nursing facility	0.69 (0.65–0.74)	<0.001

*Multivariable logistic regression was performed with empirical standard-error estimates, after accounting for clustering within the hospital.
†Information on race was obtained from Medicare data and is based on self-reporting by patients at the time of enrollment.
‡The odds ratio is that seen with an increase from one category of Deyo–Charlson score (0, 1, 2, or 3 or more) to the next. This score ranges from 0 to 33, with higher scores indicating a higher burden of chronic illness.
§The odds ratio is that seen with an increase of 100 hospital beds.
¶Logistic regression was used to model survival to discharge, with the inclusion of an indicator variable for each of the 6033 hospitals at which patients underwent CPR.

home than in the past with an increase in hospice admissions. This is an interesting finding in that hospice is designed to provide support for terminal patients, so we are effectively saving them from arrest to then send them elsewhere to die. Of course, it is hard to know if part of the reason they are sent to hospice is because the arrest created the patient status from which longer term survival was in doubt or from which quality of life was deemed less than ideal. Importantly, Table 2 shows the multivariate analysis that confirms much of what clinicians would expect in that lower rates of survival are associated with higher degrees of severity of illness, male sex, and admission from a skilled nursing facility (frailty). What may have surprised some is the association of higher rates with black race. Although this finding is extremely important in the health care debate, it does not appear to be a direct health care issue but a social issue of baseline health status and timeliness of seeking initial care.

T. Dorman, MD

Cardiac arrest survival after implementation of automated external defibrillator technology in the in-hospital setting
Forcina MS, Farhat AY, O'Neill WW, et al (Depts of Cardiovascular Medicine and Medicine, Royal Oak, MI; Miller School of Medicine at the Univ of Miami, FL)
Crit Care Med 37:1229-1236, 2009

Background.—Survival from ventricular tachycardia (VT) or ventricular fibrillation (VF) arrest is inversely related to delay to defibrillation. The automated external defibrillator (AED) has improved survival after out-of-hospital VT/VF arrest by decreasing time to defibrillation. The purpose of this study was to determine whether survival to discharge after in-hospital cardiac arrest caused by VT/VF could be improved via an institution-wide change from a standard monophasic defibrillator to a biphasic defibrillator with AED capability.

Methods and Results.—After extensive staff education, all standard defibrillators were replaced by AEDs at a single institution. Outcomes were analyzed for 1 year before the change and 1 year after the change using a prospective database. In patients whose initial rhythm was VT/VF, AEDs were not associated with improvement in time to first shock (median 1 minute for both cohorts, $p = 0.79$) or survival to discharge (31% vs. 29%, $p = 0.8$) compared with standard defibrillators. In patients whose initial rhythm was asystole or pulseless electrical activity, AEDs were associated with a significant decrease in survival (15%) compared with standard defibrillators (23%, $p = 0.04$). The overall AED cohort showed no difference in survival to discharge compared with the standard cohort (18% vs. 23%, $p = 0.09$).

Conclusions.—Replacement of standard monophasic defibrillators with biphasic AEDs was associated with unchanged survival after in-hospital

VT/VF arrest and decreased survival after in-hospital asystole or pulseless electrical activity arrest.

▶ Automated external defibrillators (AED) have been shown to increase survival after out-of-hospital cardiac arrest. This impact on survival has been most closely related to decreasing the time to cardiac defibrillation. Whether or not AEDs could also improve outcome for cardiac arrest victims in the hospital setting has been unclear, but is an important question to answer.

Forcina and colleagues performed a prospective single-center before and after study that aimed to test the impact of AED implementation throughout a single institution. The "before" period was one year in which standard defibrillators were used. The "after" period was one year in which AEDs were implemented.

There were 561 cardiac arrest patients enrolled in the study. Of those, only 87 were "shockable" rhythms (ie, pulseless ventricular tachycardia/ventricular fibrillation). However, of the 474 that were initially either asystole or pulseless electrical activity, 111 developed a late shockable rhythm. The number of subjects in the before and after groups were well matched. There was no measurable improvement in survival in the AED group. However, there was a slightly lower survival in the AED patients who initially had pulseless electrical activity or asystole.

In this single-center experience, AED-capable defibrillators failed to improve survival compared with standard defibrillators. The authors identified that the time to first defibrillation was not shorter in the AED group compared with standard defibrillators, and that may be responsible for the absence in difference in survival between the groups. As AEDs clearly decrease time to first defibrillation and subsequently improve clinical outcome in out-of-hospital cardiac arrest, future research should continue to test other settings in which AED implementation may be of benefit.

S. Trzeciak, MD, MPH

Prehospital therapeutic hypothermia for comatose survivors of cardiac arrest: a randomized controlled trial
Kämäräinen A, Virkkunen I, Tenhunen J, et al (Univ of Tampere, Finland; Tampere Univ Hosp, Finland; et al)
Acta Anaesthesiol Scand 53:900-907, 2009

Background.—Intravenous infusion of ice-cold fluid is considered a feasible method to induce mild therapeutic hypothermia in cardiac arrest survivors. However, only one randomized controlled trial evaluating this treatment exists. Furthermore, the implementation rate of prehospital cooling is low. The aim of this study was to evaluate the efficacy and safety of this method in comparison with conventional therapy with spontaneous cooling often observed in prehospital patients.

Methods.—A randomized controlled trial was conducted in a physician-staffed helicopter emergency medical service. After successful initial resuscitation, patients were randomized to receive either +4°C Ringer's solution with a target temperature of 33°C or conventional fluid therapy. As an endpoint, nasopharyngeal temperature was recorded at the time of hospital admission.

Results.—Out of 44 screened patients, 19 were analysed in the treatment group and 18 in the control group. The two groups were comparable in terms of baseline characteristics. The core temperature was markedly lower in the hypothermia group at the time of hospital admission (34.1 ± 0.9°C vs. 35.2 ± 0.8°C, $P < 0.001$) after a comparable duration of transportation. Otherwise, there were no significant differences between the groups regarding safety or secondary outcome measures such as neurological outcome and mortality.

Conclusion.—Spontaneous cooling alone is insufficient to induce therapeutic hypothermia before hospital admission. Infusion of ice-cold fluid after return of spontaneous circulation was found to be well tolerated and effective. This method of cooling should be considered as an important first link in the 'cold chain' of prehospital comatose cardiac arrest survivors.

▶ Therapeutic hypothermia has been shown to improve survival after resuscitation from cardiac arrest. Presumably, the earlier the intervention is initiated after return of spontaneous circulation, the better the chance for impact on the degree of anoxic brain injury. However, data is lacking on the feasibility of prehospital induction of therapeutic hypothermia. The significance of the research is that if prehospital induction of hypothermia is feasible and well tolerated, it could be initiated before emergency department care and delays in reaching target temperature could be avoided.

The authors performed their randomized trial of induced hypothermia with ice-cold saline versus conventional therapy. The trial was conducted in a helicopter emergency medical service. The primary outcome measure was body temperature at the time of hospital admission.

Forty-three patients were randomized. The body temperature was significantly lower in the hypothermia induction group at the time of hospital admission. The mean temperature was 34.1°C, which is very close to the typical 33-34°C target range for therapeutic hypothermia. There were no major hemodynamic changes or metabolic changes, indicating that the intervention was well tolerated.

As therapeutic hypothermia is a critical intervention for neuroprotection after cardiac arrest, studies such as this provide important information about the feasibility of earlier induction, even outside the hospital setting. Future research should aim to determine the optimal manner in which to deliver therapeutic hypothermia in the out-of-hospital setting, now that feasibility has been demonstrated.

S. Trzeciak, MD, MPH

Outcome, timing and adverse events in therapeutic hypothermia after out-of-hospital cardiac arrest
Nielsen N, for the Hypothermia Network (Lund Univ, Sweden; et al)
Acta Anaesthesiol Scand 53:926-934, 2009

Background.—Therapeutic hypothermia (TH) after cardiac arrest protects from neurological sequels and death and is recommended in guidelines. The Hypothermia Registry was founded to the monitor outcome, performance and complications of TH.

Methods.—Data on out-of-hospital cardiac arrest (OHCA) patients admitted to intensive care for TH were registered. Hospital survival and long-term outcome (6–12 months) were documented using the Cerebral Performance Category (CPC) scale, CPC 1–2 representing a good outcome and 3–5 a bad outcome.

Results.—From October 2004 to October 2008, 986 TH-treated OHCA patients of all causes were included in the registry. Long-term outcome was reported in 975 patients. The median time from arrest to initiation of TH was 90 min (interquartile range, 60–165 min) and time to achieving the target temperature ($\leq 34°C$) was 260 min (178–400 min). Half of the patients underwent coronary angiography and one-third underwent percutaneous coronary intervention (PCI). Higher age, longer time to return of spontaneous circulation, lower Glasgow Coma Scale at admission, un-witnessed arrest and initial rhythm asystole were all predictors of bad outcome, whereas time to initiation of TH and time to reach the goal temperature had no significant association. Bleeding requiring transfusion occurred in 4% of patients, with a significantly higher risk if angiography/PCI was performed (2.8% vs. 6.2% $P = 0.02$).

Conclusions.—Half of the patients survived, with >90% having a good neurological function at long-term follow-up. Factors related to the timing of TH had no apparent association to outcome. The incidence of adverse events was acceptable but the risk of bleeding was increased if angiography/PCI was performed.

▶ This was a descriptive analysis of registry data obtained over a 4-year period (2004-2008) of patients treated with therapeutic hypothermia after out-of-hospital cardiac arrest. The strength of this article is in the size of the sample ($n = 986$). Hypothermia was induced by a variety of techniques, including ice packs, cold intravenous fluid infusion, air cooling, circulating water blankets, and intravascular cooling devices. In this sample there were remarkably good outcomes, especially in the subjects with an initial "shockable" rhythm (ventricular fibrillation/pulseless ventricular tachycardia). Overall, half the patients survived. A high proportion of these patients had favorable neurologic outcome. The most common clinically significant adverse events were cardiac arrhythmia, infection, and hyperglycemia.

The efficacy of therapeutic hypothermia for neuroprotection has been demonstrated in clinical trials. This study represents important data on clinical effectiveness, ie, can similar favorable clinical outcomes be demonstrated when the intervention of therapeutic hypothermia is introduced in routine clinical practice (rather than within the confines of a clinical trial)? Although this is registry data without a comparison group, the high rate of survival to hospital discharge and favorable neurologic outcome are promising and lend further support to the effectiveness of this intervention for postresuscitation care.

S. Trzeciak, MD, MPH

Anion gap as a screening tool for elevated lactate in patients with an increased risk of developing sepsis in the Emergency Department
Berkman M, Ufberg J, Nathanson LA, et al (Harvard Univ School of Medicine, Boston, MA; Temple Univ School of Medicine, Philadelphia, PA)
J Emerg Med 36:391-394, 2009

Objectives.—Serum lactate levels are a useful tool in monitoring critically ill patients, especially those who are septic. However, lactate levels are often not routinely drawn or rapidly available in some institutions. The objective of this study was to determine if a readily available anion gap (AG) could be used as a surrogate marker for abnormal lactate level in Emergency Department (ED) patients at risk for sepsis.

Methods.—Prospective, observational cohort study of consecutive ED patients seen at an urban university tertiary care referral center with 46,000 annual ED visits. ED patients aged 18 years or older presenting with clinically suspected infection were eligible for enrollment if a serum chemistry and lactate levels were drawn during the ED visit. During the 9-month study period, 1419 patients were enrolled. The initial basic chemistry panels, calculated AG, and lactate levels drawn in the ED were collected. We defined, a priori, an AG > 12 and a lactate > 4 mmol/L to be abnormal. Analysis was performed with Student's t-test, operating characteristics with 95% confidence intervals, and logistic regression.

Results.—The mean AG was 11.8 (SD 3.6) and the mean lactate was 2.1 (SD 1.3). For an AG > 12, the mean lactate was 2.9 (SD 1.7), compared with 1.8 (SD 0.8) for an AG < 12. The sensitivity of an elevated AG (> 12) in predicting elevated lactate levels (>4 mmol/L) was 80% (72–87%) and the specificity was 69% (66–71%). Patients with a gap > 12 had a 7.3-fold (4.6–11.4) increased risk of having a lactate > 4 mmol/L. The area under the curve was 0.84.

Conclusion.—This study suggests that an elevated AG obtained in the ED is a moderately sensitive and specific means to detect elevated lactate levels in ED patients at risk for sepsis. This information may be somewhat helpful to Emergency Physicians to risk-stratify their patients to provide more aggressive early resuscitation.

▶ Serum lactate concentration has been identified as an important and independent predictor of death in patients with sepsis. Particularly lactate concentration ≥4 mmol/L identifies a population at an increased risk of death, and this threshold has been advocated for indicating the need for aggressive resuscitation. Not all emergency departments or ICUs routinely measure serum lactate in patients with sepsis. Whether or not the presence or absence of increased anion gap can be substituted for lactate measurement, or whether the absence of elevated anion gap can be used as rationale to not obtain a lactate measurement in these patients is unknown.

The authors found that anion gap > 12 was only 80% sensitive (95% confidence interval [CI] 72%-87%) for predicting a lactate level > 4 mmol/L. Although the presence of a major lactic acidosis should in theory increase anion gap, this study shows that anion gap may be insensitive for detecting lactate > 4 mmol/L. Therefore, anion gap may not be a reasonable surrogate for the measurement of serum lactate levels in this population.

S. Trzeciak, MD, MPH

Inadequate Blood Glucose Control Is Associated With In-Hospital Mortality and Morbidity in Diabetic and Nondiabetic Patients Undergoing Cardiac Surgery

Ascione R, Rogers CA, Rajakaruna C, et al (Univ of Bristol, UK)
Circulation 118:113-123, 2008

Background.—Derangement of glucose metabolism after surgery is not specific to patients with diabetes mellitus. We investigated the effect of different degrees of blood glucose control (BGC) on clinical outcomes after cardiac surgery.

Methods and Results.—We analyzed 8727 adults operated on between April 1996 and March 2004. The highest blood glucose level recorded over the first 60 hours postoperatively was used to classify patients as having good (<200 mg/dL), moderate (200 to 250 mg/dL), or poor (>250 mg/dL) BGC; 7547 patients (85%) had good, 905 (10%) had moderate, and 365 (4%) had poor BGC. Patients with inadequate BGC were more likely to present with advanced New York Heart Association class, congestive heart failure, hypertension, renal dysfunction, and ejection fraction <50% ($P \leq 0.001$). We found that 52% of patients with poor, 31% with moderate, and 8% with good BGC had diabetes mellitus. Inadequate BGC, but not diabetes mellitus ($P = 0.79$), was associated with in-hospital mortality (good, 1.8%; moderate, 4.2%; poor, 9.6%; adjusted odds ratio: poor versus good BGC, 3.90 [95% confidence interval, 2.47 to 6.15]; moderate versus good BGC, 1.68 [95% confidence interval, 1.25 to 2.25]). Inadequate BGC also was associated with postoperative myocardial infarction (eg, odds ratio, poor versus good BGC: 2.73 [95% confidence interval, 1.74 to 4.26]) and with pulmonary and renal complications in patients without known diabetes mellitus (eg, odds ratio, poor versus good BGC: 2.27 [95% confidence interval, 1.65 to 3.12] and 2.82 [95% confidence interval, 1.54 to 5.14] respectively).

Conclusions.—More than 50% of patients with moderate to poor BGC after cardiac surgery were not previously identified as diabetic. Inadequate postoperative BGC is a predictor of in-hospital mortality and morbidity.

▶ Glycemic control in the acute care of critically ill patients has become a key topic over the last decade. There are longstanding data that diabetes has been an independent risk factor for morbidity and mortality among critically ill patients and important for cardiac surgical patients specifically. Furnary and colleagues have shown that there is an association with glycemic control in diabetics and improved outcomes.[1] Importantly, they showed that with glycemic control, the mortality rate of diabetics merged with those of nondiabetics. Importantly, with increasing obesity in our populations, more patients with the metabolic syndrome are presenting for cardiac surgery and may not carry the diagnosis of diabetes, but certainly exhibit insulin resistance following surgery. In this retrospective, observational study by Ascione, they take an in-depth look at the association of inadequate glycemic control in both diabetic and nondiabetic patients undergoing cardiac surgery. They showed that glycemic control, and not history of diabetes, is independently associated with mortality and other complications, but not with perioperative infections. They report that of those with moderate to poor glycemic control, less than 50% were previously diagnosed as having diabetes. These findings can have important implications for the development and implementation of an insulin protocol in cardiac surgical patients.

Strengths of their analyses are that they took into account any associations between the surgeon of record by using a clustered analysis and that they looked for interactions between blood glucose levels and history of diabetes for each outcome of interest. However, as with many studies evaluating glycemic control, we are left with uncertainty as to what is the best measure of adequate glucose control. These authors looked at glucose values immediately after surgery, and at 12, 48, and 60 hours after surgery and used the single highest value of glucose to classify patients as having good, moderate, or poor glucose control. This definition contrasts with Furnary's method and others in the literature. This method, plus the high threshold for what they categorized as good control, introduces a great risk of misclassification of what the patient's overall course of glucose control looks like. However, most likely this misclassification would bias the results toward the null hypothesis. That is, such misclassification would have stacked the deck in favor of finding no association between glycemic control and outcomes. Furthermore, because they classified patients into good, moderate, and poor control, we do not have insight into what the most appropriate glucose is to target. Finally, they report no data on hypoglycemic events and the potential impact of these on the outcomes of interest. Despite these limitations, this article gives us more evidence that perioperative glycemic control in cardiac surgical patients is important and we need to continue to tease out what the ideal glucose target is, what patients should be included in our insulin protocols, and how we can protect against the unintended consequences of hypoglycemia. Finally, it also points out the power of the use of established databases and linking to other electronic databases to begin to answer these important questions that are key to us developing best practices for the care of our cardiac surgical patients.

E. A. Martinez, MD, MHS

Reference

1. Furnary AP, Wu Y, Bookin SO. Effect of hyperglycemia and continuous intravenous insulin infusions on outcomes of cardiac surgical procedures: the Portland diabetic project. *Endocr Pract.* 2004;2:21-33.

Improved Patient Survival Using a Modified Resuscitation Protocol for Out-of-Hospital Cardiac Arrest
Garza AG, Gratton MC, Salomone JA, et al (Georgetown Univ School of Medicine, Washington, DC; Health Department, Kansas City, MO; et al)
Circulation 119:2597-2605, 2009

Background.—Cardiac arrest continues to have poor survival in the United States. Recent studies have questioned current practice in resuscitation. Our emergency medical services system made significant changes to the adult cardiac arrest resuscitation protocol, including minimizing chest compression interruptions, increasing the ratio of compressions to ventilation, deemphasizing or delaying intubation, and advocating chest compressions before initial countershock.

Methods and Results.—This retrospective observational cohort study reviewed all adult primary ventricular fibrillation and pulseless ventricular tachycardia cardiac arrests 36 months before and 12 months after the protocol change. Primary outcome was survival to discharge; secondary outcomes were return of spontaneous circulation and cerebral performance category. Survival of out-of-hospital arrest of presumed primary cardiac origin improved from 7.5% (82 of 1097) in the historical cohort to 13.9% (47 of 339) in the revised protocol cohort (odds ratio, 1.80; 95% confidence interval, 1.19 to 2.70). Similar increases in return of spontaneous circulation were achieved for the subset of witnessed cardiac arrest patients with initial rhythm of ventricular fibrillation from 37.8% (54 of 143) to 59.6% (34 of 57) (odds ratio, 2.44; 95% confidence interval, 1.24 to 4.80). Survival to hospital discharge also improved from an unadjusted survival rate of 22.4% (32 of 143) to 43.9% (25 of 57) (odds ratio, 2.71; 95% confidence interval, 1.34 to 1.59) with the protocol. Of the 25 survivors, 88% (n = 22) had favorable cerebral performance categories on discharge.

Conclusions.—The changes to our prehospital protocol for adult cardiac arrest that optimized chest compressions and reduced disruptions increased the return of spontaneous circulation and survival to discharge in our patient population. These changes should be further evaluated for improving survival of out-of-hospital cardiac arrest patients.

▶ Quality of cardiopulmonary resuscitation (CPR), including (1) minimization of chest compression interruptions, (2) more compressions and less ventilations, and (3) chest compressions before initial countershock, have been identified as important factors related to successful return of spontaneous circulation. This was a retrospective observational cohort study in one emergency medical service (EMS) system. It was a before and after study that aimed to determine whether or not changes to standard practice that were focused on improving CPR quality would be associated with improved outcome after ventricular fibrillation or pulseless ventricular tachycardia cardiac arrest. The "before" period consisted of 36 months before a profound change, and the "after" period consisted of 12 months after the protocol change. The protocol change involved minimization of chest compression interruptions, increasing the frequency of chest compressions, and the ratio of compressions to ventilation, de-emphasizing the need for immediate intubation (and favoring chest compressions), and advocating chest compressions before the initial defibrillation attempt. The primary outcome measure was survival to hospital discharge, and the secondary outcome measure was achievement of return of spontaneous circulation.

There were 1097 subjects in the historical group and 339 in the new protocol group. The authors found that the new protocol period was significantly associated improved survival and return of spontaneous circulation.

In this before and after trial, the authors identified that an EMS-based protocol targeting the optimization of chest compression and reduced disruptions of CPR was associated with improved outcome from cardiac arrest. Although causality cannot be inferred from this methodology, the results are quite compelling that the protocol change was responsible for the observed differences in outcome. Given the historically abysmal survival of out-of-hospital cardiac arrest, data such as this is promising and suggests that there is in fact something that can be done to improve outcome from this disease.

S. Trzeciak, MD, MPH

Myocardial Infarction/Cardiogenic Shock/Cardiogenic Pulmonary Edema

Early versus Delayed, Provisional Eptifibatide in Acute Coronary Syndromes

Giugliano RP, White JA, Bode C, et al (Brigham and Women's Hosp, Boston, MA; Duke Univ Med Ctr, Durham, NC; Universitätsklinikum Freiburg, Germany; et al)
N Engl J Med 360:2176-2190, 2009

Background.—Glycoprotein IIb/IIIa inhibitors are indicated in patients with acute coronary syndromes who are undergoing an invasive procedure. The optimal timing of the initiation of such therapy is unknown.

Methods.—We compared a strategy of early, routine administration of eptifibatide with delayed, provisional administration in 9492 patients who had acute coronary syndromes without ST-segment elevation and who were assigned to an invasive strategy. Patients were randomly assigned to receive either early eptifibatide (two boluses, each containing 180 μg per kilogram of body weight, administered 10 minutes apart, and a standard infusion ≥12 hours before angiography) or a matching placebo infusion with provisional use of eptifibatide after angiography (delayed eptifibatide). The primary efficacy end point was a composite of death, myocardial infarction, recurrent ischemia requiring urgent revascularization, or the occurrence of a thrombotic complication during percutaneous coronary intervention that required bolus therapy opposite to the initial study-group assignment ("thrombotic bailout") at 96 hours. The key secondary end point was a composite of death or myocardial infarction within the first 30 days. Key safety end points were bleeding and the need for transfusion within the first 120 hours after randomization.

Results.—The primary end point occurred in 9.3% of patients in the early-eptifibatide group and in 10.0% in the delayed-eptifibatide group (odds ratio, 0.92; 95% confidence interval [CI], 0.80 to 1.06; P = 0.23). At 30 days, the rate of death or myocardial infarction was 11.2% in the early-eptifibatide group, as compared with 12.3% in the delayed-eptifibatide group (odds ratio, 0.89; 95% CI, 0.79 to 1.01; P = 0.08). Patients in the early-eptifibatide group had significantly higher rates of bleeding and red-cell transfusion. There was no significant difference between the two groups in rates of severe bleeding or nonhemorrhagic serious adverse events.

Conclusions.—In patients who had acute coronary syndromes without ST-segment elevation, the use of eptifibatide 12 hours or more before angiography was not superior to the provisional use of eptifibatide after angiography. The early use of eptifibatide was associated with an increased risk of non–life-threatening bleeding and need for transfusion. (ClinicalTrials.gov number, NCT00089895.)

▶ The American College of Cardiology/American Heart Association 2007 Guidelines for the Management of Unstable Angina/Non-ST-Elevation Myocardial Infarction (UA/NSTEMI) include several class I and class II recommendations regarding treatment with glycoprotein (GP) IIb/IIIa inhibitors and other antiplatelet agents.[1] One of the 6 class I recommendations for antiplatelet therapy is that for UA/NSTEMI patients in whom an initial invasive strategy is selected, antiplatelet therapy in addition to aspirin should be initiated before diagnostic angiography (upstream) with either clopidogrel or an intravenous GP IIb/IIa inhbitor.[1] One of the 3 class IIa recommendations for antiplatelet therapy is that for UA/NSTEMI patients in whom an initial invasive strategy is selected, it is reasonable to initiate antiplatelet therapy with both clopidogrel and an intravenous GP IIb/IIIa inhibitor.[1] Numerous clinical trials have shown beneficial effects of abciximab, eptifibatide, and tirofiban in patients with acute coronary syndromes (ACS), but several recent studies suggest that the increased bleeding risk of upstream administration of a GP IIb/IIIa inhibitor before coronary angiography may outweigh the potential benefits.

The Acute Catheterization and Urgent Intervention Triage Strategy (ACUITY) trial randomized 13 819 patients with ACS to 1 of 3 antithrombotic regimens: (1) bivalirudin, a direct thrombin inhibitor; (2) bivalirudin plus a GP IIb/IIIa inhibitor; or (3) a GP IIb/IIIa inhibitor plus either unfractionated heparin (UFH) or enoxaparin.[2] Bivalirudin alone, as compared with heparin plus a GP IIb/IIIa inhibitor, was associated with a noninferior rate of the composite ischemia end point (7.8% and 7.3%, respectively; $P = .32$; relative risk, 1.08; 95% confidence interval [CI], 0.93–1.24) and a significantly reduced rate of major bleeding (3.0% vs 5.7%; $P < .001$; relative risk, 0.53; 95% CI, 0.43–0.65). The American College of Cardiology/American Heart Association 2007 Guidelines for the Management of UA/NSTEMI include the following class IIa recommendation—for UA/NSTEMI patients in whom an initial invasive strategy is selected, and it is reasonable to omit upstream administration of an intravenous GP IIb/IIIa antagonist before diagnostic angiography if bivalirudin is selected as the anticoagulant and at least 300 mg of clopidogrel was administered at least 6 hours earlier than planned catheterization or percutaneous coronary intervention (PCI)."[1]

The Early Glycoprotein IIb/IIIa Inhibition in Non-ST-Segment Elevation ACS (EARLY ACS) trial compared early routine administration of eptifibatide before coronary angiography with delayed provisional administration after coronary angiography in 9492 patients with high-risk ACS without ST-segment elevation. There was no significant difference in the frequency of the primary efficacy end point, a composite of death, MI, recurrent ischemia requiring urgent revascularization, or the occurrence of a thrombotic complication during PCI that required bolus therapy opposite to the initial study group assignment at 96 hours. These rates of bleeding and red-cell transfusion were significantly greater among the patients in the early-eptifibatide group.

Recent studies have suggested that bleeding is an independent risk factor for death in patients with ACS.[3-5] Among patients who were enrolled in the ACUITY trial, the risk of death was slightly greater among patients with major bleeding (hazard ratio 3.5) than among patients with MI (hazard ratio 3.1).[5] Major bleeding was associated with a 4-fold increased hazard of death, MI, or stroke during the first 30 days among patients who were enrolled in the Fifth Organization to Assess Strategies in Ischemic Syndromes (OASIS 5) trial, a double-blind study that randomized 20 078 patients with non-ST-segment elevation ACS to either subcutaneous fondaparinux 2.5 mg daily or subcutaneous enoxaparin 1 mg/kg twice daily.[4] At the discretion of the treating physician, 18% of patients also received a GP IIb/IIIa inhibitor and 67% received a thienopyridine.[6] Among patients who were treated with a GP IIb/IIIa inhibitor, treatment with fondaparinux was associated with a 40% reduction in major bleeding at 30 days after enrollment compared with treatment with enoxaparin (5.2% vs 8.3%, hazard ratio 0.61, $P < .001$).[6]

Thus, the results of randomized clinical trials suggest that the following treatment strategies appear to be associated with the least risk of bleeding in patients with ACS who are treated with aspirin and a thienopyridine: (1) fondaparinux plus delayed provisional administration of a GP IIb/IIIa inhibitor

after coronary angiography or (2) bivalirudin plus delayed provisional administration of a GP IIb/IIIa inhibitor. The role of upstream administration of a GP
IIb/IIIa inhibitor before coronary angiography is unclear. The 2009 Focused
Updates of the ACC/AHA guidelines for the Management of Patients with
STEMI state that "...an argument can be made against the routine upstream
use of GP IIb/IIIa therapy in all non-ST-elevation ACS patients intended for
an invasive strategy."[7] Furthermore, the updated guidelines state that "...a
high-risk group that would clearly benefit from the early administration of
eptifibatide upstream before cardiac catheterization has not been identified."[7]

S. W. Werns, MD

References

1. Anderson JL, Adams CD, Antman EM, et al. ACC/AHA 2007 guidelines for the management of patients with unstable angina/non-ST-elevation myocardial infarc-tion: a report of the American College of Cardiology/American Heart Association Task Force on Practice Guidelines. *Circulation.* 2007;116:e148-e304.
2. Stone GW, McLaurin BT, Cox DA, et al. Bivalirudin for patients with acute coro-nary syndromes. *N Engl J Med.* 2006;355:2203-2216.
3. Yan AT, Yan RT, Huynh T, et al. Bleeding and outcome in acute coronary syndrome: insights from continuous electrocardiogram monitoring in the Integrilin and Enoxaparin Randomized Assessment of Acute Coronary syndrome Treatment (INTERACT) trial. *Am Heart J.* 2008;156:769-775.
4. Budaj A, Eikelboom JW, Mehta SR, et al. Improving clinical outcomes by reducing bleeding in patients with non-ST-elevation acute coronary syndromes. *Eur Heart J.* 2009;30:655-661.
5. Mehran R, Pocock SJ, Stone GW, et al. Associations of major bleeding and myocardial infarction with the incidence and timing of mortality in patients pre-senting with non-ST-elevation acute coronary syndromes: a risk model from the ACUITY trial. *Eur Heart J.* 2009;30:1457-1466.
6. Jolly SS, Faxon DP, Fox KAA, et al. Efficacy and safety of fondaparinux versus enoxaparin in patients with acute coronary syndromes treated with glycoprotein IIb/IIIa inhibitors or thienopyridines: results from the OASIS 5 (Fifth Organization to Assess Strategies in Ischemic Syndromes) trial. *J Am Coll Cardiol.* 2009;54: 468-476.
7. Kushner FG, Hand M, Smith SC Jr, et al. 2009 Focused updates: ACC/AHA guide-lines for the management of patients with ST-elevation myocardial infarction (updating the 2004 guideline and 2007 focused update) and ACC/AHA/SCAI guidelines on percutaneous coronary intervention (updating the 2005 guidelines and 2007 focused update): a report of the American College of Cardiology Foundation/American Heart Association Task Force on Practice Guidelines. *Circulation.* 2009;120:2271-2306.

Adding intravenous unfractionated heparin to standard enoxaparin causes excessive anticoagulation not detected by activated clotting time: Results of the STACK-on to ENOXaparin (STACKENOX) study

Drouet L, Bal dit Sollier C, Martin J (Hôpital Lariboisière, Paris, France; Sharpe-Strumia Res Foundation of the Bryn Mawr Hosp, PA)
Am Heart J 158:177-184, 2009

Background.—The STACKENOX study assessed the cumulative anticoagulation effect of administering stack-on intravenous unfractionated heparin (UFH) to subjects already receiving enoxaparin.

Methods.—Seventy-two healthy subjects aged 40 to 60 years received subcutaneous enoxaparin (1 mg/kg every 12 hours) for 2.5 days (steady state) and were randomized to receive a 70 IU/kg intravenous UFH bolus 4, 6, or 10 hours after the final enoxaparin dose. Anticoagulation levels were assessed in subjects receiving enoxaparin alone and after the UFH bolus by monitoring activated clotting time (ACT), anti-Xa and anti-IIa activities, and thrombin generation (endogenous thrombin potential [ETP]).

Results.—After the final enoxaparin dose, ETP levels decreased by 40%; anti-Xa and anti-IIa activities increased, as expected; and ACT levels did not indicate any anticoagulation effect. Stack-on UFH at 4, 6, or 10 hours after the last enoxaparin dose significantly increased anti-Xa and anti-IIa activities ($P < .0001$) to well above accepted therapeutic levels and resulted in total inhibition of thrombin generation for ≥ 2 hours; ACT levels remained within the range commonly observed in subjects receiving UFH.

Conclusions.—The administration of stack-on UFH to subjects already receiving recommended enoxaparin dosing may result in over-anticoagulation, and should be avoided. Activated clotting time assessment did not detect the over-anticoagulation resulting from co-administration of enoxaparin and UFH.

▶ A combination of potent antiplatelet and anticoagulant drugs is recommended for patients who undergo elective percutaneous coronary intervention (PCI) and for patients with acute coronary syndromes (ACS) or ST-segment elevation myocardial infarction (MI). Antiplatelet therapy includes aspirin plus a thienopyridine, eg, clopidogrel or prasugrel. The options for anticoagulant therapy include unfractionated heparin (UFH), low molecular weight heparin (LMWH), bivalirudin, and fondaparinux, a factor Xa inhibitor. Although the recommended regimens have been shown to reduce the risk of death, MI, and coronary stent thrombosis, they increase the risk of bleeding. Recent studies have suggested that bleeding is an independent risk factor for death after PCI or MI.[1,2]

Compared with UFH, treatment with enoxaparin, a LMWH, is associated with a lower risk of death, MI, and urgent revascularization in patients with ACS.[3] When patients with ACS undergo PCI it is common practice to administer a dose of UFH despite ongoing treatment with LMWH, presumably because a prompt, bedside assessment of the extent of anticoagulation during treatment with LMWH is not readily available. There is evidence, however, that there is an increased incidence of bleeding in patients who cross-over from LMWH to UFH.[4] Therefore, the study conducted by Drouet et al is interesting and important. The results indicate that measurement of the activated clotting time does not detect over-anticoagulation that results from coadministration of enoxaparin and UFH. The implications of the study are that adding UFH to enoxaparin in patients who undergo PCI results in over-anticoagulation and probably increases the risk of bleeding.

This study has 2 minor limitations. One is that the subjects were healthy rather than patients with ACS or MI or patients undergoing PCI. The second limitation is that the bleeding risk associated with the observed levels of over-anticoagulation is unknown.

S. W. Werns, MD

References

1. Budaj A, Eikelboom JW, Mehta SR, et al. Improving clinical outcomes by reducing bleeding in patients with non-ST-elevation acute coronary syndromes. *Eur Heart J.* 2009;30:655-661.
2. Mehran R, Pocock SJ, Stone GW, et al. Associations of major bleeding and myocardial infarction with the incidence and timing of mortality in patients presenting with non-ST-elevation acute coronary syndromes: a risk model from the ACUITY trial. *Eur Heart J.* 2009;30:1457-1466.
3. Murphy SA, Gibson CM, Morrow DA, et al. Efficacy and safety of the low-molecular weight heparin enoxaparin compared with unfractionated heparin across the acute coronary syndrome spectrum: a meta-analysis. *Eur Heart J.* 2007;28: 2077-2086.
4. SYNERGY Trial Investigators. Enoxaparin vs unfractionated heparin in high-risk patients with non-ST-segment elevation acute coronary syndromes managed with an intended early invasive strategy. *JAMA.* 2004;292:45-54.

Efficacy and Safety of Fondaparinux Versus Enoxaparin in Patients With Acute Coronary Syndromes Treated With Glycoprotein IIb/IIIa Inhibitors or Thienopyridines: Results From the OASIS 5 (Fifth Organization to Assess Strategies in Ischemic Syndromes) Trial

Jolly SS, Faxon DP, Fox KAA, et al (McMaster Univ, Hamilton, Ontario, Canada; Brigham and Women's Hosp and Harvard Med School, Boston, MA; Royal Infirmary and Univ of Edinburgh, Scotland; et al)

J Am Coll Cardiol 54:468-476, 2009

Objectives.—This study sought to evaluate the relative safety and efficacy of fondaparinux and enoxaparin in patients with acute coronary syndromes (ACS) treated with glycoprotein (GP) IIb/IIIa inhibitors or thienopyridines.

Background.—The OASIS 5 (Fifth Organization to Assess Strategies in Ischemic Syndromes) trial showed that fondaparinux reduced major bleeding by 50% compared with enoxaparin while preserving similar efficacy. Whether this benefit is consistent in the presence or absence of concurrent antiplatelet therapy with clopidogrel and GP IIb/IIIa inhibitors is unknown.

Methods.—Patients with ACS (n = 20,078) were randomized as a part of the OASIS 5 trial to receive either fondaparinux or enoxaparin. The use of GP IIb/IIIa inhibitors or thienopyridines was at the discretion of the treating physician. A Cox proportional hazard model was used to compare outcomes.

Results.—Of the 20,078 patients randomized, 3,630 patients received GP IIb/IIIa and 13,531 received thienopyridines. There was a 40% reduction in major bleeding with fondaparinux compared with enoxaparin in those treated with GP IIb/IIIa (5.2% vs 8.3%, hazard ratio [HR]: 0.61, p < 0.001). A similar reduction was found in those treated with thienopyridines (3.4% vs 5.4%, HR: 0.62, p < 0.001). Ischemic events were similar between the groups, resulting in a superior net clinical outcome (death, myocardial infarction, refractory ischemia, or major bleeding) favoring fondaparinux (GP IIb/IIIa subgroup 14.8% vs 18.9%, HR: 0.77, p = 0.001 and thienopyridines subgroup 11.0% vs 13.2%, HR: 0.82, p < 0.001).

Conclusions.—In patients receiving GP IIb/IIIa inhibitors or thienopyridines, fondaparinux reduces major bleeding and improves net clinical outcome compared with enoxaparin.

▶ Various antiplatelet and anticoagulant agents have been shown to reduce the risk of death, MI, and coronary stent thrombosis in patients with non-ST-segment elevation acute coronary syndromes (ACS) or ST-segment elevation myocardial infarction (MI), but they increase the risk of bleeding. Recent studies have suggested that bleeding is an independent risk factor for death after percutaneous coronary intervention (PCI) or MI.[1,2] Therefore, it is important to examine the rates of bleeding that have been reported in clinical trials that compared different antithrombin drugs.

Clinical trials have not supported the hypothesis that treatment with low molecular weight heparin (LMWH) would cause less bleeding than treatment with unfractionated heparin (UFH). The Superior Yield of the New Strategy of Enoxaparin, Revascularization and Glycoprotein IIb/IIIa Inhibitors (SYNERGY) trial was a prospective, randomized, open-label, multicenter trial that enrolled a total of 10 027 high-risk patients with non-ST–segment elevation ACS to be treated with an intended early invasive strategy.[3] More bleeding was observed with enoxaparin, with a statistically significant increase in thrombolysis in MI (TIMI) major bleeding (9.1% vs 7.6%, $P = .008$) but a nonsignificant excess in global utilization of streptokinase and t-PA for occluded arteries (GUSTO) severe bleeding (2.7% vs 2.2%, $P = .08$) and transfusions (17.0% vs 16.0%, $P = .16$). Petersen et al[4] analyzed the outcomes of 21 946 patients with non-ST–segment elevation ACS who were enrolled in 6 randomized trials that compared enoxaparin with UFH. There was no significant difference in the frequency of blood transfusion (OR, 1.01; 95% CI, 0.89-1.14) or major bleeding (OR, 1.04; 95% CI, 0.83-1.30) at 7 days after randomization.

Jolly et al analyzed the frequency of bleeding complications among patients who were enrolled in the OASIS 5 (Fifth Organization to Assess Strategies in Ischemic Syndromes) trial, a double-blind study that randomized 20 078 patients with non-ST–segment elevation ACS to either subcutaneous fondaparinux 2.5 mg daily or subcutaneous enoxaparin 1 mg/kg twice daily. At the discretion of the treating physician, 18% of patients also received a glycoprotein (GP) IIb/IIIa inhibitor and 67% received a thienopyridine. Among patients who were treated with a GP IIb/IIIa inhibitor treatment, fondaparinux was associated with a 40% reduction in major bleeding at 30 days after enrollment. Fondaparinux also was associated with a 40% reduction in major bleeding among patients who were treated with a thienopyridine. Among patients who underwent PCI there was an increase in the rate of guiding-catheter thrombus formation with fondaparinux (29 episodes [0.9%], vs 8 episodes with enoxaparin [0.3%]).[5]

Bivalirudin, a direct thrombin inhibitor, also has been shown to reduce the risk of bleeding in patients with ACS or ST-segment elevation MI. The Acute Catheterization and Urgent Intervention Triage Strategy (ACUITY) trial randomized 13 819 patients with ACS to 1 of 3 antithrombotic regimens: UFH or enoxaparin plus a GP IIb/IIIa inhibitor, bivalirudin plus a GP IIb/IIIa inhibitor, or bivalirudin alone.[6] Bivalirudin alone, as compared with heparin plus a GP IIb/IIIa inhibitor, was associated with a noninferior rate of the composite ischemia end point (7.8% and 7.3%, respectively; $P = .32$; relative risk, 1.08; 95% confidence interval [CI], 0.93-1.24) and a significantly reduced rate of major bleeding (3.0% vs 5.7%; $P < .001$; relative risk, 0.53; 95% CI, 0.43-0.65). The HORIZONS-AMI trial enrolled 3602 patients who were anticipated to undergo primary PCI for ST-segment elevation MI.[7] The rate of major bleeding unrelated to coronary artery bypass graft surgery 30 days after randomization was significantly lower among patients assigned to treatment with bivalirudin compared with patients who were treated with UFH and a GP IIb/IIIa inhibitor (4.9% vs 8.3%; relative risk, 0.60; 95% CI, 0.46-0.77; $P < .001$).

There are no published studies that directly compared bivalirudin with fondaparinux in patients with ACS or MI. The most recent ACC/AHA Practice Guidelines include class I indications for both bivalirudin and fondaparinux in patients with ACS or ST-segment elevation MI. The results of the study by Jolly et al provide strong support for choosing fondaparinux instead of UFH or a LWMH to anticoagulate patients with ACS or STEMI. Bivalirudin is an excellent alternative that is not associated with an increased risk of catheter thrombosis. Therefore, unlike fondaparinux, supplemental treatment with LMWH or UFH is unnecessary in patients who are treated with bivalirudin and undergo PCI.

S. W. Werns, MD

References

1. Budaj A, Eikelboom JW, Mehta SR, et al. Improving clinical outcomes by reducing bleeding in patients with non-ST-elevation acute coronary syndromes. *Eur Heart J.* 2009;30:655-661.

2. Mehran R, Pocock SJ, Stone GW, et al. Associations of major bleeding and myocardial infarton with the incidence and timing of mortality in patients presenting with non-ST-elevation acute coronary syndromes: a risk model from the ACUITY trial. *Eur Heart J.* 2009;30:1457-1466.
3. SYNERGY Trial Investigators. Enoxaparin vs unfractionated heparin in high-risk patients with non-ST-segment elevation acute coronary syndromes managed with an intended early invasive strategy. *JAMA.* 2004;292:45-54.
4. Petersen JL, Mahaffey KW, Hasselblad V, et al. Efficacy and bleeding complications among patients randomized to enoxaparin or unfractionated heparin for antithrombin therapy in non-ST-segment elevation acute coronary syndromes. *JAMA.* 2004;292:89-96.
5. The Fifth Organization to Assess Strategies in Acute Ischemic Syndromes Investigators. Comparison of fondaparinux and enoxaparin in acute coronary syndromes. *N Engl J Med.* 2006;354:1464-1476.
6. Stone GW, McLaurin BT, Cox DA, et al. Bivalirudin for patients with acute coronary syndromes. *N Engl J Med.* 2006;355:2203-2216.
7. Stone GW, Witzenbichler B, Guagliumi G, et al. Bivalirudin during primary PCI in acute myocardial infarction. *N Engl J Med.* 2008;358:2218-2230.

Pharmacodynamic effect and clinical efficacy of clopidogrel and prasugrel with or without a proton-pump inhibitor: an analysis of two randomized trials

O'Donoghue ML, Braunwald E, Antman EM, et al (Brigham and Women's Hosp, Boston, MA)
Lancet 374:989-997, 2009

Background.—Proton-pump inhibitors (PPIs) are often prescribed in combination with thienopyridines. Conflicting data exist as to whether PPIs diminish the efficacy of clopidogrel. We assessed the association between PPI use, measures of platelet function, and clinical outcomes for patients treated with clopidogrel or prasugrel.

Methods.—In the PRINCIPLE-TIMI 44 trial, the primary outcome was inhibition of platelet aggregation at 6 h assessed by light-transmission aggregometry. In the TRITON-TIMI 38 trial, the primary endpoint was the composite of cardiovascular death, myocardial infarction, or stroke. In both studies, PPI use was at physician's discretion. We used a multivariable Cox model with propensity score to assess the association of PPI use with clinical outcomes.

Findings.—In the PRINCIPLE-TIMI 44 trial, 201 patients undergoing elective percutaneous coronary intervention were randomly assigned to prasugrel (n=102) or high-dose clopidogrel (n=99). Mean inhibition of platelet aggregation was significantly lower for patients on a PPI than for those not on a PPI at 6 h after a 600 mg clopidogrel loading dose ($23 \cdot 2 \pm 19 \cdot 5\%$ *vs* $35 \cdot 2 \pm 20 \cdot 9\%$, p=$0 \cdot 02$), whereas a more modest difference was seen with and without a PPI after a 60 mg loading dose of prasugrel ($69 \cdot 6 \pm 13 \cdot 5\%$ *vs* $76 \cdot 7 \pm 12 \cdot 4\%$, p=$0 \cdot 054$). In the TRITON-TIMI 38 trial, 13 608 patients with an acute coronary syndrome were randomly assigned to prasugrel (n=6813) or clopidogrel (n=6795). In this study, 33% (n=4529) of patients were on a PPI at randomisation. No association existed between PPI use and risk of the primary endpoint for patients treated with clopidogrel (adjusted hazard ratio [HR] 0·94, 95% CI 0·80–1·11) or prasugrel (1·00, 0·84–1·20).

Interpretation.—The current findings do not support the need to avoid concomitant use of PPIs, when clinically indicated, in patients receiving clopidogrel or prasugrel.

▶ The American College of Cardiology/American Heart Association 2007 guidelines for the management of unstable angina/non-ST-rlevation myocardial infarction include the following class I recommendation: "in unstable angina/non-ST-segment elevation myocardial infarction patients with a history of gastrointestinal bleeding, when aspirin and clopidogrel are administered alone or in combination, drugs to minimize the risk of recurrent gastrointestinal bleeding (eg, proton-pump inhibitors) should be prescribed concomitantly."[1] A 2008 expert consensus document on reducing the gastrointestinal risk of antiplatelet therapy and NSAID use reiterated the same recommendation.[2] Therefore, the Public Health Advisory that was announced by the United States Food and Drug Administration (FDA) on November 17, 2009 is somewhat problematic. It stated that FDA is alerting the public to new safety information concerning an interaction between clopidogrel (Plavix), an anticlotting medication, and omeprazole (Prilosec/Prilosec OTC), a proton pump inhibitor...New data show that when clopidogrel and omeprazole are taken together, the effectiveness of clopidogrel is reduced.

The presumed stimulus for the revised labeling of clopidogrel is a retrospective cohort study of 8205 patients with acute coronary syndrome (ACS) who were taking clopidogrel after discharge from 127 Veterans Affairs hospitals between October 2003 and January 2006.[3] The use of clopidogrel plus a proton pump inhibitor (PPI) was associated with an increased risk of death or rehospitalization for ACS compared with the use of clopidogrel without a PPI (adjusted odds ratio [AOR], 1.25; 95% confidence interval [CI], 1.11-1.41). Among patients taking clopidogrel after hospital discharge and prescribed a PPI at any point during follow-up ($n = 5244$), periods of use of clopidogrel plus a PPI (compared with periods of use of clopidogrel without a PPI) were associated with a greater risk of death or rehospitalization for ACS (adjusted hazard ratio, 1.27; 95% CI, 1.10-1.46).

Proton pump inhibitors may interact with clopidogrel because they inhibit the activity of cytochrome P450 CYP2C19, one of the enzymes involved in the conversion of clopidogrel, an inactive prodrug, to an active metabolite. Coadministration of clopidogrel and omeprazole has been shown to reduce the conversion of clopidogrel to an active metabolite. O'Donoghue et al found that inhibition of platelet aggregation was significantly lower for patients on a PPI than for those not on a PPI at 6 hours after a 600 mg loading dose of clopidogrel. Nevertheless, among the 13 608 patients with an ACS who were enrolled in the Trial to Assess Improvement in Therapeutic Outcomes by Optimizing Platelet Inhibition with Prasugrel-Thrombolysis in Myocardial Infarction (TRITON-TIMI) 38 study and randomly assigned to prasugrel or clopidogrel, there was no association between PPI use and the risk of the primary endpoint, a composite of cardiovascular death, MI, or stroke. The COGENT trial was a multicenter, international, randomized, double-blind, double-dummy, placebo-controlled, parallel group, phase 3 efficacy and safety study of CGT-2168, a fixed-dose combination of clopidogrel (75 mg) and omeprazole (20 mg), compared with clopidogrel. After enrollment of 3627 patients the study was terminated prematurely due to lack of funding. There was no difference in the frequency of cardiovascular events but the median follow-up was only 133 days.

A recent study provided evidence that omeprazole inhibits the metabolism of clopidogrel to a greater extent than other PPIs. A total of 104 patients who underwent coronary stenting for non-ST-segment elevation ACS were randomized to omeprazole or pantoprazole 20 mg daily. After treatment with aspirin 75 mg daily and clopidogrel 150 mg daily for 1 month, patients receiving pantoprazole had a significantly better platelet response to clopidogrel and there were more clopidogrel nonresponders in the omeprazole group than in the pantoprazole group: 44% versus 23% ($P = .04$), odds ratio: 2.6 (95% confidence interval: 1.2 to 6.2).[4]

A post-hoc analysis of a trial of clopidogrel therapy after PCI found that the use of PPI was associated with a worse clinical outcome independent of the use of clopidogrel.[5] Therefore, the results of observational studies may be confounded because patients who need a PPI may have more comorbidities. Nevertheless, the interaction between clopidogrel and a PPI may be important in selected patients, especially those with a mutant allele of the cytochrome P450 genes that convert clopidogrel to its active metabolite. One approach is to prescribe pantoprazole instead of omeprazole when a PPI is indicated in a patient taking clopidogrel. A second approach is to prescribe prasugrel when a PPI is indicated although some studies have found that the frequency of major bleeding is greater during treatment with prasugrel compared with clopidogrel.[6] Another recommendation, based on the short plasma half-lives of clopidogrel and PPI, is to separate the doses of clopidogrel and a PPI by 12 to 20 hours to minimize competitive inhibition of cytochrome P450 metabolism.[7]

S. W. Werns, MD

References

1. Anderson JL, Adams CD, Antman EM, et al. ACC/AHA 2007 guidelines for the management of patients with unstable angina/non-ST-elevation myocardial infarction: a report of the American College of Cardiology/American Heart Association Task Force on Practice Guidelines. *Circulation.* 2007;116:e148-e304.
2. Bhatt DL, Scheiman J, Abraham NS, et al. ACCF/ACG/AHA 2008 expert consensus document on reducing the gastrointestinal risk of antiplatelet therapy and NSAID use. *Circulation.* 2008;118:1894-1909.
3. Ho PM, Maddox TM, Wang L, et al. Risk of adverse outcomes associated with concomitant use of clopidogrel and proton pump inhibitors following acute coronary syndrome. *JAMA.* 2009;301:937-944.
4. Cuisset T, Frere C, Quilici J, et al. Comaprison of omeprazole and pantoprazole influence on a high 150-mg clopidogrel maintenance dose. *J Am Coll Cardiol.* 2009;54:1149-1153.

5. Dunn SP, Macaulay TE, Brennan DM, et al. Baseline proton pump inhibitor use is associated with increased cardiovascular events with and without the use of clopidogrel in the CREDO trial [abstract]. *Circulation.* 2008;118:815A.
6. Wiviott SD, Braunwald E, McCabe CH, et al. Prasugrel versus clopidogrel in patients with acute coronary syndromes. *N Engl J Med.* 2007;347:2001-2015.
7. Laine L, Hennekens C. Proton pump inhibitor and clopidogrel interaction: fact or fiction? [published online ahead of print November 10 2009]. *Am J Gastroenterol.* 2010;105:34-41.

Effects of aspirin dose on ischaemic events and bleeding after percutaneous coronary intervention: insights from the PCI-CURE study

Jolly SS, Pogue J, Haladyn K, et al (McMaster Univ and Population Health Res Inst, Hamilton, Canada; et al)
Eur Heart J 30:900-907, 2009

Aims.—In the setting of percutaneous coronary intervention (PCI), due to a paucity of data, the optimal dose of aspirin is uncertain. We evaluated the safety of different doses of aspirin after PCI.

Methods and Results.—In the PCI-CURE study, 2658 patients with acute coronary syndromes undergoing PCI were stratified into three aspirin dose groups $\geq$200 mg (high, $n = 1064$), 101–199 mg (moderate, $n = 538$), and $\leq$100 mg (low, $n = 1056$). For efficacy, the moderate- (7.4%) and high-dose groups (8.6%) had similar rates of cardiovascular death, myocardial infarction, or stroke compared with the low-dose group (7.1%). For safety, major bleeding was increased with high-dose aspirin [3.9, 1.5, and 1.9% in the high-, moderate-, and low-dose groups; hazard ratio (HR) of high vs. low dose 2.05 (95% CI 1.20–3.50], $P = 0.009$]. The net adverse clinical events (death, MI, stroke, major bleeding) favoured low-over high-dose aspirin (8.4 vs. 11.0, HR 1.31, 95% CI 1.00–1.73 $P = 0.056$).

Conclusion.—In this large observational analysis of patients undergoing PCI, low-dose aspirin appeared to be as effective as higher doses in preventing ischaemic events but was also associated with a lower rate of major bleeding and an improved net efficacy to safety balance.

▶ There is uncertainty regarding the optimal dose of aspirin for a patient with an acute coronary syndrome (ACS) or ST-segment elevation myocardial infarction (MI). Four small randomized trials of aspirin in patients with non-ST-segment elevation ACS demonstrated a 50% or greater reduction in the risk of death or MI by aspirin doses ranging from 75 mg daily to 1200 mg daily. Among 20 521 patients with ACS who were enrolled in the Global Utilization of Streptokinase and t-PA for Occluded Coronary Arteries (GUSTO) IIb and Platelet Glycoprotein IIb/IIIa in Unstable Angina: Receptor Suppression Using Integrilin Therapy (PURSUIT) trials, an aspirin dose of 150 mg or greater was associated with a lower risk of MI at 6 months compared with an aspirin dose less than 150 mg (hazard ratio 0.79; 95% CI 0.64-0.98; $P = .03$).[1] The Second International Study of Infarct Survival (ISIS-2) demonstrated that aspirin 160 mg daily for 1 month reduced vascular mortality at 35 days by 23% in patients who were enrolled within 24 hours of suspected acute MI.[2]

Several retrospective analyses have been performed to determine whether the dose of aspirin affects clinical outcomes in patients with ST-segment elevation MI[3] or ACS.[4,5] Berger et al[3] analyzed the outcomes for 48 422 patients with ST-segment elevation MI who were enrolled in the GUSTO I and III trials and treated with fibrinolytic therapy. The dose of aspirin was left to the discretion of the treating physician. The initial dose of aspirin was 325 mg for 24.4% of patients and 162 mg for 75.6% of patients. Aspirin dose was not associated with 24-hour, 7-day, or 30-day adjusted mortality rates. Compared with an initial aspirin dose of 162 mg, an initial dose of 325 mg was associated with a significant increase in moderate or severe bleeding in-hospital.

Peters et al[4] analyzed the outcomes of 12 562 patients with ACS who were enrolled in the Clopidogrel in Unstable Angina to Prevent Recurrent Events (CURE) trial, a randomized comparison of aspirin plus clopidogrel versus aspirin alone. Patients were divided into 3 aspirin dose groups: ≤100 mg /day, 101 to 199 mg/day, and ≥200 mg/day. Higher doses of aspirin increased the risk of major bleeding in patients who were randomized to both arms of the study. Higher doses of aspirin were not associated with lower clinical event rates. Percutaneous coronary intervention (PCI)-CURE was a substudy of the CURE trial that consisted of the 2658 patients who underwent PCI.[5] A post-hoc analysis of the patients who were enrolled in PCI-CURE found that the moderate-dose (101-199 mg) and high-dose (≥200 mg) aspirin groups had similar rates of cardiovascular death, MI, or stroke compared with the low-dose (≤100 mg) aspirin group. Major bleeding was increased with high-dose aspirin.

The clopidogrel optimal loading dose usage to reduce recurrent events-Organization to Assess Strategies in Ischemic Syndromes (CURRENT OASIS)-7 trial is the first randomized trial to compare 2 different doses of aspirin in patient with ACS.[6] It was a phase II, multicenter, randomized, 2×2 factorial design trial that compared 2 clopidogrel regimens in a double-blind fashion and 2 aspirin doses in an open-label fashion. All patients received a loading dose of ≥300 mg of aspirin on day one of the trial. The low-dose aspirin group received 75 to 100 mg/day on days 2 to 30 while the high-dose group received 300 to 325 mg/day. A total of 25 087 ACS patients (70.8% non-ST-segment elevation ACS, 29.2% ST-segment elevation MI) were enrolled. Ninety-nine percent of the patients underwent coronary angiography and PCI was performed in 70% of the patients. There was no significant difference between the high-dose and low-dose aspirin groups in the primary efficacy end point: cardiovascular death, MI, and stroke at 30 days. Also, there were no significant differences between the 2 aspirin groups in the frequency of major or severe bleeding.

The American College of Cardiology/American Heart Association (ACC/AHA) 2007 guidelines for the management of unstable angina/non-ST-elevation MI (UA/NSTEMI) include the following class I recommendation regarding aspirin: "aspirin should be administered to UA/NSTEMI patients as soon as possible after hospital presentation and continued indefinitely in patients not known to be intolerant of that medication." The guidelines recommend that the initial dose of aspirin should be between 162 and 325 mg daily.[7]

The ACC/AHA/SCAI 2007 Focused Update for PCI recommended the following aspirin regimens after PCI: 162 to 325 mg daily for at least one month after a bare-metal stent, 3 months after a sirolimus-eluting stent, and 6 months after a pacli-taxel-eluting stent, followed by 75 to 162 mg/day indefinitely.[8]

As noted in the editorial by Steinhubl and Berger[9] that accompanied the article by Jolly et al, there is no pharmacologic basis for the most commonly prescribed dose of aspirin, 325 mg daily. Based on the results reported by Jolly et al and the other studies discussed above, and recent evidence that bleeding is an independent risk factor for death in patients with ACS,[10-12] it seems reasonable to conclude that the lower doses of aspirin (75-162 mg daily) confer equal benefit and less harm than the higher doses.

S. W. Werns, MD

References

1. Quinn MJ, Aronow HD, Califf RM, et al. Aspirin dose and six-month outcome after an acute coronary syndrome. *J Am Coll Cardiol*. 2004;43:972-978.
2. ISIS-2 (Second International Study of Infarct Survival) Collaborative Group. Randomised trial of intravenous streptokinase, oral aspirin, both, or neither among 17,187 cases of suspected acute myocardial infarction. *Lancet*. 1988;2: 349-360.
3. Berger JS, Stebbins A, Granger CB, et al. Initial aspirin dose and outcome among ST-elevation myocardial infarction patients treated with fibrinolytic therapy. *Circulation*. 2008;117:192-199.
4. Peters RJG, Mehta SR, Fox KAA, et al. Effects of aspirin dose when used alone or in combination with clopidogrel in patients with acute coronary syndromes. Observations from the clopidogrel in unstable angina to prevent recurrent events (CURE) study. *Circulation*. 2003;108:1682-1687.
5. Mehta SR, Yusuf S, Peters RJ, et al. Effects of pretreatment with clopoidogrel and aspirin followed by long-term therapy in patients undergoing percutaneous coronary intervention: the PCI-CURE study. *Lancet*. 2001;358:527-533.
6. Mehta SR, et al. CURRENT OASIS-7: A 2X2 factorial randomized trial of optimal clopidogrel and aspirin dosing in patients with ACS undergoing an early invasive strategy with intent for PCI, ClinicalTrialResults.org.
7. Anderson JL, Adams CD, Antman EM, et al. ACC/AHA 2007 guidelines for the management of patients with unstable angina/non-ST-elevation myocardial infarction: a report of the American College of Cardiology/American Heart Association Task Force on Practice Guidelines. *Circulation*. 2007;116:e148-e304.
8. King SB III, Smith SC Jr, Hirshfeld JW Jr. 2007 focused update of the ACC/AHA/SCAI 2005 Guideline Update for Percutaneous Coronary Intervention: a report of the American College of Cardiology/American Heart Association Task Force on Practice Guidelines. *Circulation*. 2008;117:261-295.
9. Steinhubl SR, Berger PB. Aspirin following PCI: too much of a good thing? *European Heart Journal*. 2009;30:882-884.
10. Yan AT, Yan RT, Huynh T, et al. Bleeding and outcome in acute coronary syndrome: insights from continuous electrocardiogram monitoring in the Integrilin and Enoxaparin Randomized Assessment of Acute Coronary syndrome Treatment (INTERACT) trial. *Am Heart J*. 2008;156:769-775.
11. Budaj A, Eikelboom JW, Mehta SR, et al. Improving clinical outcomes by reducing bleeding in patients with non-ST-elevation acute coronary syndromes. *Eur Heart J*. 2009;30:655-661.
12. Mehran R, Pocock SJ, Stone GW, et al. Associations of major bleeding and myocardial infarction with the incidence and timing of mortality in patients presenting with non-ST-elevation acute coronary syndromes: a risk model from the ACUITY trial. *Eur Heart J*. 2009;30:1457-1466.

Impact of Chronic Kidney Disease on Major Bleeding Complications and Mortality in Patients With Indication for Oral Anticoagulation Undergoing Coronary Stenting

Manzano-Fernández S, Marín F, Pastor-Pérez FJ, et al (Univ Hosp Virgen de la Arrixaca, Murcia, Spain; et al)

Chest 135:983-990, 2009

Background.—Patients with indications for oral anticoagulation (OAC) undergoing percutaneous coronary artery stenting (PCI-S) represent a high-risk population for major bleeding complications. Chronic kidney disease (CKD) is also associated with poor outcome after PCI-S. Limited data are available regarding the impact of CKD on the frequency of major bleeding and mortality in this population.

Methods.—We investigated the influence of CKD on major bleeding and all-cause mortality in patients with indication for OAC who undergo PCI-S. Patients were grouped according to calculated creatinine clearance (CrCl): CrCl > 60 mL/min, (n = 98) and CrCl ≤ 60 mL/min, (n = 68). Major bleeding and major adverse vascular events (all-cause mortality, myocardial infarction, repeat revascularization, stent thrombosis, or stroke) were collected during follow-up.

Results.—We analyzed 166 consecutive patients with indication(s) for OAC (77% men; mean age, 71 years; range, 66 to 76 years) after undergoing PCI-S. CKD was associated with higher risk for major bleeding (hazard ratio [HR], 3.44; 95% confidence interval [CI], 1.50 to 7.93; $P = 0.004$) and all-cause mortality (HR, 3.50; 95% CI, 1.53 to 7.99; $P = 0.003$). In multivariate analyses, age > 75 years (HR, 2.75; 95% CI, 1.15 to 6.56; $P = 0.023$), CKD (HR, 2.59; 95% CI, 1.00 to 6.95; $P = 0.049$), anemia (HR, 2.36; 95% CI, 1.00 to 5.54; $P = 0.049$), and triple antithrombotic therapy (HR, 3.29; 95% CI, 1.23 to 8.84; $P = 0.018$) were independent predictors for major bleeding, whereas age > 75 years (HR, 2.38; 95% CI, 1.03 to 5.59; $P = 0.046$) and CKD (HR, 2.44; 95% CI, 1.03 to 5.82; $P = 0.044$) were predictors for all-cause mortality.

Conclusion.—In this high-risk population, CKD is independently associated with increased major bleeding and all-cause mortality following PCI-S.

▶ The study by Manzano-Fernandez et al[1] is relevant to 2 important patient subsets: patients with chronic kidney disease (CKD) and patients with indications for both chronic antiplatelet and oral anticoagulant therapy. Previous studies have shown that CKD is associated with both an increased prevalence of coronary artery disease and an increased risk of adverse outcomes, including death, after an acute coronary syndrome (ACS)[2] and after percutaneous coronary intervention (PCI).[3,4] A compilation of 4 large ACS trial databases included 18 621 patients with ST-segment elevation myocardial infarction (STEMI) and 19 304 patients with non-ST-segment elevation ACS.[2] Renal function was abnormal, defined as a creatinine clearance < 70 mL/min, in

41% of patients with STEMI and 42% of patients with non ST-segment elevation ACS. Despite the exclusion of patients with end-stage renal disease (ESRD) from all 4 studies, abnormal renal function was an independent predictor of mortality at 30 days and 180 days in patients with either STEMI or non-ST-segment elevation ACS.

There are conflicting data regarding the impact of CKD on restenosis and other outcomes after PCI, partly because most randomized PCI trials have excluded patients with CKD.[5] Lemos et al[6] analyzed a series of 1080 consecutive patients who underwent PCI during the 6 months before and 6 months after the introduction of sirolimus-eluting stents. Baseline impairment of renal function, defined as a creatinine clearance < 60 mL/min, was not an independent predictor of target vessel revascularization. Target vessel revascularization was lower among patients with impaired renal function who received sirolimus-eluting coronary stents compared with those who received bare-metal stents.[6] Appleby et al[4] analyzed the effect of renal function on the late outcomes of a cohort of 11 953 consecutive patients who underwent their first PCI at one cardiac center. Renal impairment, defined as a creatinine clearance < 60 mL/min, was present in 3070 patients (25.7%). Multivariate analysis showed that the use of drug-eluting stents was associated with reduced subsequent revascularization (hazard ratio 0.68; confidence interval 0.53–0.88; $P = .004$) but not lower mortality.

Bleeding is an independent risk factor for death after PCI or MI.[7,8] There is evidence that patients with CKD have an increased risk of bleeding after PCI. Among 4623 patients who were treated with a glycoprotein IIb/IIIa inhibitor during PCI, creatinine clearance < 70 mL/min was associated with increased rates of minor and major bleeding and transfusion compared with creatinine clearance ≥70 mL/min.[9] Furthermore, several studies found that patients with CKD often receive excessive doses of antithrombotic drugs during PCI.[10-12] Among 30 136 patients who were enrolled in a registry of patients who were hospitalized for ACS, renal insufficiency, defined as a serum creatinine > 2.0 mg/dL, creatinine clearance < 30 mL/min, or need for dialysis, was associated with excess dosing of antiplatelet and antithrombin agents.[10] Forty-two percent of patients who were administered antithrombotic agents received at least one dose of unfractionated heparin, low-molecular weight heparin, or a glycoprotein IIb/IIIa inhibitor outside the recommended range, and 15% of major bleeding events could be attributed to excess dosing. In one clinical trial, the maintenance infusion of eptifibatide was not adjusted for a creatinine clearance ≤50 mL/min in 15 of 33 patients (45%), resulting in a bleeding rate of 20%.[11] Among 22 778 dialysis patients who were enrolled in a PCI registry, 5084 patients (22.3%) received an antithrombotic medication that is contraindicated in dialysis patients; 2375 (46.7%) received enoxaparin, 3261 (64.4%) received eptifibatide, and 552 (10.9%) received both.[12] After risk adjustment, there was a significant association of enoxaparin with in-hospital major bleeding and death.

Clearly, patients with CKD may benefit from strategies that minimize the intensity and duration of exposure to anticoagulant and antiplatelet agents both during and after PCI. It is critical to recognize that enoxaparin and eptifibatide require dose adjustment in patients with CKD and should not be used in dialysis patients. Bivalirudin was found to cause less bleeding than heparin in patients with CKD and may be a better option.[13] Although current guidelines recommend dual antiplatelet therapy, that is, aspirin plus a thienopyridine (clopidogrel or prasugrel) for a minimum of 1 month after a bare-metal stent and 12 months after a drug-eluting stent, the optimal duration of dual antiplatelet therapy after a drug-eluting stent is uncertain.[14,15] Premature discontinuation of clopidogrel within 6 months after implantation of a drug-eluting stent is associated with an increased risk of stent thrombosis, an event that may result in MI or sudden death.[16] Therefore, the selection of bare-metal versus drug-eluting stents in patients with CKD should consider the relative risks of increased target revascularization versus an increased risk of bleeding. It is somewhat reassuring that the increased bleeding risk associated with clopidogrel therapy after PCI was similar for patients with normal and impaired renal function who were enrolled in the Clopidogrel for the Reduction of Events During Observation (CREDO) trial.[17]

Indications for chronic oral anticoagulation, for example, atrial fibrillation and deep vein thrombosis, are unpredictable and fairly common in patients with or without CKD. Among 40 812 patients who were discharged after hospitalization for acute MI, the combination of aspirin, clopidogrel, and a vitamin K antagonist or dual therapy with clopidogrel plus a vitamin K antagonist was associated with an increased risk of rehospitalization for bleeding.[18] CKD was present in 2.5% of patients who had bleeding compared with 1.1% who had no bleeding. The 2007 Focused Update of the ACC/AHA/SCAI 2005 Guideline Update for PCI recommends a lower international normalized ratio target (2.0–2.5), a low dose of aspirin (75–81 mg), and a clopidogrel dose of 75 mg daily in patients who require all 3 drugs.[14] If bleeding occurs or the risk of bleeding is unacceptable, the options are to stop clopidogrel, which increases the risk of stent thrombosis, or withhold warfarin, which increases the risk of a thromboembolic event.

The publication by Manzano-Fernandez et al[1] underscores the risk of bleeding and death in patients with CKD who are treated with triple antithrombotic therapy. It is unfortunate that it does not report the percentage of patients who were receiving hemodialysis because several recent articles have concluded that aspirin, clopidogrel, and warfarin may be especially hazardous in patients with CKD who are treated with hemodialysis. Chan et al[19,20] reported that prescription of aspirin, clopidogrel, or warfarin was associated with higher mortality among hemodialysis patients, and warfarin use increased the risk of stroke in patients who had both ESRD and atrial fibrillation. Consequently, the occurrence of an indication for warfarin in a patient with CKD, especially a patient who requires hemodialysis, creates a dilemma. Further studies are needed to determine the relative efficacy and safety of bare-metal and drug-eluting coronary stents in patients with CKD.

S. W. Werns, MD

References

1. Manzano-Fernandez S, Marin F, Pastor-Perez FJ, et al. Impact of chronic kidney disease on major bleeding complications and mortality in patients with indication

for oral anticoagulation undergoing coronary stenting. *Chest.* 2009;135: 983-990.

2. Al Suwaidi J, Reddan DN, Williams K. Prognostic implications of abnormalities in renal function in patients with acute coronary syndromes. *Circulation.* 2002; 106:974-980.

3. Best PJM, Lennon R, Ting HH, et al. The impact of renal insufficiency on clinical outcomes in patients undergoing percutaneous coronary interventions. *J Am Coll Cardiol.* 2002;39:1113-1119.

4. Appleby CE, Ivanov J, Lavi S, et al. The adverse long-term impact of renal impairment in patients undergoing percutaneous coronary intervention in the drug-eluting stent era. *Circ Cardiovasc Intervent.* 2009;2:309-316.

5. Gupta R, Birnbaum Y, Uretsky BF. The renal patient with coronary artery disease. *J Am Coll Cardiol.* 2004;44:1343-1353.

6. Lemos PA, Arampatzis CA, Hoye A. Impact of baseline renal function on mortality after percutaneous coronary intervention with sirolimus-eluting stents or bare metal stents. *Am J Cardiol.* 2005;95:167-172.

7. Budaj A, Eikelboom JW, Mehta SR, et al. Improving clinical outcomes by reducing bleeding in patients with non-ST-elevation acute coronary syndromes. *Eur Heart J.* 2009;30:655-661.

8. Mehran R, Pocock SJ, Stone GW, et al. Associations of major bleeding and myocardial infarction with the incidence and timing of mortality in patients presenting with non-ST-elevation acute coronary syndromes: a risk model from the ACUITY trial. *Eur Heart J.* 2009;30:1457-1466.

9. Berger PB, Best PJM, Topol EJ, et al. The relation of renal function to ischemic and bleeding outcomes with 2 different glycoprotein IIb/IIIa inhibitors: the do Tirofiban and ReoPro Give Similar Efficacy Outcome (TARGET) trial. *Am Heart J.* 2005;149:869-875.

10. Alexander KP, Chen AY, Roe MT. Excess dosing of antiplatelet and antithrombin agents in the treatment of non-ST-segment elevation acute coronary syndromes. *JAMA.* 2005;294:3108-3116.

11. Kirtane AJ, Piazza G, Murphy SA. Correlates of bleeding events among moderate-to-high risk patients undergoing percutaneous coronary intervention and treated wth eptifibatide. Observations from the PROTECT-TIMI 30 trial. *J Am Coll Cardiol.* 2006;47:2374-2379.

12. Tsai TT, Maddox TM, Roe MT, et al. Contraindicated medication use in dialysis patients undergoing percutaneous coronary intervention. *JAMA.* 2009;302: 2458-2464.

13. Chew DP, Bhatt DL, Kimball W, et al. Bivalirudin provides increasing benefit with decreasing renal function: a meta-analysis of randomized trials. *Am J Cardiol.* 2003;92:919-923.

14. King SB III, Smith SC Jr, Hirshfeld JW Jr. 2007 focused update of the ACC/AHA/SCAI 2005 guideline update for percutaneous coronary intervention: a report of the American College of Cardiology/American Heart Association Task Force on Practice Guidelines. *Circulation.* 2008;117:261-295.

15. Kandzari DE, Angiolillo DJ, Price MJ, Teirstein PS. Identifying the "optimal" duration of dual antiplatelet therapy after drug-eluting stent revascularization. *J Am Coll Cardiol Intv.* 2009;2:1279-1285.

16. Schulz S, Schuster T, Mehilli J, et al. Stent thrombosis after drug-eluting stent implantation: incidence, timing, and relation to discontinuation of clopidogrel therapy over a 4 year period. *Eur Heart J.* 2009;30:2714-2721.

17. Best PJM, Steinhubl SR, Berger PB, et al. The efficacy and safety of short- and long-term dual antiplatelet therapy in patients with mild or moderate chronic kidney disease: results from the Clopidogrel for the Reduction of Events During Observation (CREDO) trial. *Am Heart J.* 2008;155:687-693.

18. Sorensen R, Hansen ML, Abildstrom SZ, et al. Risk of bleeding in patients with acute myocardial infarction treated with different combinations of aspirin, clopidogrel, and vitamin K antagonists in Denmark: a retrospective analysis of nationwide registry data. *Lancet.* 2009;374:1967-1974.

19. Chan KE, Lazarus JM, Thadhani R, Hakim RM. Anticoagulation and antiplate-let usage associates with mortality among hemodialysis patients. *J Am Soc Nephrol.* 2009;20:872-881.
20. Chan KE, Lazarus JM, Thadhani R, Hakim RM. Warfarin use associates with increased risk for stroke in hemodialysis patients with atrial fibrillation. *J Am Soc Nephrol.* 2009;20:2223-2233.

Cytochrome P450 Genetic Polymorphisms and the Response to Prasugrel: Relationship to Pharmacokinetic, Pharmacodynamic, and Clinical Outcomes

Mega JL, Close SL, Wiviott SD, et al (Brigham and Women's Hosp and Harvard Med School, Boston, MA; Eli Lilly and Company, Indianapolis, IN; et al)
Circulation 119:2553-2560, 2009

Background.—Both clopidogrel and prasugrel require biotransforma-tion to active metabolites by cytochrome P450 (CYP) enzymes. Among persons treated with clopidogrel, carriers of reduced-function *CYP2C19* alleles have significantly lower levels of active metabolite, diminished platelet inhibition, and higher rates of adverse cardiovascular events. The effect of CYP polymorphisms on the clinical outcomes in patients treated with prasugrel remains unknown.

Methods and Results.—The associations between functional variants in CYP genes, plasma concentrations of active drug metabolite, and platelet inhibition in response to prasugrel were tested in 238 healthy subjects. We then examined the association of these genetic variants with cardiovas-cular outcomes in a cohort of 1466 patients with acute coronary syndromes allocated to treatment with prasugrel in the Trial to Assess Improvement in Therapeutic Outcomes by Optimizing Platelet Inhibition With Prasugrel–Thrombolysis in Myocardial Infarction 38 trial. Among the healthy subjects, no significant attenuation of the pharmacokinetic or the pharmacodynamic response to prasugrel was observed in carriers versus noncarriers of at least 1 reduced-function allele for any of the CYP genes tested (*CYP2C19, CYP2C9, CYP2B6, CYP3A5,* and *CYP1A2*). Consistent with these findings, in subjects with acute coronary syndromes treated with prasugrel, no significant associations were found between any of the tested CYP genotypes and risk of cardiovascular death, myocardial infarction, or stroke.

Conclusions.—Common functional CYP genetic variants do not affect active drug metabolite levels, inhibition of platelet aggregation, or clinical cardiovascular event rates in persons treated with prasugrel. These pharmacogenetic findings are in contrast to observations with clopidogrel, which may explain, in part, the different pharmacological and clinical responses to the 2 medications.

▶ Administration of a thienopyridine results in inhibition of the platelet $P2Y_{12}$ receptor, the predominant receptor involved in adenosine diphosphate (ADP)-stimulated activation of the glycoprotein (GP) IIb/IIIa receptor. Clinical trials have established the efficacy of thienopyridines, such as ticlopidine, clopidogrel, and prasugrel, in patients with stable coronary artery disease (CAD), non-ST-segment elevation acute coronary syndromes (ACS), and ST-segment elevation myocardial infarction (MI). Clopidogrel decreases ischemic complications when added to aspirin in patients who undergo percutaneous coronary intervention (PCI),[1] patients with ACS,[2] and patients with ST-elevation MI who are treated with fibrinolytic therapy.[3] The Trial to Assess Improvement in Therapeutic Outcomes by Optimizing Platelet Inhibition with Prasugrel-Thrombolysis in Myocardial Infarction (TRITON-TIMI) 38 study compared the effects of 2 thienopyridines, clopidogrel, and prasugrel, in patients with either ACS or ST-segment elevation MI.[4] In patients with acute coronary syndromes with scheduled PCI, prasugrel therapy was associated with significantly reduced rates of ischemic events, including stent thrombosis. Although the overall risk of major bleeding was increased among patients who were randomized to prasugrel, there was no apparent excess bleeding among the cohort of patients who underwent PCI for ST-segment elevation MI.[5]

Both clopidogrel and prasugrel are prodrugs that are transformed to active metabolites by cytochrome P450 (CYP) enzymes. A number of studies have examined the effect of CYP polymorphisms on the pharmacokinetic and pharmacodynamic responses to clopidogrel and prasugrel. Patients with reduced-function alleles of the gene encoding *CYP2C19* were found to have decreased plasma concentrations of the active metabolite of clopidogrel and less inhibition of the $P2Y_{12}$ receptor as determined by in vitro assays.[6] The response to prasugrel, however, was not affected by the presence of a reduced function allele. Additional studies have examined the relationship between the CYP 450 2C19 genotype and the clinical efficacy of clopidogrel and prasugrel.[7-9] Shuldiner et al [7] reported that the loss-of-function allele *CYP2C19*2* was associated with diminished platelet response to clopidogrel therapy and increased frequency of cardiovascular ischemic events or death during 1 year of follow-up. The same allele has been associated with an increased risk of stent thrombosis after coronary artery stenting.[8] Among patients who were taking clopidogrel in the TRITON-TIMI 38 trial, carriers of the *CYP2C19* reduced-function allele were found to have an increased risk of the primary study endpoint, cardiovascular death, MI, or stroke, and an increased risk of stent thrombosis. The allele did not affect active drug metabolite levels, inhibition of platelet function, or the rates of clinical cardiovascular events in the subjects who were randomized to prasugrel.[10]

Currently, there is no readily available means to determine whether a patient is a carrier of a reduced function allele that may affect clopidogrel metabolism and the risk of coronary stent thrombosis. Therefore, it may be tempting to conclude that the increased bleeding risk associated with prasugrel is outweighed by the reduced risk of stent thrombosis. Increasing the dose of clopidogrel may an alternative approach to reduce the risk of stent thrombosis. The CURRENT OASIS 7 investigators reported that the risk of stent thrombosis was decreased by doubling the dose of clopidogrel during the first week after PCI[10]; 25 087 patients with ACS (71% non-ST-segment elevation MI, 29% ST-segment elevation MI) who were undergoing an early invasive strategy with intended PCI were randomized to standard dose clopidogrel (300 mg loading dose, then 75 mg daily) or double-dose clopidogrel (600 mg loading dose, then 150 mg/day for 7 days, followed by 75 mg daily). The rate of definite stent thrombosis after 30 days was 42% lower among the patients who were randomized to the double-dose arm of the study.

S. W. Werns, MD

References

1. Steinhubl SR, Berger PB, Mann JT, et al. Early and sustained dual oral antiplatelet therapy following percutaneous coronary intervention. *JAMA.* 2002;288:2411-2420.
2. The Clopidogrel in Unstable Angina to Prevent Recurrent Events Trial Investigators. Effects of clopidogrel in addition to aspirin in patients with acute coronary syndromes without ST-segment elevation. *N Engl J Med.* 2001;345:494-502.
3. Sabatine MS, Cannon CP, Gibson CM, et al. Addition of clopidogrel to aspirin and fibrinolytic therapy for myocardial infarction with ST-segment elevation. *N Engl J Med.* 2005;352:1179-1189.
4. Wiviott SD, Braunwald E, McCabe CH, et al. Prasugrel versus clopidogrel in patients with acute coronary syndromes. *N Engl J Med.* 2007;347:2001-2015.
5. Montalescot G, Wiviott SD, Braunwald E, et al. Prasugrel compared with clopidogrel in patients undergoing percutaneous coronary intervention for ST-elevation myocardial infarction (TRITON-TIMI 38): double-blind, randomized controlled trial. *Lancet.* 2009;373:723-731.
6. Varenhorst C, James S, Erlinge D, et al. Genetic variation of CYP2C19 affects both pharmacokinetic and pharmacodynamic responses to clopidogrel but not prasugrel in aspirin-treated patients with coronary artery disease. *Eur Heart J.* 2009;30:1744-1752.
7. Shuldiner AR, O'Connell JR, Bliden KP, et al. Association of cytochrome P4502C19 genotype with the antiplatelet effect and clinical efficacy of clopidogrel therapy. *JAMA.* 2009;302:849-858.
8. Sibbing D, Stegherr J, Latz W, et al. Cytochrome P450 2C19 loss-of-function polymorphism and stent thrombosis following percutaneous coronary intervention. *Eur Heart J.* 2009;30:916-922.
9. Simon T, Verstuyft C, Mary-Krause M, et al. Genetic determinants of response to clopidogrel and cardiovascular events. *N Engl J Med.* 2009;360:363-375.
10. Mehta SR. CURRENT OASIS 7: A 2X2 Factorial Randomized Trial of Optimal Clopidogrel and Aspirin Dosing in Patients with ACS Undergoing an Early Invasive Strategy with Intent for PCI. Available at: http://www.clinicaltrialresults.org/, accessed Jan 10, 2010.

A systematic review and meta-analysis of intra-aortic balloon pump therapy in ST-elevation myocardial infarction: should we change the guidelines?
Sjauw KD, Engström AE, Vis MM, et al (Univ of Amsterdam, The Netherlands)
Eur Heart J 30:459-468, 2009

Aims.—Intra-aortic balloon counterpulsation (IABP) in ST-segment elevation myocardial infarction (STEMI) with cardiogenic shock is strongly recommended (class IB) in the current guidelines. We performed meta-analyses to evaluate the evidence for IABP in STEMI with and without cardiogenic shock.

Methods and Results.—Medical literature databases were scrutinized to identify randomized trials comparing IABP with no IABP in STEMI. In absence of randomized trials, cohort studies of IABP in STEMI with cardiogenic shock were identified. Two separate meta-analyses were performed respectively. The first meta-analysis included seven randomized trials ($n = 1009$) of STEMI. IABP showed neither a 30-day survival benefit nor improved left ventricular ejection fraction, while being associated with significantly higher stroke and bleeding rates. The second meta-analysis included nine cohorts of STEMI patients with cardiogenic shock ($n = 10529$). In patients treated with thrombolysis, IABP was associated with an 18% [95% confidence interval (CI), 16–20%; $P < 0.0001$] decrease in 30 day mortality, albeit with significantly higher revascularization rates compared to patients without support. Contrariwise, in patients treated with primary percutaneous coronary intervention, IABP was associated with a 6% (95% CI, 3–10%; $P < 0.0008$) increase in 30 day mortality.

Conclusion.—The pooled randomized data do not support IABP in patients with high-risk STEMI. The meta-analysis of cohort studies in the setting of STEMI complicated by cardiogenic shock supported IABP therapy adjunctive to thrombolysis. In contrast, the observational data did not support IABP therapy adjunctive to primary PCI. All available observational data concerning IABP therapy in the setting of cardiogenic shock is importantly hampered by bias and confounding. There is insufficient evidence endorsing the current guideline recommendation for the use of IABP therapy in the setting of STEMI complicated by cardiogenic shock. Our meta-analyses challenge the current guideline recommendations.

▶ Cardiogenic shock is the most common cause of death in patients hospitalized with acute myocardial infarction (MI). There is no evidence that fibrinolytic therapy improves the survival of patients with acute MI and cardiogenic shock. Most fibrinolytic trials excluded patients with cardiogenic shock. The Gruppo Italiano per lo Studio della Streptochinasi nell'Infarto Miocardico (GISSI) trial randomized 280 patients with cardiogenic shock to intravenous streptokinase or placebo.[1] The 30-day mortality rates were 69.9% among 146 patients treated with streptokinase, compared with 70.1% among 134 patients who received placebo. Retrospective observational reports and a prospective randomized trial have provided evidence that revascularization via either percutaneous coronary intervention (PCI) or coronary artery bypass graft surgery improves outcome in patients with acute MI complicated by cardiogenic shock.[2-6] The Should We Emergently Revascularize Occluded Coronaries for Cardiogenic Shock (SHOCK) trial was a landmark randomized trial to evaluate early revascularization in patients with cardiogenic shock.[4-6] Although 30-day survival was not significantly different, both 6-month and 1-year survivals were greater among the patients randomized to early revascularization.[4,5]

Intra-aortic balloon pumping (IABP) often improves blood pressure and cardiac output in patients with cardiogenic shock. An IABP was inserted in

86% of patients who were enrolled in the randomized SHOCK trial.[4] The use of an IABP before PCI was associated with a significantly lower incidence of cardiac arrest or ventricular fibrillation in the cardiac catheterization laboratory among a series of 89 patients with acute MI and cardiogenic shock who underwent PCI.[7] Unfortunately, no randomized trials of IABP in cardiogenic shock have been completed.[8] Nevertheless, cardiogenic shock is a class I indication for insertion of an IABP according to the ACC/AHA guidelines for the management of patients with ST-segment elevation MI (STEMI).[9]

Sjauw et al[10] performed 2 separate meta-analyses of cohort studies of IABP therapy, one for high-risk patients with ST-segment elevation MI (STEMI) and one for STEMI patients with cardiogenic shock. Adjunctive IABP therapy was associated with an absolute decrease in 30-day mortality of 18% in patients who were treated with fibrinolytic therapy, but there was a 6% absolute increase in 30-day mortality in patients who were treated with primary PCI. The authors reached 2 principal conclusions: (1) the lower mortality of the patients who received IABP as an adjunct to fibrinolytic therapy can be explained by confounding and bias and (2) "one cannot reliably distinguish between an unexpected truly detrimental effect of IABP therapy as an adjunct to primary PCI in STEMI complicated by cardiogenic shock and the influence of bias and confounding inherent to cohort studies."

Left ventricular assist devices (LVADs) that can be inserted percutaneously are an alternative means of hemodynamic support in patients with STEMI complicated by cardiogenic shock. One prospective randomized study randomized 26 patients with cardiogenic shock to an IABP (n = 13) or the Impella LP2.5 (Abiomed Europe GmbH, Aachen, Germany).[11] The increase in cardiac index 30 minutes after the onset of hemodynamic support was significantly greater for the Impella than the IABP (0.48 L/min/m^2 vs. 0.11 L/min/m^2; P = .02). A recent meta-analysis of controlled trials comparing percutaneous LVAD with IABP found that the use of LVAD to treat cardiogenic shock provided better hemodynamic support, but 30-day survival was not improved.[12] Further studies are needed to evaluate the effects of both IABP and LVAD therapy on the outcomes of patients with cardiogenic shock.

S. W. Werns, MD

References

1. Gruppo Italiano per lo Studio della Streptochinasi nell'Infarto Miocardico (GISSI). Effectiveness of intravenous thrombolytic treatment in acute myocardial infarction. *Lancet.* 1986;1:397-402.
2. Berger PB, Holmes DR, Stebbins AL, Bates ER, Califf RM, Topol EJ. Impact of an aggressive invasive catheterization and revascularization strategy on mortality in patients with cardiogenic shock in the global utilization of streptokinase and tissue plasminogen activator for occluded coronary arteries (GUSTO-1) trial. An observational study. *Circulation.* 1997;96:122-127.
3. Berger PB, Tuttle RH, Holmes DR, et al. One-year survival among patients with acute myocardial infarction complicated by cardiogenic shock, and its relation to early revascularization. Results from the GUSTO-1 trial. *Circulation.* 1999;99:873-878.

4. Hochman JS, Sleeper LA, Webb JG, et al. Early revascularization in acute myocardial infarction complicated by cardiogenic shock. *N Engl J Med.* 1999; 341:625-634.
5. Hochman JS, Sleeper LA, White HD, et al. One-year survival following early revascularization for cardiogenic shock. *JAMA.* 2001;285:190-192.
6. Hochman JS, Sleeper LA, Webb JG, et al. Early revascularization and long-term survival in cardiogenic shock complicating acute myocardial infarction. *JAMA.* 2006;295:2511-2515.
7. Brodie BR, Stuckey TD, Hansen C, Muncy D. Intra-aortic balloon counterpulsation before primary percutaneous transluminal coronary angioplasty reduces catheterization laboratory events in high-risk patients with acute myocardial infarction. *Am J Cardiol.* 1999;84:18-23.
8. Ohman EM, Hochman JS. Aortic counterpulsation in acute myocardial infarction: physiologically important but does the patient benefit? *Am Heart J.* 2001; 141:889-892.
9. Antman EM, Anbe DT, Armstrong PW, et al. ACC/AHA guidelines for the management of patients with ST-elevation myocardial infarction: a report of the American College of Cardiology/American Heart Association Task Force on Practice Guidelines. *Circulation.* 2004;110:e82-e293.
10. Sjauw KD, Engstrom AE, Vis MM, et al. A systematic review and meta-analysis of intra-aortic balloon pump therapy in ST-elevation myocardial infarction: should we change the guidelines? *Eur Heart J.* 2009;30:459-468.
11. Seyfarth M, Sibbing D, Bauer I, et al. A randomized clinical trial to evaluate the safety and efficacy of a percutaneous left ventricular assist device versus intra-aortic balloon pumping for treatment of cardiogenic shock caused by myocardial infarction. *J Am Coll Cardiol.* 2008;52:1584-1588.
12. Cheng JM, den Uil CA, Hoeks SE. Percutaneous left ventricular assist devices vs. intra-aortic balloon pump counterpulsation for treatment of cardiogenic shock: a meta-analysis of controlled trials. *Eur Heart J.* 2009;30:2102-2108.

Routine Early Angioplasty after Fibrinolysis for Acute Myocardial Infarction

Cantor WJ, Fitchett D, Borgundvaag B, et al (Southlake Regional Health Centre, Newmarket, Ontario, Canada; The Univ of Toronto, Ontario, Canada; et al)
N Engl J Med 360:2705-2718, 2009

Background.—Patients with a myocardial infarction with ST-segment elevation who present to hospitals that do not have the capability of performing percutaneous coronary intervention (PCI) often cannot undergo timely primary PCI and therefore receive fibrinolysis. The role and optimal timing of routine PCI after fibrinolysis have not been established.

Methods.—We randomly assigned 1059 high-risk patients who had a myocardial infarction with ST-segment elevation and who were receiving fibrinolytic therapy at centers that did not have the capability of performing PCI to either standard treatment (including rescue PCI, if required, or delayed angiography) or a strategy of immediate transfer to another hospital and PCI within 6 hours after fibrinolysis. All patients received aspirin, tenecteplase, and heparin or enoxaparin; concomitant clopidogrel was recommended. The primary end point was the composite of death, reinfarction, recurrent ischemia, new or worsening congestive heart failure, or cardiogenic shock within 30 days.

Results.—Cardiac catheterization was performed in 88.7% of the patients assigned to standard treatment a median of 32.5 hours after randomization and in 98.5% of the patients assigned to routine early PCI a median of 2.8 hours after randomization. At 30 days, the primary end point occurred in 11.0% of the patients who were assigned to routine early PCI and in 17.2% of the patients assigned to standard treatment (relative risk with early PCI, 0.64; 95% confidence interval, 0.47 to 0.87; P=0.004). There were no significant differences between the groups in the incidence of major bleeding.

Conclusions.—Among high-risk patients who had a myocardial infarction with ST-segment elevation and who were treated with fibrinolysis, transfer for PCI within 6 hours after fibrinolysis was associated with significantly fewer ischemic complications than was standard treatment. (ClinicalTrials.gov number, NCT00164190.)

▶ Numerous studies have been performed to determine the optimal management of patients with ST-segment elevation myocardial infarction (STEMI) who receive fibrinolytic therapy because they present to hospitals that do not have the capability of performing timely primary percutaneous coronary intervention (PCI). Management strategies that have been investigated include so-called "facilitated PCI" and "rescue PCI." The 2009 Focused Updates of the ACC/AHA Guidelines for the Management of Patients with STEMI recommend that these terms should be abandoned.[1] The revised guidelines referred to a "pharmacoinvasive strategy" that is exemplified by the Trial of Routine Angioplasty and Stenting after Fibrinolysis to Enhance Reperfusion in Acute Myocardial Infarction (TRANSFER-AMI) study, which entails the routine and early transfer of high-risk patients to a PCI center for early PCI after receiving fibrinolytic therapy at a hospital that does not perform PCI.[2] Patients with STEMI were eligible for enrollment in the TRANSFER-AMI study if they had at least one of the following high-risk characteristics: systolic blood pressure < 100 mm Hg, heart rate > 100, Killip class II or III, ≥2 mm of ST-segment depression in the anterior leads, or ≥1 mm of ST-segment elevation in right-sided lead V4 (V4R).[2] The patients who were randomly assigned to a strategy of immediate transfer to a PCI-capable hospital underwent PCI a median of 2.8 hours after randomization, resulting in a significant lower rate of ischemic complications compared with the standard strategy of medical management for at least 24 hours unless there was hemodynamic instability or persistent ST-segment elevation and chest pain.[2]

The revised guidelines recommend that patients with a STEMI who present to a PCI-capable facility should undergo immediate catheterization and PCI if appropriate, while patients with a STEMI who present to a non-PCI-capable facility should be managed with either fibrinolytic therapy or immediate transfer for PCI. Furthermore, the guidelines recommend that management after fibrinolytic therapy should be determined by an assessment of the patient's risk. Cardiogenic shock, severe heart failure and/or pulmonary edema, and hemodynamically compromising arrhythmias after fibrinolytic therapy are designated class I indications for prompt transfer to a PCI-capable facility for coronary angiography with intent to perform PCI or emergency coronary artery bypass surgery.[1,3] Among patients who lack certain electrocardiographic or hemodynamic features that are deemed to confer "high-risk," persistent ischemic symptoms or suspected failure to reperfuse after fibrinolytic therapy is regarded as a class IIb indication for transfer to a PCI-capable facility.

S. W. Werns, MD

References

1. Kushner FG, Hand M, Smith SC Jr, et al. 2009 focused updates: ACC/AHA guidelines for the management of patients with ST-elevation myocardial infarction (updating the 2004 guideline and 2007 focused update) and ACC/AHA/SCAI guidelines on percutaneous coronary intervention (updating the 2005 guidelines and 2007 focused update): a report of the American College of Cardiology Foundation/American Heart Association Task Force on Practice Guidelines. *Circulation.* 2009;120:2271-2306.
2. Cantor WJ, Fitchett D, Borgundvaag B, et al. Routine early angioplasty after fibrinolysis for acute myocardial infarction. *N Engl J Med.* 2009;360:2705-2718.
3. Antman EM, Hand M, Armstrong PW, et al. 2007 focused update of the ACC/AHA 2004 guidelines for the management of patients with ST-elevation myocardial infarction: a report of the American College of Cardiology/American Heart Association Task Force on Practice Guidelines. *J Am Coll Cardiol.* 2008; 51:210-247.

Pulmonary Embolism/Pulmonary Artery Hypertension

Negative Predictive Value of Computed Tomography Pulmonary Angiography With Indirect Computed Tomography Venography in Intensive Care Unit Patients

Ravenel JG, Northam MC, Nguyen SA (Med Univ of South Carolina, Charleston)
J Comput Assist Tomogr 33:739-742, 2009

Purpose.—The aim of the study was to evaluate the negative predictive value (NPV) of combined computed tomography (CT) pulmonary angiography (CTPA) and indirect CT venography (CTV) in the intensive care unit (ICU) setting.

Materials and Methods.—We retrospectively reviewed the records of 181 consecutive ICU patients who underwent CTPA/CTV. Radiology reports were examined to determine whether the study was positive for pulmonary embolism (PE), PE and deep venous thrombosis (DVT), or DVT alone; indeterminate; or negative. Results that were reported as negative were further evaluated for evidence of PE or DVT within 30 days by imaging, clinical evaluation, or autopsy data. The outcomes were evaluated for significance by calculating the rate ratio and 95% confidence interval.

Results.—A total of 41 patients (22.7%) were diagnosed with venous thromboembolism, 29 (70.7%) with PE, 8 (19.5%) with PE and DVT, and 4 (9.8%) with DVT. Seven studies were considered nondiagnostic. Seventeen deaths occurred within 30 days of CTA/CTV, of which none was felt to be related to PE/DVT. Of the 140 studies read as negative or nondiagnostic, 4 were determined to have venous thromboembolism (3 PEs and 1 DVT) within 30 days of the initial study (NPV = 97.1%). If patients who received prophylactic anticoagulation or inferior vena cava interruption (n = 25) were excluded, NPV decreases to 96.5%.

Conclusion.—A negative CTPA/CTV is reliable for the exclusion of significant venous thromboembolism in ICU patients.

▶ This article is important to discuss as it supports the value of combining negative CT venography (CTV) with negative CT pulmonary angiography (CTPA) in the ICU setting to increase negative predictive value of the combined test. Although this is a significant addition to the literature this is still a retrospective study and does not conclusively establish this as a firm policy that can be followed. For example, in the Prospective Investigation of Pulmonary Embolism Disease II (PIOPED II) study[1] although negative CTV did add to the negative predictive value of CTPA, other testing, such as perfusion scanning or ultrasound, was used; in areas of high discordance between pretest clinical probability and test results, neither negative nor positive test could be totally reliable.

R. P. Dellinger, MD

Reference

1. Stein PD, Fowler SE, Goodman LR, et al. Multidetector computed tomography for acute pulmonary embolism. *N Engl J Med.* 2006;354:2317-2327.

64-MDCT Pulmonary Angiography and CT Venography in the Diagnosis of Thromboembolic Disease
Nazaroğlu H, Özmen CA, Akay HÖ, et al (Dicle Univ School of Medicine, Diyarbakir, Turkey)
AJR Am J Roentgenol 192:654-661, 2009

Objective.—The purpose of our study was to investigate whether CT venography (CTV) performed after CT pulmonary angiography (CTPA) using 64-MDCT provides additional findings in the diagnosis of thromboembolic disease.

Materials and Methods.—Three hundred six consecutive patients in whom pulmonary embolism (PE) was clinically suspected were included in the study. The study group was classified according to the diagnostic quality of the CTPA examinations, the presence or absence of PE and deep venous thrombosis (DVT), and the most proximal localization that the embolus could lodge in the pulmonary artery.

Results.—The diagnostic quality of CTPA was insufficient in 5.9%, acceptable in 8.2%, and excellent in 85.9% of the patients. The diagnostic quality of CTV was insufficient in 11.4%, acceptable in 47.4%, and excellent in 41.2%. The percentages of nondiagnostic examinations for CTPA and CTV were 5.2% and 10.8%, respectively. Acute PE and acute DVT were observed in 25.2% and 18.0%, respectively. The percentage of subsegmental emboli among patients with acute PE was 15.6%. The percentage of patients with thromboembolic disease was 29.1%. Of patients who were diagnosed as having thromboembolic disease, 13.5% (12 of 89 patients) had DVT only. Of all patients, 3.9% (12 of 306) had only isolated DVT. The number of patients with subsegmental PE who had DVT was two (0.7% all patients).

Conclusion.—As in MDCT scanning with a smaller number of slices, the combination of CTV with CTPA in 64-MDCT results in a small but definitive increase in the percentage of patients with a diagnosis of thromboembolic disease.

▶ First there was ventilation perfusion lung scanning for diagnosis of pulmonary embolism (PE), then there was computed angiographic tomography. These primary diagnostic tests are supplemented with D-dimer, leg ultrasound, and pretest clinical probability to form the primary basis of our PE diagnostic testing regimens. The most recent addition to our armamentarium is adding CT venography (CTV) to CT pulmonary angiography (CTPA). In this study, an additional 4% of patients were diagnosed with thromboembolic disease by the addition of CTV. This additional diagnostic capability must be weighed against additional radiation exposure. The dye load would be the same. It should also be noted that tests of insufficient quality for analysis are more likely to occur with CTV as opposed to CTPA. Perhaps the best approach would be to make a decision in advance as to additional CTV study if CTPA is negative in patients pre-identified with higher pretest probability of PE (intermediate or high pretest probability).

R. P. Dellinger, MD

D-**Dimers and Efficacy of Clinical Risk Estimation Algorithms: Sensitivity in Evaluation of Acute Pulmonary Embolism**
Gupta RT, Kakarla RK, Kirshenbaum KJ, et al (Duke Univ Med Ctr, Durham, NC; Advocate Illinois Masonic Med Ctr, Chicago, IL)
AJR Am J Roentgenol 193:425-430, 2009

Objective.—The goal of this study was to test the efficacy of clinical risk algorithms and a quantitative immunoturbidimetric D-dimer assay in the evaluation of patients undergoing pulmonary CT angiography for suspected acute pulmonary embolism.

Subjects and Methods.—From April 1, 2007, to March 31, 2008, emergency department evaluations for clinically suspected pulmonary embolism were performed with the revised Geneva score, a quantitative D-dimer assay, and pulmonary CT angiography.

Results.—Evaluations for pulmonary embolism were performed for 745 consecutively registered patients, 627 of whom were included in the study.

The other 118 patients were excluded because a D-dimer assay was not performed. According to the revised Geneva score, 281 patients had low clinical probability of having pulmonary embolism; 330, intermediate probability; and 16, high probability. CT angiography showed that 28 patients had pulmonary embolism (six in the low-probability group, 17 in the intermediate-probability group, and five in the high-probability group). The sensitivity, negative predictive value, and specificity of the D-dimer assay were 100%, 100%, and 25% (low-clinical-probability group); 100%, 100%, and 33% (intermediate-probability group); and 80%, 80%, and 37% (high-probability group).

Conclusion.—The data appear to support the use of a quantitative D-dimer assay as a first-line test in evaluation for pulmonary embolism when the clinical probability of the presence of pulmonary embolism is low or intermediate. The sensitivity and negative predictive value were 100% for these cases. More than 26% of CT angiographic examinations might have been avoided if the D-dimer assay had been used as a first-line test in the care of patients at low or intermediate risk. Because of the small sample size, the D-dimer assay is not recommended as a first-line test in the evaluation of patients at high risk.

▶ The newer quantitative D-dimer assays are proving to be a significant addition to our diagnostic armamentarium for making pulmonary embolism very unlikely. A positive D-dimer is not of clinical value because it may be positive due to a wide variety of other patient factors in comorbidities, such as postoperative state, older age, inflammatory states, and pregnancy. However, in the emergency department where patients present, often with fewer comorbidities in hospitalized patients, it is of particular value. It is, however, important for the caregiver to establish pretest clinical probability of PE before knowing the test results so that they will not be influenced in patients with a characterization of low or intermediate risk. The primary gain from not proceeding to additional testing in the presence of low or intermediate risk in the emergency department and nonelevated D-dimer is the avoidance of dyes, and radiographic and x-ray exposure for patients who are being considered for pulmonary embolism.

R. P. Dellinger, MD

Removal of the G2 Filter: Differences between Implantation Times Greater and Less than 180 Days

Lynch FC, Kekulawela S (Penn State Univ College of Medicine, Hershey, PA)
J Vasc Interv Radiol 20:1200-1209, 2009

Purpose.—To investigate whether filters implanted for longer periods are more difficult or hazardous to remove.

Materials and Methods.—A retrospective review of G2 inferior vena cava filter removals was performed. Objective measures reflecting the difficulty of the removal procedure were evaluated for differences required to remove a filter with an implantation period greater or less than 180 days.

Results.—One hundred seventy of 174 G2 filters were successfully removed (97.7% success rate). There was no significant difference in the success rate ($P = .86$), total procedure time ($P = .87$), fluoroscopy time ($P = .13$), or contrast medium use ($P = .22$) required to remove filters implanted for more than 180 days compared to those implanted for a shorter period of time. There was no significant difference in the frequency of filter movement ($P = .90$), tilt ($P = .87$), and caval penetration ($P = .41$) between the two groups. Six filter fractures were observed, all with implantation times greater than 180 days.

Conclusions.—The removal of a G2 filter that has been in place for more than 180 days can be performed as easily, as safely, and with a similar degree of success as one that has been in place for less time. Movement, tilt, and penetration are early events after implantation that may have an effect on successful filter removal.

▶ As more and more retrievable filters are placed, an understanding of safety as well as characteristics that influence removal cap ability are surfacing. Indications for retrievable filter placement are primarily when pulmonary embolism or deep vein thrombosis is diagnosed in patients who at the time have contraindications to anticoagulation but within the short-term with these contraindications will abate. When the patient will be ambulatory in the long-term and would benefit from the improved venous drainage with filter removal, a retrievable filter makes sense. Anticoagulation is begun when the contraindication is no longer present; following successful anticoagulation the filter is removed. Time has been identified as one factor that influences ability to remove retrievable filter. Likewise, tilt and imbedding in inferior vena cava (IVC) wall are previously recognized factors for failure to retrieve. Previous literature has suggested 180 days as an outside time range for attempting filter removal. This article demonstrates that filters considerably out from 180 days can still be removed. Furthermore, filters with clot in place were not necessarily a contraindication to removal. The aggressive approach taken by the authors of this article included anticoagulation in patients with large clot burden followed by filter removal. Even filter fracture was not necessarily an absolute contraindication to removal. The results from this article are likely related to the high expertise and high interest in this particular area by this group of interventional radiologists.

R. P. Dellinger, MD

Relationship between the extent of deep venous thrombosis and the extent of acute pulmonary embolism as assessed by CT angiography

Ghaye B, Willems V, Nchimi A, et al (Univ Hosp of Liege, Belgium; et al)
Br J Radiol 82:198-203, 2009

The aim of our study is to investigate prospectively the quantitative relationship between deep venous thrombosis (DVT) and acute pulmonary embolism (PE). 110 patients clinically suspected of having venous thromboembolic disease underwent combined CT pulmonary angiography (CTPA) and venography of lower limb veins. 44 patients presented with clinical signs of DVT and positive ultrasonography or ascending venography, but no clinical sign of PE (Group 1). 66 patients presented with clinical signs of PE and positive CTPA (Group 2). Clot load in lower limb veins and pulmonary arteries were scored by two independent readers, each using two separate systems for DVT and two for PE. 27 (61%) patients in Group 1 also had PE, and 55 (83%) patients in Group 2 also had DVT. Correlations between PE and DVT scores were weak but statistically significant in Group 2 (r_s ranging from 0.470–0.520; $p \leq 0.001$), but only some were significant in Group 1 (r_s ranging from 0.253–0.318; p-values ranging from 0.035–0.097). In conclusion, although PE occurs in a majority of patients with DVT, and *vice versa*, the amount/burden of clot load in one condition does not necessarily indicate — or indicates only weakly — the degree of burden in the other condition.

▶ This study supports logic that already existed but nevertheless, is important to confirm. When evaluating a patient for possible pulmonary embolism (PE), the finding of negative leg ultrasound (primary diagnostic test for deep venous thrombosis [DVT] in this study) does not exclude the diagnosis of PE. It is well known that dye or computed tomography angiography may be positive in the absence of DVT. This may be because the ultrasound test is not sensitive enough, as it is known to be the case if a single clot had formed and dislodged traveling into the pulmonary circulation. In the case, the patient should be treated identically as if the patient would have been treated with documented PE in DVT. The patient is at risk to reform leg clot and re-embolize. The presence of acute DVT in the absence of PE by angiography has minimal effect on treatment plan. It is also reasonable to assume that almost any combination of leg clot and chest clot would be possible with thromboembolic disease.

R. P. Dellinger, MD

3 Hemodynamics and Monitoring

Assessment of Left Ventricular Function by Intensivists Using Hand-Held Echocardiography
Melamed R, Sprenkle MD, Ulstad VK, et al (Hennepin County Med Ctr, Minneapolis, MN)
Chest 135:1416-1420, 2009

Background.—Bedside transthoracic echocardiography (TTE) provides rapid and noninvasive hemodynamic assessment of critically ill patients but is limited by the immediate availability of experienced sonographers and cardiologists.

Methods.—Forty-four patients in the medical ICU underwent near-simultaneous limited TTE performed by intensivists with minimal training in echocardiography, and a formal TTE that was performed by certified sonographers and was interpreted by experienced echocardiographers. Intensivists, blinded to the patient's diagnosis and the results of the formal TTE, were asked to determine whether left ventricular (LV) function was grossly normal or abnormal and to place LV function into one of the following three categories: 1, normal; 2, mildly to moderately decreased; and 3, severely decreased.

Results.—Using the formal TTE as the "gold standard," intensivists correctly identified normal LV function in 22 of 24 cases (92%) and abnormal LV function in 16 of 20 cases (80%). The κ statistic for the agreement between intensivist and echocardiographer for any abnormality in LV function was 0.72 (95% confidence interval [CI], 0.52 to 0.93; $p < 0.001$). Intensivists correctly placed LV function into one of three categories in 36 of 44 cases (82%); in 6 of the 8 cases that were misclassified, the error involved an overestimation of LV function. The κ statistic for agreement between the intensivist and echocardiographer with regard to placement into one of three categories of LV function was 0.68 (95% CI, 0.48 to 0.88; $p < 0.001$).

Conclusions.—Intensivists were able to estimate LV function with reasonable accuracy using a hand-held unit in the ICU, despite having undergone minimal training in image acquisition and interpretation.

▶ Management of hemodynamically unstable patients can be quite difficult. The most common strategy is to start with fluid administration and then add

TABLE 1.—Normal vs Abnormal LV Function

	Formal TTE by Echocardiographer	
Limited TTE by Intensivist	Normal Findings	Abnormal Findings
Normal findings	22	4
Abnormal findings	2	16

TABLE 2.—LV Function by Category*

	Formal TTE by Echocardiographer		
Limited TTE by Intensivist	Category 1	Category 2	Category 3
Category 1	22	4	0
Category 2	2	9	2
Category 3	0	0	5

*Category 1, normal LV function; category 2, mild-to-moderate decrease in LV function; category 3, severe decrease in LV function.

titration of vasoactive medications. Echocardiograms or more invasive monitoring usually is ordered in patients who are not responsive or in those whose response is less robust that expected. With the advent of more portable echo devices, earlier evaluation might impact patient care paradigms. This study evaluated whether with a short course of training, intensivists could make the correct diagnosis regarding left ventricular (LV) function. The gold standard used was LV function as assessed by a classically trained and experienced echocardiographer from images attained by transthoracic echocardiography (TTE). Table 1 shows the comparison data for which intensivists identified normal LV function correctly 92% of the time and abnormal LV function correctly only 80% of the time. Table 2 shows were the discordant readings occurred and demonstrates that intensivists when discordant with the gold standard were typically off by a single category. Thus, this study demonstrates that intensivists can be taught to acquire and interpret images from a bedside hand-held echocardiography. Where the study doesn't help the clinician is in several areas. First, which hand-held device is adequate for obtaining the correct images? If one uses these hand-held devices, will one miss other important findings that would have been obtained by classic TTE such as valvular abnormalities? If one uses hand-held echocardiography, will these findings impact patient care paradigms? Importantly, in most discordant interpretations the discordance stemmed from the intensivists making the wrong read. Can this be corrected by additional training or experience? Will these discordant interpretations translate into harm that might offset gains? Clearly, more research is needed in this domain.

T. Dorman, MD

Dynamic preload indicators fail to predict fluid responsiveness in open-chest conditions

de Waal EEC, Rex S, Kruitwagen CLJJ, et al (Univ Med Ctr, Utrecht, The Netherlands; Univ Hosp, Germany)
Crit Care Med 37:510-515, 2009

Objective.—Dynamic preload indicators like pulse pressure variation (PPV) and stroke volume variation (SVV) are increasingly being used for optimizing cardiac preload since they have been demonstrated to predict fluid responsiveness in a variety of perioperative settings. However, in open-chest conditions, the value of these indices has not been systematically examined yet. We, therefore, evaluated the ability of PPV and SVV to predict fluid responsiveness under open- and closed-chest conditions.

Design.—Prospective, controlled, clinical study.

Setting.—University hospital.

Patients.—Twenty-two patients scheduled for elective coronary artery bypass graft surgery.

Interventions.—Defined volume loads (VL) (10 mL kg^{-1} hydroxyethyl starch 6%) intra- and postoperatively.

Measurements and Main Results.—Stroke volume index was measured 1) before and after a VL intraoperatively in open-chest conditions, and 2) under closed-chest conditions within 1 hour after arrival in the intensive care unit. Central venous pressure and global end diastolic volume were assessed as static preload indicators. In addition, PPV and SVV (both obtained with PiCCO system) were recorded. Fluid-responders were defined by an

TABLE 5.—Receiver Operating Characteristic and Pearson's Correlation Analysis for Several Preload Indicators as Predictors of Increase in Stroke Volume Index by more than 12% after Volume Loading in Open and Closed Chest Conditions

Baseline Hemodynamic Indices	Receiver Operating Characteristic Curves Predicting Increase in Stroke Volume Index ≥12%				Pearsons' Correlation with Increase in Stroke Volume Index	
	Area Under the Curve	Standard Error	*p* Value	95% Confidence Interval	R^2	*p* Value
Open chest						
Central venous pressure	0.578	0.168	0.678	0.248–0.907	0.0742	0.274
Global end diastolic volume index	0.756	0.130	0.173	0.500–1.011	0.4949	0.001[a]
Intrathoracic blood volume index	0.756	0.130	0.173	0.500–1.011	0.4944	0.001[a]
Pulse pressure variation	0.556	0.126	0.767	0.308–0.803	0.1046	0.190
Stroke volume variation	0.489	0.134	0.953	0.225–0.752	0.0419	0.4156
Closed chest						
Central venous pressure	0.636	0.124	0.279	0.393–0.880	0.0043	0.087
Global end diastolic volume index	0.700	0.123	0.121	0.460–0.940	0.0977	0.168
Intrathoracic blood volume index	0.682	0.123	0.159	0.441–0.923	0.0986	0.166
Pulse pressure variation	0.884	0.075	0.004[a]	0.736–1.032	0.5620	0.000[a]
Stroke volume variation	0.911	0.069	0.003[a]	0.776–1.046	0.5554	0.000[a]

[a]$p < 0.05$.

increase in stroke volume index ≥12% subsequent to the VL. Receiver operating characteristic analysis showed that all preload indicators failed to predict fluid responsiveness in open-chest conditions. Under closed-chest conditions, the areas under the receiver operating characteristic curve for PPV and SVV were 0.884 ($p = 0.004$) and 0.911 ($p = 0.003$), respectively, whereas the static and volumetric preload parameters failed to predict fluid responsiveness. A PPV of ≥10% identified fluid-responders with a sensitivity of 64% and a specificity of 100%, while a SVV of > 8% identified fluid-responders with a sensitivity of 100% and a specificity of 78%.

Conclusions.—Our results suggest that the dynamic preload indicators PPV and SVV are able to predict fluid responsiveness under closed-chest conditions, whereas all static and dynamic preload indicators fail to predict fluid responsiveness under open-chest conditions.

▶ Practitioners are more frequently using less invasive methods of determining cardiac parameters. Use of these devices requires the clinician to understand the limitations of such devices. In this study, the authors studied whether an open chest impacted variables commonly thought to reflect intravascular volume. Specifically, the dynamic response of these variables to a fluid challenge has been shown to correlate with improvements in stroke volume/stroke volume index. Thus, fluid responsiveness is a marker of a Starling response and emboldens to clinicians to provide additional fluid for ongoing hypotension. Surprisingly, these authors found that in the same patient these parameters did indeed differentiate fluid responsiveness defined as an increase in stroke volume index of at least 12% when the chest was closed. However, the predictive nature of these variables was lost when the chest was opened. Table 5 demonstrates the significant area under the curve (AUC) for the receiver operating characteristics (ROCs) in these 2 conditions. Thus, use of these variables in the open chest is fraught with erroneous interpretation. These findings of the impact of an open chest beg the question as to what is the relationship of these numbers to stroke index when the abdomen is open?

T. Dorman, MD

Uncalibrated Stroke Volume Variations Are Able to Predict the Hemodynamic Effects of Positive End-Expiratory Pressure in Patients with Acute Lung Injury or Acute Respiratory Distress Syndrome after Liver Transplantation
Biais M, Nouette-Gaulain K, Quinart A, et al (Centre Hospitalier Universitaire de Bordeaux, France; Université Victor Segalen Bordeaux 2 and Centre Hospitalier Universitaire de Bordeaux, France)
Anesthesiology 111:855-862, 2009

Background.—Positive end-expiratory pressure (PEEP) may reduce cardiac output and total hepatic blood flow after liver transplantation. Pulse pressure variation is useful in predicting the PEEP-induced decrease in cardiac output. The aim of the study was to examine the relationships between stroke volume variations (SVV) obtained with the Vigileo monitor (Edwards Lifesciences, Irvine, CA), and the hemodynamic effects of PEEP.

Methods.—Over 2 yr, patients presenting an acute lung injury or an acute respiratory distress syndrome in the 72 h after liver transplantation were prospectively enrolled. Patients were monitored with a pulmonary artery catheter (stroke volume) and with the Vigileo system (stroke volume and SVV). Measurements were performed in duplicate, first during zero end-expiratory pressure and then 10 min after the addition of 10 cm H_2O PEEP.

Results.—Twenty-six patients were included. Six patients were excluded from analysis. On PEEP, SVV and pulse pressure variation increased significantly and stroke volume decreased significantly. PEEP-induced changes in stroke volume measured by pulmonary artery catheter were significantly correlated with SVV ($r^2 = 0.69$; $P < 0.001$) and pulse pressure variation on zero end-expiratory pressure ($r^2 = 0.66$, $P < 0.001$). PEEP-induced decrease in stroke volume measured by pulmonary artery catheter $\geq$ 15% was predicted by an SVV > 7% (sensitivity = 100%, specificity = 80%) and by a pulse pressure variation > 8% (sensitivity = 80%, specificity = 100%). PEEP-induced changes in stroke volume measured by pulmonary artery catheter and Vigileo device were correlated ($r^2 = 0.51$, $P < 0.005$).

Conclusions.—SVV obtained with Vigileo monitor is useful to predict decrease in stroke volume induced by PEEP. Moreover, this device is able to track changes in stroke volume induced by PEEP.

▶ Stroke volume variation as well as systolic pressure and pulse pressure variations are clearly underutilized in the ICU. Three different technologies exist to quantify the area under the arterial pressure waveform as it correlates with increases and decreases in stroke volume. Although these techniques require some invasiveness, similar information can also be gained from information that is already available in mechanically ventilated patients using the arterial pressure waveform. The greater the effect of PEEP on intravascular volume as it is linked to decrease in stroke volume, the greater the delta will be with these 2 measurements.

R. P. Dellinger, MD

Routine transthoracic echocardiography in a general Intensive Care Unit: An 18 month survey in 704 patients
Marcelino PA, Marum SM, Fernandes APM, et al (Hosp Curry Cabral, Lisbon, Portugal)
Eur J Intern Med 20:e37-e42, 2009

The authors analyzed 704 transthoracic echocardiographic (TTE) examinations, performed routinely to all admitted patients to a general

16-bed Intensive Care Unit (ICU) during an 18-month period. Data acquisition and prevalence of abnormalities of cardiac structures and function were assessed, as well as the new, previously unknown severe diagnoses.

A TTE was performed within the first 24 h of admission on 704 consecutive patients, with a mean age of 61.5 ± 17.5 years, ICU stay of 10.6 ± 17.1 days, APACHE II 22.6 ± 8.9, and SAPS II 52.7 ± 20.4. In four patients, TTE could not be performed. Left ventricular (LV) dimensions were quantified in 689 (97.8%) patients, and LV function in 670 (95.2%) patients. Cardiac output (CO) was determined in 610 (86.7%), and mitral E/A in 399 (85.9% of patients in sinus rhythm).

TABLE 3.—Echocardiographic Abnormalities Detected

TTE Alterations		Severe Previously Unknown TTE Diagnoses	
Left ventricular enlargement (n)	65	Severe left ventricular systolic dysfunction	23
Right ventricular enlargement (*n*)	99	Severe valvular disease	10
Left atrium enlargement (*n*)	163	Tamponade	4
Left ventricular systolic dysfunction (*n*)	132	Endocarditis	8
LV hypertrophy (*n*)	41	Others:	
		Hypertrophic cardiomyopathy	2
		Intracardiac Mass	6
Pericardial effusion (*n*)	15		
Total (*n* and %)	234 (33%)[a]		53 (7.5%)

[a]Note: Many patients presented more than one echocardiographic alteration, thus, the number of patients with these alterations does not correspond to the sum of all alterations.

TABLE 4.—Differences Between Patients with and without Echocardiographic Alterations

Parameter	Patients Without Echocardiographic Alterations	Patients With Echocardiographic Alterations	*p* value
N	470	234	
Age (years)	58.1 ± 17.4 (21–92)	66 ± 16.5 (18–92)	<0.001
ICU stay (days)	10.9 ± 18.4 (0.4–119.3)	10.9 ± 16.5 (0.4–177)	ns
APACHE II	21.1 ± 8.9 (9–45)	24.4 ± 8.7 (9–47)	<0.001
SAPS II	48.7 ± 21 (9–115)	57.4 ± 18.8 (27–105)	ns
Mortality	84 (25.4%)	94 (40.1%)	<0.001
MAP (mm Hg)	82.7 ± 20.9 (32–141)	77.2 ± 22 (35–134)	<0.001
HR (bpm)	99.6 ± 18.8 (66–137)	99.4 ± 20.8 (63–134)	ns
CVP (mm Hg)	9.4 ± 4.6 (−2 to 22)	12.4 ± 4.8 (4–27)	<0.001
IVC maximum dimension (mm)	14.7 ± 4.4 (5–30)	18.3 ± 4.6 (9–28)	<0.001
IVC index (%)	33 ± 26 (0–100)	23 ± 23 (0–100)	<0.001
Cardiac index (l/min/m^2)	3.89 ± 0.93	3.34 ± 0.95 (1.3–6.97)	<0.001

Legend: ICU. Intensive Care Unit; MAP, mean arterial pressure; HR, heart rate; CVP, central venous pressure; IVC, inferior vena cava; l/min/m^2, liters per minute per squared meter; mm Hg, millimeters of mercury; ns, nonsignificant.

TABLE 5.—Prevalence of Echocardiographic Alterations in Different Diagnostic Groups

	n	Detected Echocardiographic Alterations (*n* and %)
All patients	704	234 (33.2%)
Medical patients	426	191 (44.8%)
Surgical patients	181	45 (24.8%)
Liver transplant patients	97	8 (8.2%)

Echocardiographic abnormalities were detected in 234 (33%) patients, the most common being left atrial (LA) enlargement ($n = 163$), and LV dysfunction ($n = 132$). Patients with these alterations were older (66 ± 16.5 vs 58.1 17.4, $p < 0.001$), presented a higher APACHE II score (24.4 ± 8.7 vs 21.1 ± 8.9, $p < 0.001$), and had a higher mortality rate (40.1% vs 25.4%, $p < 0.001$). Severe, previously unknown echocardiographic diagnoses were detected in 53 (7.5%) patients; the most frequent condition was severe LV dysfunction. Through a multivariate logistic regression analysis, it was determined that mortality was affected by tricuspid regurgitation ($p = 0.016$, CI 1.007–1.016) and ICU stay ($p < 0.001$, CI 1–1.019). We conclude that TTE can detect most cardiac structures in a general ICU. One-third of the patients studied presented cardiac structural or functional alterations and 7.5% severe previously unknown diagnoses.

▶ This is an observational trial with no control group of routine transthoracic echocardiography performed in the first 24 hours of admission to an intensive care unit (ICU). Not surprisingly, the authors found that one can indeed perform such a routine exam. The overall rate of echocardiographic abnormalities, whether important to care during the period of critical illness was fairly high and varied by patient type (Table 5). The majority of these abnormalities were not considered severe (Table 3). Older patients and those with lower blood pressure and cardiac index were more likely to have an abnormal echocardiogram (Table 4). This study is important because it shows that echocardiograms in the ICU have use. What the study lacks however is the ability to understand that use from a clinical relevance and a fiscal standpoint. For instance, how many of the valve abnormalities were identifiable by auscultation? Would the echocardiograms that identified severe abnormalities have been based upon clinical variables such as presence of a murmur or shock resistant to volume resuscitation and thus are not really findings supportive of a routine exam? The finding of endocarditis, although important principally, impacts duration of antibiotic therapy and not acute care management and thus again may not be a finding supportive of routine exam.

T. Dorman, MD

Ultrasound evidence of the optimal wrist position for radial artery cannulation
Mizukoshi K, Shibasaki M, Amaya F, et al (Kyoto Prefectural Univ of Medicine, Japan)
Can J Anesth 56:427-431, 2009

Purpose.—Radial artery cannulation is a common medical procedure for anesthesia and critical care. To establish the ideal wrist position for radial artery cannulation, we performed ultrasound examinations of the radial artery to investigate the effect of the angle of wrist extension on radial artery dimensions.

Clinical Features.—Measurements were performed in 17 healthy subjects and 17 surgical patients scheduled for coronary artery bypass graft (CABG) surgery. The radial artery was echographically visualized near the styloid process of the radius at the wrist. Radial artery dimensions were measured at wrist joint angles of 0, 15, 30, 45, 60 and 75°.

Observations.—In both groups, radial artery height was affected by the wrist joint angle. Vessel height was decreased at 60° (one way ANOVA $P = 0.027$ vs 0°) and 75° ($P < 0.001$ vs 0, 15, 45°) in healthy subject and at 75° in CABG patients ($P < 0.001$ vs 0°). The mean differences in radial artery height at 0 and 75° were 0.33 ± 0.09 mm and 0.20 ± 0.06 mm for

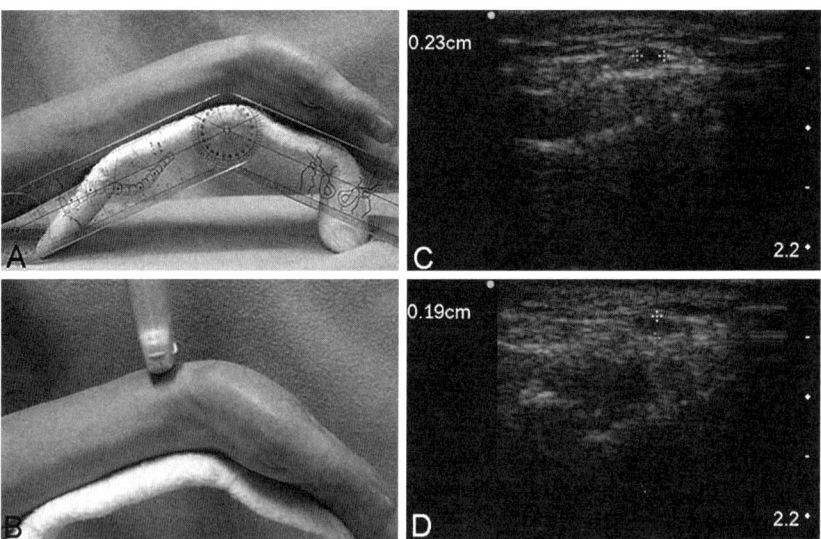

FIGURE 1.—Ultrasound examination of the radial artery. a The wrist board and arthrometer used in the study. The wrist joint angulation was maintained at 45° in this figure. b The sonography probe was placed over the point at which arterial pulsations were palpated most prominently. c, d Ultrasound images of the radial artery. The radial artery was visualized as a small, pulsatile, echolucent area. Vessel width was measured in (c), and vessel height was measured in (d). (Courtesy of Mizukoshi K, Shibasaki M, Amaya F, et al. Ultrasound evidence of the optimal wrist position for radial artery cannulation. *Can J Anesth.* 2009;56:427-431.)

TABLE 1.—Radial Artery Size in Male and Female Subjects

	Male	Female
Height (mm)	$2.50 \pm 0.57**$	1.94 ± 0.46
Width (mm)	$3.01 \pm 0.63*$	2.70 ± 0.67

$*P < 0.05.$
$**P < 0.01.$

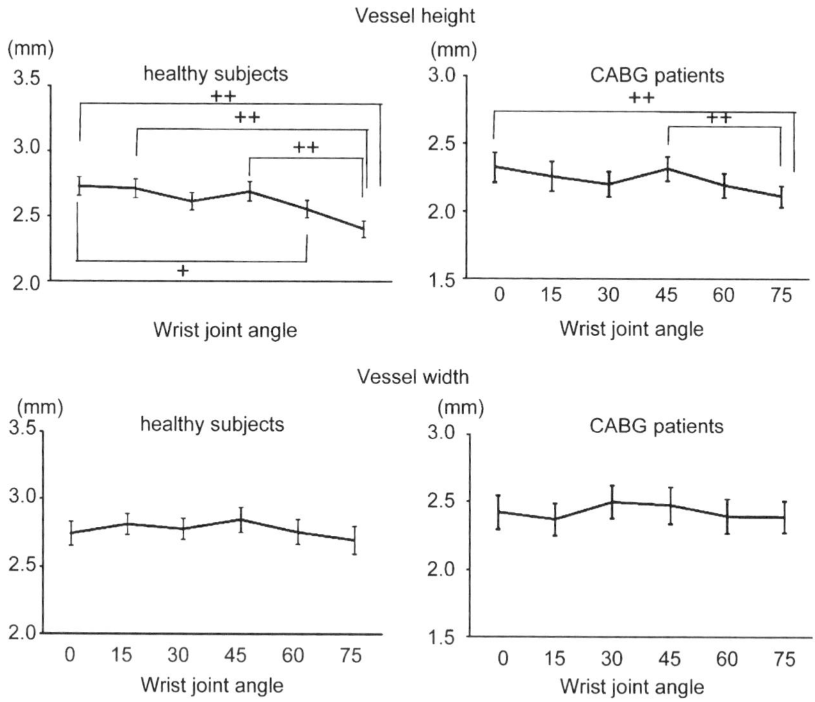

FIGURE 3.—Effect of wrist joint angle on radial artery height and width. Vessel height (*upper panels*) and width (*lower panels*) are shown. Vessel height decreased as wrist joint angulation increased, while vessel width remained unchanged. Vessel height decreased in healthy subjects when the angle of the wrist joint was positioned at 60° and in CABG patients when positioned at 75°. [+] $P = 0.015$; [++] $P < 0.001$ by Tukey's test. (Courtesy of Mizukoshi K, Shibasaki M, Amaya F, et al. Ultrasound evidence of the optimal wrist position for radial artery cannulation. *Can J Anesth*. 2009;56:427-431.)

healthy and CABG patients, respectively. Vessel width was not affected by wrist joint angulation up to 75° of extension.

Conclusion.—Our results demonstrate that in healthy subjects, radial artery dimensions are unaltered when the wrist joint is extended up to an angle of 45°. Extension at 60° for healthy subjects and 75° for

CABG patients, however, results in a decrease in the height of the radial artery, which could possibly render arterial catheterization more difficult.

▶ This is a simple yet important evaluation of the optimal wrist angle for insertion of a radial arterial catheter as determined by maximal height of an ultrasound attained image. Fig 1 shows the manner in which measuring the wrist angle was standardized and controlled. The study evaluated the radial artery in an equal number of healthy volunteers and patients 2 to 3 days before coronary artery bypass (CAB) surgery. The authors controlled for distortion related to the probe before measurements were obtained, and the final measurements were calculated by a blinded team member. The mean heights and widths were not different between these 2 groups. Differences were identified by gender with men having large radial arteries (Table 1). On average the width of the vessel was greater then the height, and importantly the height was significantly lessened once the wrist angle exceed 45° (Fig 3). The implications of this are that placement of arterial lines would be easier in men than women as there is greater discrepancy between the external diameter of the needle and the vessel in men. In addition, placement would be easier when the height is not negatively impacted by more extreme angles of extension. These findings are important enough to impact one's practice immediately by avoiding angles greater than 45°. Confirmation of these findings should occur through subsequent studies that should also include attempts to cannulate so that real world difficulties can be compared with the end point in this article of vessel height.

T. Dorman, MD

Influence of Respiratory Rate on Stroke Volume Variation in Mechanically Ventilated Patients

De Backer D, Taccone FS, Holsten R, et al (Université libre de Bruxelles, Belgium)
Anesthesiology 110:1092-1097, 2009

Background.—Heart-lung interactions are used to evaluate fluid responsiveness in mechanically ventilated patients, but these indices may be influenced by ventilatory conditions. The authors evaluated the impact of respiratory rate (RR) on indices of fluid responsiveness in mechanically ventilated patients, hypothesizing that pulse pressure variation and respiratory variation in aortic flow would decrease at high RRs.

Methods.—In 17 hypovolemic patients, thermodilution cardiac output and indices of fluid responsiveness were measured at a low RR (14–16 breaths/min) and at the highest RR (30 or 40 breaths/min) achievable without altering tidal volume or inspiratory/expiratory ratio.

Results.—An increase in RR was accompanied by a decrease in pulse pressure variation from 21% (18–31%) to 4% (0–6%) ($P < 0.01$) and in respiratory variation in aortic flow from 23% (18–28%) to 6% (5–8%)

($P < 0.01$), whereas respiratory variations in superior vena cava diameter (caval index) were unaltered, i.e., from 38% (27–43%) to 32% (22–39%), P = not significant. Cardiac index was not affected by the changes in RR but did increase after fluids. Pulse pressure variation became negligible when the ratio between heart rate and RR decreased below 3.6.

Conclusions.—Respiratory variations in stroke volume and its derivates are affected by RR, but caval index was unaffected. This suggests that right and left indices of ventricular preload variation are dissociated. At high RRs, the ability to predict the response to fluids of stroke volume

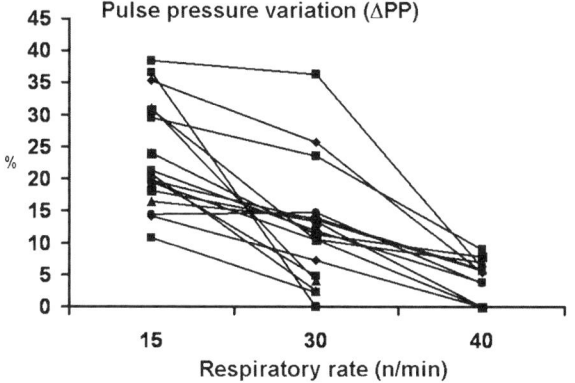

FIGURE 1.—Evolution of pulse pressure variation ($\triangle$PP) at each respiratory rate. Data from individual patients are reported. (Courtesy of De Backer D, Taccone FS, Holsten R, et al. Influence of respiratory rate on stroke volume variation in mechanically ventilated patients. *Anesthesiology.* 2009;110:1092-1097.)

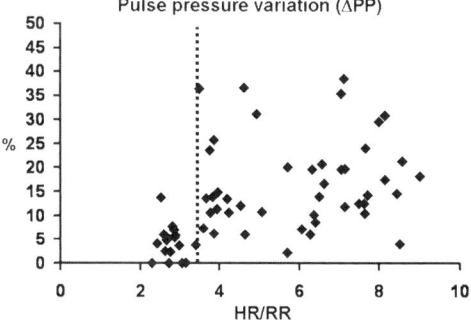

FIGURE 2.—Relationship between pulse pressure variation ($\triangle$PP) and heart rate to respiratory rate ratio (HR/RR). During increases in respiratory rate, $\triangle$PP became negligible when HR/RR ratio was less than or equal to 3.6. Below this cutoff, $\triangle$PP can no longer be used to predict fluid responsiveness. In this figure, 12 patients contributed with 4 points, and 5 patients contributed with 3 points, depending on the maximal RR achieved. (Courtesy of De Backer D, Taccone FS, Holsten R, et al. Influence of respiratory rate on stroke volume variation in mechanically ventilated patients. *Anesthesiology.* 2009;110:1092-1097.)

variations and its derivate may be limited, whereas caval index can still be used (Figs 1 and 2).

▶ The importance of adequate volume resuscitation in the hemodynamic management of the critically ill patient is a well-accepted principle of care. As we move further away from the use of pulmonary artery catheters to assess the pulmonary artery occlusion pressure and rely on noninvasive measures to assess hemodynamic function, it is important for us to know the limits on their usefulness. Assessment of the arterial pulse pressure during passive leg raising or with positive pressure ventilation have been accepted methods to determine a volume responsive patient.[1,2] This study helps to refine our interpretation of pulse pressure changes based on the underlying respiratory rate. Knowing that high respiratory rates may limit the usefulness of this technique is an important observation for the critical care community to acknowledge. It was also interesting to note that the superior vena cava diameter (caval index) was still able to reflect volume responsiveness with the high respiratory rates.

R. A. Balk, MD

References

1. Michard F, Teboul JL. Predicting fluid responsiveness in ICU patients: a critical analysis of the evidence. *Chest.* 2002;121:2000-2008.
2. Pinsky MR. Using ventilation induced aortic pressure and flow variation to diagnose preload responsiveness. *Intensive Care Med.* 2004;30:1008-1010.

Increased splanchnic oxygen extraction because of routine nursing procedures

Jakob SM, Parviainen I, Ruokonen E, et al (Bern Univ Hosp and Univ of Bern, Switzerland; Kuopio Univ Hosp, Finland)
Crit Care Med 37:483-489, 2009

Objective.—Multiple organ failure is a common complication of acute circulatory and respiratory failure. We hypothesized that therapeutic interventions used routinely in intensive care can interfere with the perfusion of the gut and the liver, and thereby increase the risk of mismatch between oxygen supply and demand.

Design.—Prospective, observational study.

Setting.—Interdisciplinary intensive care unit (ICU) of a university hospital.

Patients.—Thirty-six patients on mechanical ventilation with acute respiratory or circulatory failure or severe infection were included.

Interventions.—Insertion of a hepatic venous catheter.

Measurements and Main Results.—Daily nursing procedures were recorded. A decrease of $\geq 5\%$ in hepatic venous oxygen saturation (Sho_2) was considered relevant. Observation time was 64 (29–104) hours (median [interquartile range]). The ICU stay was 11 (8–15) days,

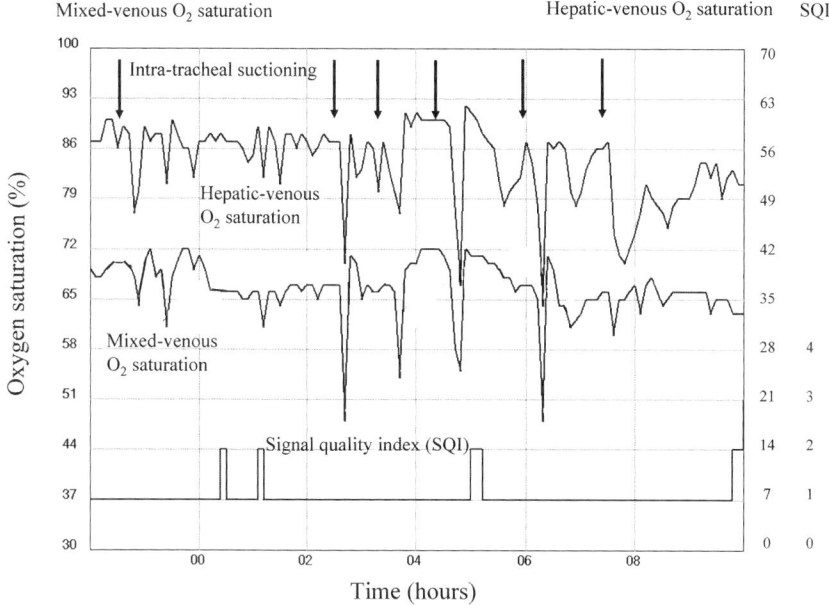

FIGURE 2.—An example of decreases in both hepatic and mixed venous oxygen saturation during repeated episodes of intratracheal suctioning. The signal quality index refers to hepatic venous oxygen saturation (1 and 2 of four possible categories indicate a sufficient signal quality according to the manufacturer). (Courtesy of Jakob SM, Parviainen I, Ruokonen E, et al. Increased splanchnic oxygen extraction because of routine nursing procedures. *Crit Care Med.* 2009;37:483-489.)

and hospital mortality was 35%. The number of periods with procedures/patient was 170 (98–268), the number of procedure-related decreases in Sho_2 was 29 (13–41), and the number of decreases in Sho_2 unrelated to procedures was 9 (4–19). Accordingly, procedure-related Sho_2 decreases occurred 11 (7–17) times per day. Median Sho_2 decrease during the procedures was 7 (5–10)%, and median increase in the gradient between mixed and hepatic venous oxygen saturation was 6 (4–9)%. Procedures that caused most Sho_2 decreases were airway suctioning, assessment of level of sedation, and changing patients' position. Sho_2 decreases were associated with small but significant increases in heart rate and intravascular pressures. Maximal Sequential Organ Failure Assessment scores in the ICU correlated with the number of Sho_2 decreases (r: .56; $p < 0.001$) and with the number of procedure-related Sho_2 decreases (r: .60; $p < 0.001$).

Conclusions.—Patients are exposed to repeated episodes of impaired splanchnic perfusion during routine nursing procedures. More research is needed to examine the correlation, if any, between nursing procedures and hepatic venous desaturation (Fig 2).

▶ This study presents an interesting observation and one worthy of further investigation. The authors used a catheter in the hepatic vein to monitor hepatic venous oxygen saturation during various patient interventions during the day as a reflection of the perfusion and oxygen use of the splanchnic bed. Several points can be made from the findings of this small study. First, the hepatic venous oxygen saturation seems to parallel the central venous oxygen saturation. Second, the observation that the venous oxygen saturation decreases during suctioning and turning is not new or unexpected. The reduction during assessment of sedation was a bit surprising. Finally, the clinical significance and impact of the observed intermittent decreases in venous oxygen saturation during various procedures and interventions still awaits definition. We will await further investigation of this hypothesis, but it is likely that the studies can be conducted with a central venous catheter and not rely on a hepatic vein catheter.

R. A. Balk, MD

Impact of shock requiring norepinephrine on the accuracy and reliability of subcutaneous continuous glucose monitoring

Holzinger U, Warszawska J, Kitzberger R, et al (Med Univ of Vienna, Austria)
Intensive Care Med 35:1383-1389, 2009

Objective.—To evaluate the impact of circulatory shock requiring norepinephrine therapy on the accuracy and reliability of a subcutaneous continuous glucose monitoring system (CGMS) in critically ill patients.

Design and Setting.—A prospective, validation study of a medical intensive care unit at a university hospital was carried out.

Methods.—Continuous glucose monitoring was performed subcutaneously in 50 consecutive patients on intensive insulin therapy (IIT), who were assessed according to the a priori strata of circulatory shock requiring norepinephrine therapy or not.

Results.—A total of 736 pairs of sensor glucose (SG)/blood glucose (BG) values were analysed (502 without and 234 with norepinephrine therapy). For all values, repeated measures Bland–Altman analysis showed a mean difference of 0.08 mmol/l (limits of agreement: -1.26 and 1.43 mmol/l). Circulatory shock requiring norepinephrine therapy did not influence the relation of arterial BG with SG in a multivariable random effects linear regression analysis. The covariates norepinephrine dose, body mass index (BMI), glucose level and severity of illness also had no influence. Insulin titration grid analysis showed that 98.6% of the data points were in the acceptable treatment zone. No data were in the life-threatening zone.

Conclusions.—Circulatory shock requiring norepinephrine therapy, as well as other covariates, had no influence on the accuracy and reliability of the CGMS in critically ill patients.

▶ Much emphasis has been placed on research regarding tight glycemic control in critically ill patients in recent years. The major adverse event associated with tight glycemic control is hypoglycemia. In order to protect patients from hypoglycemic events, better methods of glucose monitoring are desirable.

One such method is continuous subcutaneous glucose monitoring. However, it is unclear how these types of techniques would perform in patients with circulatory shock due to reduced skin perfusion by vasoconstriction. This could potentially be especially problematic in those with vasopressor-dependent shock treated with vasopressor agents such as norepinephrine. The objective of this study was to determine the accuracy of continuous subcutaneous glucose monitoring in patients with circulatory shock requiring norepinephrine.

Fifty patients were enrolled, 27 with shock requiring norepinephrine and 23 without shock. A total of 736-paired measurements were made comparing blood serum glucose with subcutaneous sensor glucose. The investigators performed Bland-Altman analysis to assess agreement. Agreement was reasonable, regardless of whether or not the patient had circulatory shock. This technique for continuous blood glucose monitoring does not appear to be impacted in a significant way by the presence of circulatory shock and holds promise for glucose monitoring during tight glycemic control therapy.

S. Trzeciak, MD, MPH

4 Burns

The Incidence and Outcome of Extubation Failure in Burn Intensive Care Patients

Smailes ST, Martin RV, McVicar AJ (St. Andrew's Centre for Plastic Surgery and Burns, Broomfield Hosp, Essex, United Kingdom; Anglia Ruskin Univ, Essex, United Kingdom)
J Burn Care Res 30:386-392, 2009

To identify the incidence and outcome of extubation failure in patients with burn. Retrospective cohort study in a tertiary burn intensive care unit. A review of the casenotes of 132 consecutive adult patients with burn admitted between 2001 and 2005, and requiring mechanical ventilation for >24 hours, was undertaken. Sixty-seven patients underwent extubation and entered data analyses. Extubation failure was defined as reintubation within 48 hours. The outcomes of interest were incidence and cause of extubation failure, duration of mechanical ventilation (DMV), length of stay (LOS), and mortality. The patients who succeeded and failed extubation were similar in terms of age, sex, burn size ($P = .3$), and incidence of inhalation injury ($P = .1$). Of 67 planned extubations, 20 (30%) failed. DMV (22.5 vs. 4 days; $P < .001$), intensive care LOS (1.20 vs. 0.41 days/% burn; $P < .001$), and hospital LOS (1.90 vs. 1.18 days/% burn; $P < .003$) were significantly longer in reintubated patients when compared with those who extubated successfully. Extubation outcome, burn size, and age provided the best predictive model for patient outcome ($P = .02$), but extubation outcome was the only predictor that operated individually ($P = .05$). The aetiology of extubation failure in 15 (75%) patients was poor pulmonary toilet. The incidence of extubation failure in this homogenous population of patients with burn is higher than general intensive care patients (30% vs. 4–23%). The DMV, lengths of intensive care, and hospital stay are significantly longer in patients who failed extubation. In addition to burn size and age, extubation outcome is an important predictor of intensive care mortality. The indication for reintubation in most patients is poor airway clearance.

▶ The authors have performed a retrospective cohort study in patients who are on mechanical ventilation > 24 hours. Only 67 of 132 patients in 5 years who underwent extubation required ventilation > 24 hours, did not require tracheostomy, survived, did not have accidental extubation, or had burns as causes for their skin loss, were eligible for study. Of those patients, 20 failed extubation within 48 hours (30% failure rate). The authors conclude that extubation outcome is the best predictor of patient outcome. Unfortunately, this study has some serious flaws that limit the generalizability of the findings to other burn patients.

The most serious flaws in this study are the subjective nature of the criteria used for extubation, such as "significant improvement in respiratory failure," and no "significant" facial/airway swelling, but most importantly "attending anesthetist made all of the decisions regarding the timing and implementation of extubation." As Dr Bessey noted in his editorial,[1] given that there are 10 different anesthetists caring for these patients, and only 13.4 patients each year, each anesthetist has limited contact with burn patients, with an average of 1.34/year. The absence of attention to secretions, either amount, or nature of, is an additional critically missing factor.

A policy of daily sedation and anxiolytic liberation guided by respiratory therapists and nurses experienced in burn care decreases ventilator-associated pneumonia while decreasing time on the ventilator for burn patients. A rapid shallow breathing index (RSBI) evaluation was not performed in these patients, nor was a 2-minute preextubation protocol, both of which have been shown to be effective screening tools to determine extubation readiness. The authors describe a 30% extubation failure rate, but their extubation criteria are subjective and variable. They also describe an on-going prospective study evaluating spontaneous breathing trial and selected weaning predictors in their patient population. I look forward to that study, but until that time, critical care clinicians caring for burn patients should rely on tried and true methods such as the RSBI, daily sedation and anxiolytic liberation, and/or the 2 minutes preextubation protocol outlined by Nisim and colleagues.[2]

B. A. Latenser, MD

References

1. Bessey PQ. Invited critique of "the incidence and outcome of extubation failure in burn intensive care patients". *J Burn Care Res*. 2009;30:393-394.
2. Nisim AA, Margulies DR, Wilson MT, et al. A 2-minute pre-extubation protocol for ventilated intensive care unit patients. *Am J Surg*. 2008;196:890-895.

Toxic Epidermal Necrolysis in Children: Medical, Surgical, and Ophthalmologic Considerations
Goyal S, Gupta P, Ryan CM, et al (Harvard Med School, Boston, MA; Shriners Burns Hosp for Children, Boston, MA)
J Burn Care Res 30:437-449, 2009

Toxic epidermal necrolysis is a rare acute inflammatory multisystem life-threatening condition characterized by widespread epidermal necrosis and profound toxic systemic reaction. Implicated etiologic agents in children include drugs, infections, and autoimmune diseases. The pathophysiology includes separation of the epidermis at the dermal–epidermal junction of both skin and extracutaneous epithelium and mucous membranes. The general consensus is that expeditious transfer to a burn center, maintenance of fluid and electrolyte balance, temperature maintenance, control of evaporative losses, avoidance of use of complicating drugs as corticosteroids and topical sulfa compounds, aggressive septic surveillance, vigorous nutritional support via nasoenteric tube, early ophthalmologic consultation, and appropriate wound care with a regimen of therapy relying on basic principles of treatment of partial-thickness epidermal wounds predict better outcome in the treatment of this disease process. The course of toxic epidermal necrolysis in children, even though dramatic at onset, leads to low mortality when managed appropriately. The current limited published evidence does not clearly delineate differences in epidemiology, pathogenesis, and prognosis of severe skin reactions in children as compared with adults. In this article, we review the available literature on the pathogenesis, clinical features, pathophysiology, treatment, and complications of this rare disease in children.

▶ This easy-to-read review article nicely covers the topic of toxic epidermal necrolysis (TEN) in children. Whether you believe that erythema multiforme, Stevens-Johnson syndrome, and TEN are distinct entities, or represent a spectrum of 1 single disease entity, the etiology and pathophysiologic derangements have been less widely debated. While in the critical care phase, children should be treated in burn centers, as wound care is the central thread that joins all these cases together. Outcomes have been shown to be markedly better for both children and adults when treated in burn centers.

Care of the patient with TEN does not end once the child is discharged from the hospital. The myriad short and long-term complications highlighted in (Table 3) help to educate the primary care practitioner that many specialists

TABLE 3.—Systemic Features and Complications

Oral cavity: Mucosal lesions (ranging from erosions to bullae), depapillation of tongue
Skin: Superficial infections, pruritis, patchy hypo/hyperpigmentation, hypertrophic scarring, punctate keloids, finger/toe nail deformities, nevi, hyperhidrosis
Respiratory: Pneumonia, mucosal sloughing, progressive respiratory failure, acute respiratory distress syndrome, pulmonary embolus, bronchiolitis obliterans, bronchiectasis, chronic bronchitis, obstructive pulmonary disease
Cardiac: Atrial fibrillation, ventricular fibrillation, chronic heart failure, myocardial infarction (rare), congestive heart failure
Gastrointestinal: Esophageal strictures, bowel obstruction/perforation, abdominal compartment syndrome, ileus, hepatitis, intestinal sloughing, rectal bleeding, stress ulcers, shock liver, pancreatitis, cholestasis, gastrointestinal bleeding
Hematological: Neutropenia, coagulopathy, anemia, disseminated intravascular coagulation, heparin induced thrombocytopenia
Infectious: Septicemia (primarily *Pseudomonas aeruginosa* and *Staphylococcus aureus*), candedemia, urinary tract infections
Genitourinary: Vaginal stenosis and ulceration, vulvovaginal synechiae, genital involvement, urethritis
Renal: Acute tubular necrosis, glomerulonephritis (rare), acute renal failure, chronic renal insufficiency
Neurological: Intracerebral hemorrhage, cerebral edema, brain stem herniation
Psychiatric: Major depression, posttraumatic stress disorder
Other: Hypoalbuminemia, SIADH, hyponatremia, hypercalcemia, hyperfibrinogenemia

SIADH, syndrome of inappropriate antidiuretic hormone.

may be needed to follow these children into adulthood. Included in the list might be: pulmonologists, cardiologists, gastroenterologists, gynecologists, ophthalmologists, and psychiatrists. If you read nothing else on TEN, this excellent review article will hit the high points and prevent you from misdiagnosing or mistreating this life-threatening disease in children (or adults).

B. A. Latenser, MD

Development and validation of a model for prediction of mortality in patients with acute burn injury
The Belgian Outcome in Burn Injury Study Group (Ghent Univ Hosp, Belgium)
Br J Surg 96:111-117, 2009

Background.—The objective was to develop a user-friendly model to predict the probability of death from acute burns soon after injury, based on burned surface area, age and presence of inhalation injury.

Methods.—This population-based cohort study included all burned patients admitted to one of the six Belgian burn centres. Data from 1999 to 2003 (5246 patients) were used to develop a mortality prediction model, and data from 2004 (981 patients) were used for validation.

Results.—Mortality in the derivation cohort was 4·6 per cent. A mortality score (0–10 points) was devised: 0–4 points according to the percentage of burned surface area (less than 20, 20–39, 40–59, 60–79 or at least 80 per cent), 0–3 points according to age (under 50, 50–64, 65–79 or at least 80 years) and 3 points for the presence of an inhalation injury. Mortality in the validation cohort was 4·3 per cent. The model predicted 40 deaths, and 42 deaths were observed ($P = 0·950$). Receiver–operator characteristic curve analysis of the model for prediction of mortality demonstrated an area under the curve of 0·94 (95 per cent confidence interval 0·90 to 0·97).

Conclusion.—An accurate model was developed to predict the probability of death from acute burn injury based on simple and objective clinical criteria.

▶ The authors have done an excellent job of taking an existing model that predicts burn mortality and created a model that is both easy to use and precise in its ability to estimate the probability of death. The use of the variables age, percentage body surface area burn, and the presence of inhalation injury are not new. Most predictors use some combination of these factors, but the ease of this scoring system allows burn care providers to make the predictions in real time, rather than after discharge, when all the data are available.

I agree that the model will have to be validated external to Belgian burn centers, and I hope the authors are in the process of doing so. A word of caution, however, using a scoring system that is not 100% accurate and basing the decision to provide or withhold care solely upon that scoring system should be discouraged. The outcomes in each burn center, and for each burn care physician, are slightly unique. Each burn care physician must use his/her best judgment when counseling a patient and family regarding decision making and futility of care. Certainly, part of that judgment should involve using some objective measure such as a scoring system. When used in conjunction with the practices in a burn center and the experiences of the physician, the patient and family will be best served, regardless of the "numbers".

B. A. Latenser, MD

Fire-related deaths in India in 2001: a retrospective analysis of data
Sanghavi P, Bhalla K, Das V (Cambridge, MA; Harvard Univ, Cambridge, MA; Johns Hopkins Univ, Baltimore, MD)
Lancet 373:1282-1288, 2009

Background.—Hospital-based studies have suggested that fire-related deaths might be a neglected public-health issue in India. However, no national estimates of these deaths exist and the only numbers reported in published literature come from the Indian police. We combined multiple health datasets to assess the extent of the problem.

Methods.—We computed age–sex-specific fire-related mortality fractions nationally using a death registration system based on medically certified causes of death in urban areas and a verbal autopsy based sample survey for rural populations. We combined these data with all-cause mortality estimates based on the sample registration system and the population census. We adjusted for ill-defined injury categories that might contain misclassified fire-related deaths, and estimated the proportion of suicides due to self-immolation when deaths were reported by external causes.

Findings.—We estimated over 163 000 fire-related deaths in 2001 in India, which is about 2% of all deaths. This number was six times that reported by police. About 106 000 of these deaths occurred in women, mostly between 15 and 34 years of age. This age–sex pattern was consistent across multiple local studies, and the average ratio of fire-related deaths of young women to young men was 3:1.

Interpretation.—The high frequency of fire-related deaths in young women suggests that these deaths share common causes, including kitchen accidents, self-immolation, and different forms of domestic violence. Identification of populations at risk and description of structural determinants from existing data sources are urgently needed so that interventions can be rapidly implemented.

▶ All accolades to the authors for finally bringing this public health issue forward with real evidence. Fire deaths related to domestic violence and self-immolation are known to exist in many parts of the world. As the authors so eloquently point out, deaths due to fire in the highest at-risk group, the 15 to 34 age group in women, are often misidentified by the family to cover a homicide or suicide. In this same time period, only $\frac{1}{2}$ as many women died during childbirth, yet that statistic places them at 22% of the world estimate.

Decreasing maternal mortality rates worldwide is a focus of many international agencies, yet deaths from fire in young women remain largely underreported. Another frightening statistic is that women are more than 3 times as likely to die of fire-related injuries than men. In cultures where women are victims of economic dependence and poverty, cultural/religious institutions often control access to the legal system.

In the United States, any disease or public health problem with 22/100000 women dying every year would garner a great deal of attention from health care providers, the media, and perhaps even the government. Other countries in Asia and Africa have much in common with the Indian subcontinent, and the problems of burning as a form of domestic violence are no exception. The authors suggest that policy measures, research, and a proactive approach will make the best use of this data.

Although not usually fatal, acid violence is prevalent in India and other countries such as Bangladesh, Pakistan, Uganda, and Malaysia. In Bangladesh, 1 group in particular has been effective in decreasing the incidence of acid throwing against young women. Using a nationwide reporting system, providing medical care, psychological support, job training, and legal counsel for the acid survivors, the assailants have been brought to trial and prison sentences imposed. Perhaps the authors should be encouraged to learn advocacy from this group. For more information on acid survivors, visit the website at: www.acidsurvivors.org.

B. A. Latenser, MD

Silver deposits in cutaneous burn scar tissue is a common phenomenon following application of a silver dressing
Wang X-Q, Chang H-E, Francis R, et al (Univ of Queensland, Brisbane, Australia; Queensland Health, Brisbane, Australia; et al)
J Cutan Pathol 36:788-792, 2009

Background.—Silver dressings have been widely and successfully used to prevent cutaneous wounds, including burns, chronic ulcers, dermatitis and other cutaneous conditions, from infection. However, in a few cases, skin discolouration or argyria-like appearances have been reported. This study investigated the level of silver in scar tissue post-burn injury following application of Acticoat™, a silver dressing.

Methods.—A porcine deep dermal partial thickness burn model was used. Burn wounds were treated with this silver dressing until completion of re-epithelialization, and silver levels were measured in a total of 160 scars and normal tissues.

Results.—The mean level of silver in scar tissue covered with silver dressings was 136 µg/g, while the silver level in normal skin was less than 0.747 µg/g. A number of wounds had a slate-grey appearance, and dissection of the scars revealed brown-black pigment mostly in the middle and deep dermis within the scar. The level of silver and the severity of the slate-grey discolouration were correlated with the length of time of the silver dressing application.

Conclusions.—These results show that silver deposition in cutaneous scar tissue is a common phenomenon, and higher levels of silver deposits and severe skin discolouration are correlated with an increase in the duration of this silver dressing application.

▶ Silver containing creams, foams, sponges, and sheets have played a major role in controlling bacterial infections in burn wounds. The latest burn and wound technologies now focus on new and improved methods of silver delivery to wounds. Although systemic absorption of silver has been a concern with the increasing popularity of silver containing dressings, no studies to date have shown elevated blood silver levels to a concerning level. I have several issues with the present study, and the authors do touch lightly on these issues. First, the wounds were left to heal for 6 weeks, with silver containing dressings in constant contact during that time. In humans, the standard of care is that a wound not anticipated to heal within 14 days should undergo excision and skin grafting. A silver dressing would not likely be in place for 6 weeks. Secondly, it is purely speculation on the authors' part that the silver deposits are not expected to diminish or disappear with time. The authors have forgotten that a scar continues to undergo changes for up to 5 years during the maturation process, and is metabolically active while undergoing changes. Finally, the authors do note that this porcine model is not the ideal one to study skin discoloration from melanin accumulation. Although of some academic interest, until the authors find a model where results are translatable to humans, I am not convinced that the authors' contention that silver deposits in burn scars "is a common phenomenon" is justifiable.

B. A. Latenser, MD

Complications of Femoral Artery Catheterization in Pediatric Burn Patients

Mourot JM, Oliveira HM, Woodson LC, et al (The Univ of Texas Med Branch and Shriners Burns Hosp for Children, Galveston)
J Burn Care Res 30:432-436, 2009

A retrospective analysis of all pediatric patients admitted for acute burn treatment during a 7-year period was conducted to examine patients who underwent femoral artery catheterization and discuss the associated complications and treatment options. The total number of femoral artery catheterizations performed, nature of vascular complications, treatment rendered, and patient outcome were reviewed. Of the 1800 acute burn pediatric patients treated during our study period (1996–2002), 234 patients underwent a total of 745 femoral artery catheterizations. There was a 1.9% incidence of significant complications as a result of catheterization, including problems during catheter insertion, diminished distal arterial pulses following catheter placement and catheter malfunction.

Eight patients (3.4%) developed occlusion or spasm of the femoral artery evidenced by loss of distal pulses. Of these, three required thrombectomy and the other five were treated nonsurgically with immediate catheter removal and systemic heparinization. Both groups showed similar overall outcome with return of distal pulses and absence of distal limb or tissue loss. Our findings indicate that femoral artery catheterization in pediatric burn patients is associated with a low occurrence of vascular complications. The majority of patients with acute distal limb ischemic symptoms can be managed nonoperatively with immediate removal of the catheter and systemic heparinization.

▶ I commend the authors for reviewing their results with pediatric burn patients undergoing femoral artery catheterization. The finding that younger children with smaller arteries had a higher complication rate is supported by previous work, yet I am forced to speculate why the authors waited 7 years from the end of their data collection to publish their work. I wonder if knowing the size of catheter placed would have impacted the authors' conclusions. I am troubled that 13% of the patients had a catheter change over a wire, a practice associated with bacteremia in burn patients, which was not discussed in this study. Finally, the authors conclude that femoral artery catheters should be placed by the most experienced clinician, yet most of the lines in this particular study seem to have been placed by residents. I agree that the complication rate in this study is low, but the complications noted were devastating, including surgical exploration, fasciotomy, and amputations. Although femoral arterial catheterization may be safe, the clinician needs to keep in mind that when these complications do occur, they may be quite injurious. Femoral artery catheters in burned children should be reserved for situations where they are absolutely required for patient care, and removed at the earliest opportunity.

B. A. Latenser, MD

Bone marrow-derived cells in the healing burn wound—More than just inflammation
Rea S, Giles NL, Webb S, et al (Royal Perth Hosp, Australia; et al)
Burns 35:356-364, 2009

Scarring after severe burn is a result of changes in collagen deposition and fibroblast activity that result in repaired but not regenerated tissue. Re-epithelialisation of wounds and dermal cell repopulation has been thought to be driven by cells in the periphery of the wound. However, recent research demonstrated that cells originating from the bone marrow contribute to healing wounds in other tissues and also after incisional injury. We investigated the contribution of bone marrow-derived cells to long-term cell populations in scar tissue (primarily fibroblasts and keratinocytes) after severe burn. Wild-type mice were lethally irradiated and then the bone marrow reconstituted by injection of chimeric bone marrow cells expressing EGFP marker protein. Mice with chimeric bone marrow were then given a burn, either an 1-cm diameter injury (to mimic minor injury) or 2-cm diameter (to mimic moderate injury). Wounds were analysed at days 1, 3, 7, 14, 21, 28, 56 and 120 using FACS and immunohistochemistry to identify the percentage and cell type within the wound originating from the bone marrow. The inflammatory cell infiltrate at the early time-points was bone marrow in origin. At later time-points, we noted that over half of the fibroblast population was bone marrow-derived; we also observed that a small percentage of keratinocytes appeared to be bone marrow in origin.

These findings support the theory that the bone marrow plays an important role in providing cells not only for inflammation but also dermal and epidermal cells during burn wound healing. This increases our understanding of cell origins in the healing wound, and has the potential to impact on clinical practice providing a potential mechanism for intervention away from conventional topical treatments and directed instead to systemic treatments affecting the bone marrow response.

▶ The authors have provided intriguing data regarding wound healing, with a specific eye toward the scarring that takes place after a burn wound heals. This is the first article that examines the role of bone marrow derived cells in response to a small burn wound. In many burn survivors, the hypertrophic scar is the leading cause of morbidity for the patient. In the short term, problems with itching and hypersensitivity to touch, heat, and cold interfere with normal daily functions such as bathing, walking, sleeping, and return to work. In the longer term, hypertrophic scarring can lead to facial deformity, joint contracture, and deformity such as neck, shoulders, elbows, wrists, fingers, hips, knees, and ankles, leading to a lifetime of limitations.

If the authors have actually discovered a relationship between the bone marrow derived cells and scarring in burn wounds, then the healing process can be altered to provide less scarring and improved outcomes. If it is possible to do, the authors' work lays the foundation to devise an intervention that will allow burn care clinicians to get involved at the source, rather than waiting for the outcome, when we treat the sequellae of hypertrophic burn scars with topical and oral antipruritic agents, compression garments, scar massage, and often years of physiotherapy. I hope the authors will continue their work, and we will finally be able to understand hypertrophic scar formation in burn patients and get this work out of the lab and at the bedside.

B. A. Latenser, MD

Acalculous cholecystitis in severely burned patients: Incidence and predisposing factors

Theodorou P, Maurer CA, Spanholtz TA, et al (Univ of Witten-Herdecke, Cologne, Germany; Hosp of Liestal, Switzerland; et al)
Burns 35:405-411, 2009

Objective.—To investigate the incidence and predisposing factors of acalculous cholecystitis (AAC) in severely burned patients.

Background Data.—Although some studies report on AAC in critically ill patients, very little is known about AAC after severe burns.

Methods.—We conducted a retrospective cohort study involving patients with burns admitted to the burn intensive care unit (BICU) of a university hospital. The patient cohort was divided into two groups (AAC group: burned patients with histological proven acalculous cholecystitis, $n = 15$; Control group: population of all other burned patients admitted to the BICU, $n = 1225$). Univariate and multivariate analyses were used to identify predisposing factors for the development of AAC.

Results.—Fifteen patients with acalculous cholecystitis were identified in the study period. This represents 1.2% of all significant burns admitted. Comparing the AAC group with the Control population the following patients' characteristics, therapeutic measures and outcome parameters were significantly different in the univariate analysis: mean age (54.0 years vs. 42.0 years), BMI (28.9 kg/m^2 vs. 25.6 kg/m^2), abbreviated burn severity index (8.3 vs. 6.4), total body surface area burn deep partial thickness (12.0% vs. 6.2%) and full thickness (10.2% vs. 6.8%), concomitant inhalation injury (80.0% vs. 28.9%), sepsis (46.7% vs. 14.9%), catecholamine (100% vs. 30.4%) and antibiotic requirement (100% vs. 58.2%), non-biliary tract operations (4.9 vs. 1.5), BICU length of stay (63.4 days vs. 21.0 days), ventilator days (50.3 vs. 11.9), packed red blood cells (PRBCs) administration (70.0 units vs.13.0 units) and mortality (53.3% vs. 19.7%). In the multivariate analysis however, only age, the number of administered units of PRBCs and the duration of mechanical ventilation turned out to be independent predictors for the occurrence of AAC.

Conclusion.—AAC is a rare complication of severely burned patients and may reflect the severity of the patient's general conditions. Predisposing factors for AAC are advanced age, the need of blood transfusions and prolonged mechanical ventilation. In the presence of these predisposing factors, early monitoring may help to detect AAC earlier and to initiate appropriate intervention.

▶ Acalculous cholecystitis is a known complication of severe illness, and severe thermal injury is no exception. The authors have shown us that several factors are associated with worse outcomes in burn patients: age, blood transfusions, and prolonged mechanical ventilation. Age, inhalation injury, and size of burn have long been known to adversely affect outcomes in patients with burn. In this study, the vast majority of patients developing acalculous cholecystitis had inhalation injury, which helps to explain the association with prolonged mechanical ventilation.

Palmieri et al[1] showed that the number of blood transfusions received adversely affected outcomes in burn patients, independent of burn size. The proposed mechanism is the immunosuppressive effect of blood transfusions, probably having more of an effect in burn patients than in other patients with critical illness. I find the amount of blood transfused to the patients in this study to be excessive, with a mean of 70 units packed red cells in each patient who developed acalculous cholecystitis. It is clear that a restrictive blood administration policy based upon demonstrated physiologic need is both economically and medically sound practice.

Another treatment modality in this burn patient population concerning to me is the amount of systemic antibiotics administered at the time of admission. Unless treatment has been delayed for days to weeks, even the most critically burned patient does not have an infection at the time of burn. I would encourage everyone to read the white paper on sepsis and infections from thought leaders of the American Burn Association.[2] Based upon the current literature, this consensus article clearly outlines definitions and criteria of sepsis and infections in patients with burn. Prophylactic antibiotics have no place in the treatment of burn patients and their routine use is condemned.

I find it perplexing that the gastrointestinal (GI) tract was not used in most patients. Most of the patients were fasting for greater than 7 days, although the reason(s) is unclear. Current literature suggests that burn patients may be fed from the time of admission. Unless on pressors, patients should be fed early, even during the initial resuscitation period. Postpyloric feeding tubes allow tube feedings to be safely continued throughout operative interventions. Coupled with anabolic steroids such as oxandrolone, the obligatory negative nitrogen balance experienced by the severely burned patients can be ameliorated. Burn patients can leave the hospital at approximately their admission weight. Parenteral nutrition does not maintain the immune function of the GI tract, another contributing factor to the increased infections seen in the patients in this present study.

Finally, although an infrequent occurrence (15 patients in 16 years), acalculous cholecystitis must be considered to be diagnosed. Early diagnosis and cholecystectomy will most certainly improve outcome for those affected patients. For patients who are intubated, a routine daily sedation vacation and physical examination during that time will provide the physician with an opportunity to make the diagnosis.

B. A. Latenser, MD

References

1. Palmieri TL, Caruso DM, Foster KN, et al. Effect of blood transfusion on outcome after major burn injury: a multicenter study. *Crit Care Med.* 2006;34:1602-1607.
2. Greenhalgh DG, Saffle JR, Holmes JH, et al. American Burn Association consensus conference to define sepsis and infection in burns. *J Burn Care Res.* 2007;28:776-790.

Abdominal Complications after Severe Burns

Markell KW, Renz EM, White CE, et al (The United States Army Inst of Surgical Res, Fort Sam Houston; et al)
J Am Coll Surg 208:940-947, 2009

Background.—Abdominal catastrophe in the severely burned patient without abdominal injury has been described. We perceived an alarming recent incidence of this complication in our burn center, both during acute resuscitation and later in the hospital course. We sought to define incidence, outcomes, and associated factors, such as excessive resuscitation volume and treatment issues.

Study Design.—We examined all severely burned military and civilian patients with abdominal pathology between March 2003 and February 2008. Data included age, gender, total body surface area burn, inhalation injury, Injury Severity Score, disposition, resuscitation volume, time from injury to diagnosis, use of recombinant factor VIIa, vasopressors, and early tube feedings. We assembled a Delphi panel of surgeons experienced in abdominal catastrophes to review these data.

Results.—Among 1,825 patients admitted to the US Army Institute of Surgical Research Burn Center, 120 (6.6%) were diagnosed with abdominal pathology (burn size 48% ± 19%), of which 51 (2.8%) had abdominal catastrophe. The majority of these occurred in the first days after injury with associated abdominal compartment syndrome (32 of 51) and increased linearly to burn size. We noted another group of patients who presented primarily with ischemic bowel later in the course, with the same clinical presentation. Resuscitation volume was 6.02 mL/kg/percent total body surface area burned. Vasopressors were used in 71% of patients and tube feedings in 57% before diagnosis.

Conclusions.—Abdominal catastrophe without abdominal trauma occurs in 2.8% of our population. Associated mortality was 78% without obvious cause. Delphi panel experts recommended more aggressive monitoring of abdominal compartment pressures and earlier operative management to improve outcomes.

▶ Wolf and colleagues have presented a primer on how to conduct a quality improvement project. They started with a fact finding mission to define the magnitude of the problem (a perceived alarming incidence of abdominal catastrophe in patients with thermal injury), collected relevant data (body surface area, presence of inhalation injury, resuscitation volumes, use of pressors, early use of tube feedings, presence of abdominal decompression), and assembled an internal panel to review their outcomes and suggest interventions to improve outcomes (more aggressive monitoring and earlier operative management).

Although the authors have drawn some interesting conclusions, they haven't taken them far enough and have missed some critical definitions. The authors have not used standard definitions of abdominal compartment syndrome that have been popularized by the World Society of the Abdominal Compartment

Syndrome.[1] It is difficult to provide comparisons with the more recent literature as the current authors fail to use standardized definitions, making it impossible to know if the comparison is really between apples and apples. Available since 2006, the free Web site offers both assessment and management algorithms. Included on the Web site are standardized definitions of abdominal hypertension and abdominal compartment syndrome.

Another issue discussed by the authors is the issue of fluids administered. It is well known that overzealous fluid administration in patients with significant thermal injury contributes to the development of abdominal compartment syndrome. The authors do not provide us with a reason(s) why patients received nearly 50% more fluid than recommended by the Consensus Formula (4 mL/kg/percent burn). It has been postulated that fluid creep in burn patients is a problem affecting burn care practitioners around the United States. Also hypothesized are the causes, including increased use of opioids, failure to adhere to protocols, failure to use a colloid when burns are large (> 20% total body surface area [TBSA], for example), or even inexperienced clinicians. The authors conclude that more vigilant observation and earlier intervention will help decrease the high rates of abdominal complications in patients with thermal injury.

The University of Utah protocol is a simple, easy to follow guidelines that allows for appropriate fluid resuscitation with appropriate monitoring and adjustment to prevent complications. I would encourage anyone not familiar with current resuscitation guidelines or anyone looking for a straightforward approach to resuscitation to look at this easy flow diagram.[2]

B. A. Latenser, MD

References

1. World Society of the Abdominal Compartment Syndrome Web site. http://www.wsacs.org. Accessed September 26, 2009.
2. Saffle JI. The phenomenon of "fluid creep" in acute burn resuscitation. *J Burn Care Res*. 2007;28:382-392.

A Survey of North American Burn and Plastic Surgeons on Their Current Attitudes Toward Facial Transplantation
Mathes DW, Kumar N, Ploplys E (Univ of Washington, Seattle)
J Am Coll Surg 208:1051-1058, 2009

Background.—Feasibility of composite tissue allotransplantation (CTA) has been substantiated by transplantations of the hand, abdominal wall, and face. CTA has the potential to reconstruct "like with like," but the risk-to-benefit ratio and clinical indications have yet to be determined. We sought to examine the current attitudes about the emerging field of CTA from those who treat complex facial injuries.

Study Design.—In 2007, a Web-based blinded survey was sent to both burn and plastic surgeons involved in facial reconstruction. We examined the practice profile with regard to complex facial injuries and asked respondents to assess the level of risk in CTA and indications for facial transplantation. Surgeons were asked to evaluate three clinical cases (two closely mirroring clinical face transplantations) for suitability for treatment with CTA.

Results.—One hundred sixty-four surgeons responded (54% response rate) and averaged 17.3 years in practice. They saw 12.1 severe facial-injury patients per year. A total of 78.7% agreed that current techniques do not provide adequate reconstruction for severe facial injuries, and 26.2% were in favor of performing CTA on immunosuppression. Acceptable indications for CTA were multiple failed reconstructions (70%), total facial burn (59%), and absence of remote tissue (55%). Ten percent saw no acceptable indication for CTA. The scenarios that mimicked recent transplantations had moderate support in favor of CTA (20.7% for the Chinese patient and 29.3% for the French patient).

Conclusions.—This survey demonstrates support for use of CTA to reconstruct complex facial deformities. Surgeons continue to be wary of immunosuppression and chronic rejection, and many want to wait for better immunologic treatment options.

▶ Since recently performed in humans, facial transplantation has garnered significant interest in the medical community. It seems that everyone in the health care industry has an opinion about the procedure. The most common indication for complete facial transplantation would be someone with severe burns, trauma, or congenital deformities where either multiple reconstructive procedures have failed, or the patient is not a candidate for reconstructive procedures. I have 3 concerns about facial transplantation. My first concern relates to the need for immunosuppression. In normal, healthy patients, creating a condition of lifelong immunosuppression is not without risks. In the patient with burns > 10% total body surface area, a condition of immunosuppression already exists. Sepsis is already the number one cause of death in burn patients, who do not receive steroids and other immunosuppressants for obvious reasons. The burn patient who would potentially benefit the most from this experimental procedure is not a candidate with today's technology. My second reservation about facial transplantation relates to the perhaps theoretical situation where a patient undergoes facial transplantation and decides at some time in the future that he or she no longer cares for the face he or she has received and wants another one. My third reservation relates to the concern about possibly changing the personae after undergoing facial transplantation. Our face is our identity, and a complete change has the potential to change a personality.

As shown in this survey of surgeons caring for patients who might benefit from facial transplantation, the answer is not clear cut. Until the transplantation technology has improved to make the process more widely applicable, the process of facial transplantation will remain an experimental procedure that a select few choose to perform. As the media sensationalizes this procedure, patients should not be given the false hope that facial transplantation is a viable option.

B. A. Latenser, MD

Oral arginine supplementation and the effect on skin graft donor sites: a randomized clinical pilot study
Debats IB, Booi DI, Wehrens KM, et al (Univ Hosp Maastricht, The Netherlands)
J Burn Care Res 30:417-426, 2009

Although arginine has been shown to improve healing in rodents and in small induced wounds in healthy volunteers, little is known about the effects of arginine supplementation on healing of clinically relevant surgical wounds. We studied 18 patients in a double-blind randomized pilot study (12 men, 6 women), who underwent skin transplantation as part of reconstructive surgery. Patients were randomly assigned to receive arginine (n = 8) or placebo (n = 10) supplementation as an enteral dose of 36.2 g of l-arginine-HCl or an isocaloric amount of placebo (51.2 g alanine), respectively. Wound healing was evaluated at the donor sites of skin grafts by measuring angiogenesis, reepithelialization, and neutrophil count. Arginine metabolism was studied by measuring plasma and wound fluid amino acid concentrations. Our results show that none of these parameters were significantly different between the oral arginine supplementation group and the placebo group. In conclusion, enteral arginine supplementation does not improve wound healing of skin donor sites.

▶ Nearly all aspects of skin graft donor site management are widely debated in burn care. Contributing factors to delayed donor site healing are malnutrition, age, diabetes, and the size of the burn (total body surface area burn [TBSA]). Another factor influencing donor site healing is administration of oxandrolone, an anabolic steroid. There is wide interest in nutritional supplementation and the effect on donor site healing, especially specific amino acids such as arginine and glutamine. Because so many factors affect donor site healing, studies that account for all confounding variables are often difficult to design and execute. This study is no exception.

The study, as designed, is impractical and fairly meaningless. The authors have chosen a random collage of unrelated diagnoses in both the 10-patient study group and 8-patient supplementation group, including trauma, various malignancies, substance abuse, trauma, chronic wounds, and even a few burns. The average size of skin graft is remarkably small in both groups, being only 67 cm^2 in the arginine treated group and 84 cm^2 in the placebo group. Just to put things in perspective, in a normal sized adult, 150 to 2002 cm corresponds to 1% TBSA. Even the most malnourished patient will be able to heal this size donor site without nutritional supplementation.

The assertion by the authors that a normal body mass index (BMI) equates with normal nutritional status is just wrong. Patients having a BMI > 40, indicating morbid obesity, may be malnourished, have normal nutrition, or be superbly nourished. Although a normal BMI may indicate a normal nutritional status, that assumption cannot be supported as a premise for this study. Additionally, the authors state that lack of weight loss in the previous 6 months also indicates a healthy, normally nutritionalized patient, is an another erroneous assumption in this study design.

The study is designed to have 1 day of nutritional supplementation before, and 4 days of nutritional supplementation after, skin grafting. Most donor sites require greater than 5 days to heal, making the 5-day supplementation choice a bit perplexing. In this study, only 3 of 18 patients had any fluid remaining in their donor site by day 10, indicating significant wound healing in these small donor sites. The study involved drinking the nutritional supplementation, yet most patients had difficulty drinking the amino acid solution because of the bad taste, and 2 of 8 patients discontinued their study participation because of this reason. So, only 6 patients in the study group completed the treatment, leaving a very small group for analysis. The authors state that patients who have not lost weight in the previous 6 months are, by definition, of normal nutritional status, another nonsupported assumption.

So, even though it is a pilot study, the authors have simply supported the notion that donor site healing studies are difficult to conduct. Arginine may or may not improve donor site healing, but this study does not prove or disprove the question under study.

B. A. Latenser, MD

Recombinant Thrombin: Safety and Immunogenicity in Burn Wound Excision and Grafting

Greenhalgh DG, Gamelli RL, Collins J, et al (Univ of California, Sacramento; Loyola Univ Med Ctr, Maywood, IL; Eastern Virginia Med School, Norfolk; et al)
J Burn Care Res 30:371-379, 2009

This study evaluated the safety, immunogenicity, and hemostatic effect of recombinant human Thrombin (rThrombin), in patients undergoing skin grafting for burns. This was a phase 2 multiple site, single-arm, open-label study in patients receiving partial- or full-thickness autologous grafts. rThrombin was applied using a spray applicator to newly excised wounds of 1 to 4% body surface area at 5 minutes intervals for up to 20 minutes, after point source bleeding was stopped. Adverse events, skin graft survival, and formation of anti-rThrombin antibodies were measured at baseline and Day 29. There were no deaths or study drug discontinuations. Adverse events occurred in 63 of 72 patients (88%), and were typical of sequelae of skin grafting. Hemostasis was achieved within 20 minutes after application of rThrombin in 65 of 71 patients (91.5%). Skin graft failure occurred in 4 patients (6%). At the day 29 evaluation, for those patients who returned, 88.9% had $\geq$90% graft survival. One patient (1 of 70, 1.4%) had specific, low titer antibodies to rThrombin at baseline, but no increase in titer posttreatment; a second patient (1 of 62, 1.6%), developed antibodies to rThrombin at day 29. None of the antibodies neutralized native human thrombin. In excised burn wounds, hemostasis at 20 minutes was achieved in 91.5% of patients and skin graft survival was excellent. There was a low rate of antibodies to rThrombin at baseline (1.4%) and a low rate of anti-rThrombin antibody formation at day 29 (1.6%). rThrombin was well tolerated when administered with a pump spray.

▶ This well-written article examines topical recombinant human thrombin (rThrombin) in small excised burn wounds in patients with small burn injuries. Not surprisingly, the authors found a statistically significant reduction in time to hemostasis compared with saline compression on a wound. All point sources of bleeding were controlled before application of rThrombin, leaving what the authors describe as "microvascular" bleeding. The definition of bleeding and methods to control bleeding were left up to the individual authors. Then, either saline or rThrombin + pressure was placed on the wound for up to 20 minutes, but the authors were not blinded to the agent they were using, leading to another potential bias source.

The most interesting fact is that topical epinephrine was not allowed in the study, and no mention of it is made in this article. If one wants to be absolutely certain that patients are not at risk for developing specific antibodies to rThrombin, then don't expose them to this product. In addition to the potential antibody development risk, rThrombin is a very expensive product to use. Telfa pads, laparotomy pads, or any other material that is inexpensive and readily available may be dipped in epinephrine solution (90 mg/L saline) and applied directly to the wound, providing very effective hemostasis in 5 minutes.

Some authors have questioned the safety of high-dose epinephrine and the potential systemic absorption of quantities of epinephrine. There is always that one case where a mislabeled drug dosage was administered, leading to an adverse outcome, and certainly, epinephrine is a "high alert" medication. Cartotto and colleagues[1] have shown that it is possible to minimize blood loss in surgery, using techniques that do not expose the patient to potential antibody development. I would recommend that article to any who want to find safe and effective methods to minimize blood loss during burn wound excision and grafting.

Although the authors in this article have shown that rThrombin is safe and effective in the short-term, there are safer and more cost-effective alternatives.

B. A. Latenser, MD

Reference

1. Cartotto R, Musgrave MA, Beveridge M, Fish J, Gomez M. Minimizing blood loss in burn surgery. *J Trauma*. 2000;49:1034-1039.

The Association Between Blood Alcohol Level and Infectious Complications Among Burn Patients

Griffin R, Poe AM, Cross JM, et al (Univ of Alabama at Birmingham)
J Burn Care Res 30:395-399, 2009

Approximately 50% of fatal and 15% of nonfatal burn-injured patients have detectable blood alcohol content (BAC) at the time of admission, and it is hypothesized that alcohol exacerbates burn-related immunosuppression. The purpose of this study was to evaluate the association between BAC and infectious complications in burn patients. The study population consisted of 1161 burn patients admitted to a large academic burn center between January 1998 and June 2007. Patients were categorized into no BAC (0.0 g/100 ml), low/ moderate BAC (>0.0 and <0.1 g/100 ml) and high BAC (≥0.1 g/100 ml) groups based on BAC at time of admission. Risk ratios (RRs) and 95% confidence intervals (CIs) were calculated for associations between pneumonia, sepsis, urinary tract infection, line infection, and wound infection and BAC, adjusted for total burn surface area and inhalation injury. Relative to no BAC patients, both low/moderate and high BAC patients had nonsignificantly increased risk for most infectious complications. High BAC patients were at significantly increased risk for any infectious complication (RR 2.06, CI 1.25–3.41) and pneumonia (RR 2.06, CI 1.04–4.09) and a nonsignificantly increased risk of urinary tract infection (RR 2.12, CI 0.0.94–4.78). Results suggest that preinjury alcohol consumption places patients at an increased risk for infectious complications, most notably pneumonia. Further studies examining the relationship between alcohol and pneumonia among burn patients will help elucidate the reason for the increased risk observed in the current study and suggest ways to prevent infection for this particular subgroup of burn patients.

▶ Alcohol intoxication has become one of the major problems in health care today. The literature is replete with animal and human studies suggesting that acute alcohol intoxication before burn injury increases susceptibility to infection when compared with patients who sustained injury in the absence of alcohol intoxication. Bacterial translocation has previously been shown to contribute to infections in patients with severe burns as intestine-derived bacteria gain access to extraintestinal sites. Another possibility to explain the increased incidence of pneumonia in these study patients is the marked leukocytic infiltration in the lungs of burn patients.

This study would be improved if all patients had their blood alcohol levels checked upon admission. It is unclear why only one-half of the patients had their blood alcohol level checked upon admission. There may have been even more patients with elevated blood alcohol levels that did not develop infections, so the data may be misleading. Data from a referring facility, if appropriate, regarding blood alcohol level should be included in the study. Additionally, chronic alcohol intake data would have been very interesting in this patient population. If nothing else, the study demonstrates that every patient with an acute burn injury should have his/her blood alcohol level checked upon admission.

B. A. Latenser, MD

Effects of candidaemia on outcome of burns
Vinsonneau C, Benyamina M, Baixench MT, et al (Paris Descartes Univ, France)
Burns 35:561-564, 2009

Aim.—To evaluate the diversity and antifungal susceptibilities of *Candida* isolates from wounds and blood of burn victims, and the associated mortality rates compared with those of controls without candidaemia.

Methods.—We performed a nested case-control study within a database of clinical data for all patients admitted to our burn unit from January 2001 to December 2005. Each candidaemic patient was compared with two matched controls. Bloodstream cultures were performed if the core temperature was >39°C, and three sites were cultured weekly for fungal identification (burn wound, pharynx, urinary tract).

Results.—At least one episode of candidaemia was diagnosed among 20 of 851 persons admitted during the study period. Isolates in bloodstream infection were *Candida albicans* (65%), *C. parapsilosis* (25%) and *C. tropicalis* (10%). The median time between admission and onset of candidaemia was greater with *C. albicans* infection (42.6 ± 31 days) than with infection by other yeasts (18 ± 12 days). Candidaemia was associated with more extensive burn and longer duration of hospital stay but with similar mortality, compared with controls.

Conclusion.—Candidaemia in burn cases is mostly due to fluconazole-susceptible *C. albicans* and is not associated with increased mortality.

▶ This is an interesting approach to *Candida* infections in burn patients. There are several aspects of this article that I find concerning, data without which I am not sure I will agree with the authors' conclusions. First, the overall approach to burn wound management is lacking. For example, we do not know if patients undergo early excision and autografting. We also do not know what the wound care protocols in this burn unit entail. The authors state that dressing changes are performed every other day. We do know that currently used topical antimicrobials such as silver sulphadiazine or mafenide acetate have an effective time of 8 to 10 hours, leading to a practice in the United States of daily dressing changes rather than every other or every third day. We do not know the methodology used to cleanse the wounds in this particular burn center. Another treatment modality that has gone by the wayside in most United States burn centers is the Hubbard tank, a large swimming pool type apparatus used to dunk the entire patient. United States burn centers have gone to a moving water technology, with the head up/feet down position, much like a car wash, where the water is always moving, preventing bacterial and fungal stagnation in a burn wound. Bacteria and fungi from the fecal fallout zone do not set up housekeeping in clean burned areas away from the perineum. This methodology alone has decreased the bacterial/fungal colonization rates for burn patients in the United States. Finally, I am concerned about the exorbitant length of stay for these burn patients. For patients who did not develop candidemia, the average burn stay was 1.7 days/% burn; for those with candidemia, the average burn stay was 2.4 days. Factors under the control of the burn care team, such as delay in early excision, lack of daily wound care, and other infection control practices might lead to the high rate of candidemia in this burn unit. Changing practices might save significant patient expense and discomfort, even if mortality rates are not affected.

B. A. Latenser, MD

5   Infectious Disease

Nosocomial/Ventilator-Acquired Pneumonia

Impact of a Monitored Program of Care on Incidence of Ventilator-Associated Pneumonia: Results of a Longterm Performance-Improvement Project

Weireter LJ Jr, Collins JN, Britt RC, et al (Eastern Virginia Med School, Norfolk)
J Am Coll Surg 208:700-705, 2009

Background.—Ventilator-associated pneumonia (VAP) remains a major source of morbidity, mortality, and expense in the ICU despite therapies directed against it.

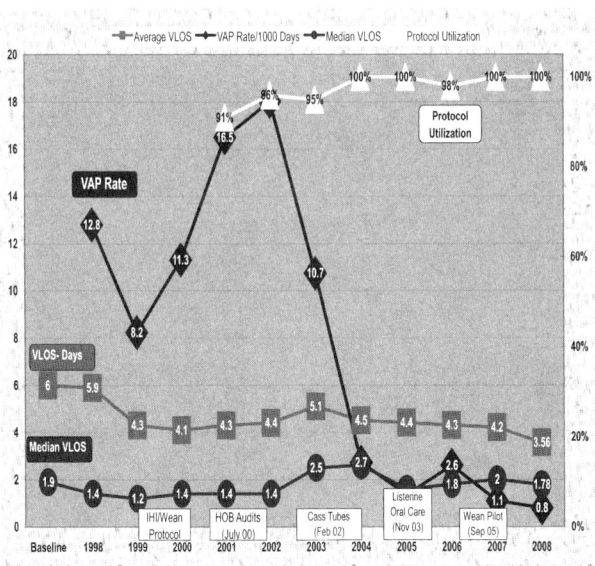

FIGURE 1.—Burn trauma unit ventilator outcomes measures. (Reprinted from Weireter LJ Jr, Collins JN, Britt RC, et al. Impact of a monitored program of care on incidence of ventilator-associated pneumonia: results of a longterm performance-improvement project. *J Am Coll Surg.* 2009;208:700-705, with permission from Elsevier.)

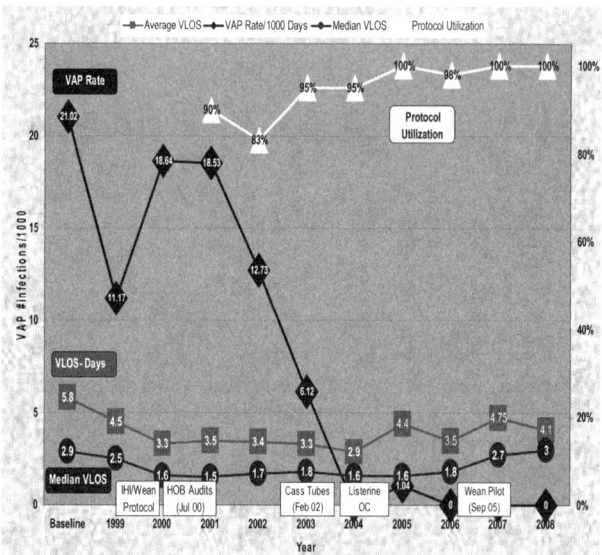

FIGURE 2.—Neurosurgical ICU ventilator outcomes measures. (Reprinted from Weireter LJ Jr, Collins JN, Britt RC, et al. Impact of a monitored program of care on incidence of ventilator-associated pneumonia: results of a longterm performance-improvement project. *J Am Coll Surg.* 2009;208:700-705, with permission from Elsevier.)

Study Design.—A retrospective review of a prospectively developed performance-improvement project monitoring the incidence of VAP in two adjacent ICUs was conducted. In response to an excessive VAP rate, weekly multidisciplinary team meetings were instituted to review data, develop care protocols, and modify care routines. Protocol compliance was monitored daily and feedback provided weekly to the care teams. VAP rates were determined by the institutional Infection Control Committee and reviewed monthly with the ICU multidisciplinary team. Duration of the investigational period was 10 years.

Results.—A standardized ventilator-weaning protocol was instituted with confirmed 95% use. Additional modifications of care, such as patient positioning, use of specific endotracheal tubes to minimize aspiration of supraglottic secretions, an oral-care regimen, and aggressive antibiotic stewardship were standardized, with a compliance rate >90%. VAP rates dropped from 12.8 per 1,000 patient-days in 1998 to 1.1 in 2007 in the burn trauma ICU and from 21.2 to <1 in the neurotrauma ICU in the same time frame. Also, mean ventilator length of stay decreased from 6 days to 4.2 and from 5.8 days to 4.75 simultaneously in the respective ICUs. Such performance improvement has been sustained since implementation of the program.

Conclusion.—A systematic, monitored program of standardized care protocols can markedly reduce VAP rate in the ICU (Figs 1 and 2).

▶ The impact of ventilator-associated pneumonia (VAP) on mortality, length of stay, and cost of care is well known among the critical care community. Various strategies have been used to decrease the development of VAP, but this study concentrates on the methodology to ensure that the critical care staff not only understand the importance of the quality improvement project, but also receive frequent feedback on their compliance rate and success with the project. This method of implementation was taken from industry where it has proved to be successful in changing performance practice. In this study, the methodology was as important as the goal of reducing the incidence of VAP, because this successful strategy can now be used to effect other needed changes in patient management or process of care. At this time where we are trying to improve quality outcomes and reduce and/or eliminate errors, this methodology may be just the tool for the job.

R. A. Balk, MD

Evaluation of the effect of diagnostic methodology on the reported incidence of ventilator-associated pneumonia

Morris AC, Kefala K, Simpson AJ, et al (Univ of Edinburgh, Scotland, UK; et al)
Thorax 64:516-522, 2009

Background.—The optimal method for diagnosing ventilator-associated pneumonia (VAP) is controversial and its effect on reported incidence uncertain. This study aimed to model the impact of using either endotracheal aspirate or bronchoalveolar lavage on the reported incidence of pneumonia and then to test effects suggested from theoretical modelling in clinical practice.

Methods.—A three-part single-centre study was undertaken. First, diagnostic performance of aspirate and lavage were compared using paired samples from 53 patients with suspected VAP. Secondly, infection surveillance data were used to model the potential effect on pneumonia incidence and antibiotic use of using exclusively aspirate or lavage to investigate suspected pneumonia (643 patients; 110 clinically suspected pneumonia episodes). Thirdly, a practice change initiative was undertaken to increase lavage use; pneumonia incidence and antibiotic use were compared for the 12 months before and after the change.

Results.—Aspirate overdiagnosed VAP compared with lavage (89% vs 21% of clinically suspected cases, p < 0.0001). Modelling suggested that changing from exclusive aspirate to lavage diagnosis would decrease reported pneumonia incidence by 76% (95% CI 67% to 87%) and antibiotic use by 30% (95% CI 20% to 42%). After the practice change initiative, lavage use increased from 37% to 58%. Although clinically suspected pneumonia incidence was unchanged, microbiologically confirmed VAP

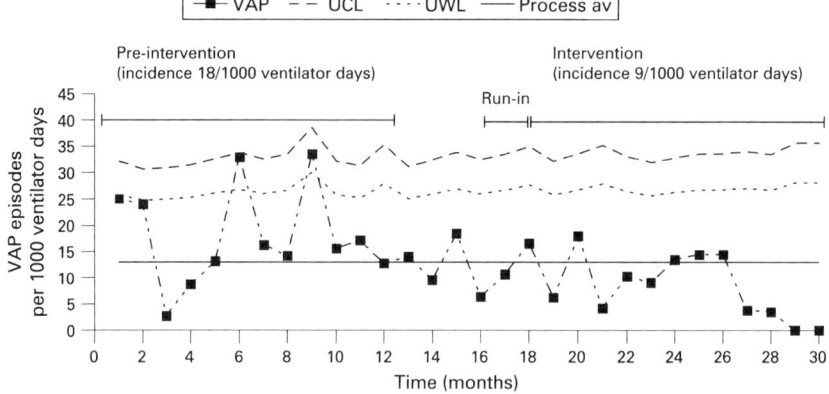

FIGURE 3.—Statistical process chart showing incidence of confirmed ventilator-associted pneumonia (VAP) in the preintervention and postintervention periods. Process av, process average; UCL, upper control line; UWL, upper warning line. Lower control line and lower warning lines are omitted for clarity. (Reprinted from Morris AC, Kefala K, Simpson AJ, et al. Evaluation of the effect of diagnostic methodology on the reported incidence of ventilator-associated pneumonia. *Thorax.* 2009;64:516-522. Reproduced with permission from the BMJ Publishing Group.)

TABLE 4.—Modelled Effect of Exclusive Use of ETA or BAL on the Reported Incidence of VAP, Using the Numbers of Clinically Suspected VAP Episodes from Infection Surveillance Occurring in the ICU Over 12 Months (fig 2; n = 110)

	BAL Mean Estimate (95% CI)	Qualitative ETA Mean Estimate (95% CI)	Quantitative ETA Mean Estimate (95% CI)
Positive culture	23 (11 to 35)	96 (85 to 106)	56 (41 to 69)
Negative culture	87 (75 to 99)	14 (4 to 25)	54 (41 to 69)
Proportion of "clinically suspected VAPs" reported as "confirmed VAP"	21% (10 to 32%)	87% (77 to 96%)	51% (37 to 63%)
Cases/1000 ventilator days	6.1 (2.9 to 9.2)	25.5 (22.5 to 28.1)	15.0 (11.0 to 18.3)

Numbers show mean estimate and upper and lower confidence limit using 95% CIs for proportions (z test) and were derived using the data from fig 1.
BAL, bronchoalveolar lavage; ETA, endotracheal aspirate; ICU, Intensive Care Unit; VAP, ventilator-associated pneumonia

decreased from 18 to 9 cases per 1000 ventilator days (p = 0.001; relative risk reduction 0.61 (95% CI 0.46 to 0.82)), and mean antibiotic use fell from 9.1 to 7.2 antibiotic days (21% decrease, p = 0.08).

Conclusions.—Diagnostic technique impacts significantly on reported VAP incidence and potentially on antibiotic use (Fig 3, Tables 4 and 5).

▶ The best method to diagnose ventilator-associated pneumonia (VAP) has been a topic of debate for decades. The current controversy centers around the choice between empiric treatment (based on guidelines and knowledge

TABLE 5.—Modelled Effect of Changing Diagnostic Strategy on the Antibiotic Load
Experienced by Patients with Suspected VAP

	BAL Mean (95% CI)	Qualitative ETA Mean (95% CI)
Positive culture "antibiotic days"	278 (133 to 424)	1104 (978 to1219)
Negative culture "antibiotic days"	505 (435 to 574)	21 (6 to 38)
Total	783 (568 to 998)	1125 (984 to 1257)
"Antibiotic days" per patient	7.1 (5.2 to 9.1)	10.2 (8.9 to 11.4)

Data obtained by combining the modelled effect on reported VAP incidence in table 4, with antibiotic load data from table 3.
The numbers in parentheses are those estimated using the 95% CIs from fig 1.
BAL, bronchoalveolar lavage; ETA, endotracheal aspirate; VAP, ventilator-associated pneumonia.

of the specific antibiogram of your institution) versus the use of an invasive diagnostic strategy (bronchoalveolar lavage [BAL] vs deep endotracheal aspirate [ETA]).[1-3] The use of an invasive strategy became easier and more acceptable with the publication of the results of ETA success by the Canadian Critical Care Trials Group.[3] This interesting single-center study illustrates the impact of using BAL and ETA, with or without quantitative cultures on the diagnosis of VAP. The diagnosis of VAP also influences the subsequent antibiotic use, which not surprisingly decreases when the diagnosis of VAP decreases. The importance of securing the diagnosis of VAP for its impact on patient management as well as antibiotic stewardship cannot be overemphasized. There may also be future financial implications if reimbursement sources decline payment for hospital-acquired infections, such as VAP.

R. A. Balk, MD

References

1. American Thoracic Society. Guidelines for the management of adults with hospital-acquired, ventilator-associated, and healthcare-associated pneumonia. *Am J Respir Crit Care Med.* 2005;171:388-416.
2. Fagon JY, Chastre J, Wolff M, et al. Invasive and noninvasive strategies for management of suspected ventilator-associated pneumonia: a randomized trial. *Ann Int Med.* 2000;132:621-630.
3. Canadian Critical Care Trials Group. A randomized trial of diagnostic techniques for ventilator-associated pneumonia. *N Engl J Med.* 2006;355:2619-2630.

Implementation of a Real-time Compliance Dashboard to Help Reduce SICU Ventilator-Associated Pneumonia With the Ventilator Bundle
Zaydfudim V, Dossett LA, Starmer JM, et al (Vanderbilt Univ Med Ctr, Nashville, TN)
Arch Surg 144:656-662, 2009

Background.—Ventilator-associated pneumonia (VAP) causes significant morbidity and mortality in critically ill surgical patients. Recent studies suggest that the success of preventive measures is dependent on compliance with ventilator bundle parameters.

Hypothesis.—Implementation of an electronic dashboard will improve compliance with the bundle parameters and reduce rates of VAP in our surgical intensive care unit (SICU).

Design.—Time series analysis of VAP rates between January 2005 and July 2008, with dashboard implementation in July 2007.

Setting.—Multidisciplinary SICU at a tertiary-care referral center with a stable case mix during the study period.

Patients.—Patients admitted to the SICU between January 2005 and July 2008.

Main Outcome Measures.—Infection control data were used to establish rates of VAP and total ventilator days. For the time series analysis, VAP rates were calculated as quarterly VAP events per 1000 ventilator days. Ventilator bundle compliance was analyzed after dashboard implementation. Differences between expected and observed VAP rates based on time series analysis were used to estimate the effect of intervention.

Results.—Average compliance with the ventilator bundle improved from 39% in August 2007 to 89% in July 2008 ($P < .001$). Rates of VAP decreased from a mean (SD) of 15.2(7.0) to 9.3(4.9) events per 1000 ventilator days after introduction of the dashboard ($P = .01$). Quarterly VAP rates were significantly reduced in the November 2007 through January 2008 and February through April 2008 periods ($P < .05$). For the August through October 2007 and May through July 2008 quarters, the observed rate reduction was not statistically significant.

Conclusions.—Implementation of an electronic dashboard improved compliance with ventilator bundle measures and is associated with reduced rates of VAP in our SICU.

▶ To decrease the incidence of ventilator-associated pneumonia (VAP) physicians and nurses have resorted to various strategies to improve both awareness and compliance. In this institution, which uses an electronic medical record, the authors incorporated a screen saver that depicts the compliance of each ventilated patient in the unit with the bundle for VAP prevention. Using simple color codes (red, green, and yellow) one can easily see who is in compliance and who is not. A sample of the screen saver is shown in Fig 1 in the original article. The effectiveness of this technique is shown in Fig 3 in the original article with a significant reduction in VAP rates after implementation. This reduction in VAP rates occurred with no change in the blood stream infection rate. It seems that a similar intervention may now be needed to decrease the rate of blood stream infections.

R. A. Balk, MD

A Randomized Trial of Dental Brushing for Preventing Ventilator-Associated Pneumonia

Pobo A, for the RASPALL Study Investigators (Univ Rovira i Virgili, Tarragona, Spain; et al)
Chest 136:433-439, 2009

Background.—Poor oral hygiene is associated with respiratory pathogen colonization and secondary lung infection. The impact of adding electric toothbrushing to oral care in order to reduce ventilator-associated pneumonia (VAP) incidence is unknown.

Methods.—The study design was a prospective, simple-blind, randomized trial of adult patients intubated for > 48 h. Controlling for exposure to antibiotic treatment, patients were randomized to oral care every 8 h with 0.12% chlorhexidine digluconate (standard group) or standard oral care plus electric toothbrushing (toothbrush group). VAP was documented by quantitative respiratory cultures. Mechanical ventilation (MV) duration, hospital ICU length of stay (LOS), antibiotic use, and hospital ICU mortality were secondary end points.

Results.—The study was terminated after randomizing 147 patients (74 toothbrush group) in a scheduled interim analysis. The two groups were comparable at baseline. The toothbrush group and standard group had similar rates of suspected VAP (20.3% vs 24.7%; p = 0.55). After adjustment for severity of illness and admission diagnosis, the incidence of microbiologically documented VAP was also similar in the two groups (hazard ratio, 0.84; 95% confidence interval, 0.41 to 1.73). The groups did not differ significantly in mortality, antibiotic-free days, duration of MV, or hospital ICU LOS.

Conclusions.—Our findings suggest that the addition of electric toothbrushing to standard oral care with 0.12% chlorhexidine digluconate is not effective for the prevention of VAP.

Trial registration.—ClinicalTrials.gov Identifier: NCT00842478.

▶ Many strategies have been investigated to discover their ability to reduce the incidence of ventilator-associated pneumonia (VAP). Among the successful strategies are elevating the head of the bed, minimizing interruptions of the ventilator circuit, silver coated endotracheal tubes, and subglottic secretion aspiration. Good mouth care has also emerged as an important contribution to maintain oral health and prevent VAP. This randomized trial evaluated the difference between good mouth care performed with chlorhexidine every 8 hours versus the same care with the addition of an electric toothbrush to clean the teeth. Unfortunately, the vast number of mechanically ventilated patients admitted to the ICU during the study period were not eligible for the trial, and the trial was stopped early for futility by the data safety monitoring board. However, it appears from this data that the addition of an electric toothbrush to the mouth care regimen used in mechanically ventilated critically ill patients did not decrease the development of VAP. For now, we will all continue to use our ventilator bundle to provide good care for our ventilated patients, and this should include adequate mouth care. The critically ill can safely leave their electric toothbrush at home because it does not appear to be needed while on mechanical ventilatory support.

R. A. Balk, MD

Effect of synbiotic therapy on the incidence of ventilator associated pneumonia in critically ill patients: a randomised, double-blind, placebo-controlled trial

Knight DJW, Gardiner D, Banks A, et al (Christchurch Hosp, New Zealand; Queen's Med Centre, Nottingham, UK; et al)
Intensive Care Med 35:854-861, 2009

Objective.—To investigate the effect of enteral Synbiotic 2000 FORTE ® (a mixture of lactic acid bacteria and fibre) on the incidence of ventilator associated pneumonia (VAP) in critically ill patients.

Design.—Prospective, randomised, double blind, placebo controlled trial.

Setting.—Tertiary referral centre, general Adult Intensive Care Unit (ICU).

Patients and Participants.—259 enterally fed patients requiring mechanical ventilation for 48 h or more were enrolled.

Intervention.—All patients were enterally fed as per a standard protocol and randomly assigned to receive either synbiotic 2000 FORTE® (twice a day) or a cellulose-based placebo for a maximum of 28 days.

Measurements and Results.—Treatment group ($n = 130$) was well matched with placebo group ($n = 129$) for age (mean 49.5 and 50 years, respectively) and APACHE II score (median 17 for both). Oropharyngeal microbial flora and colonisation rates were unaffected by synbiotics. The overall incidence of VAP was lower than anticipated (11.2%) and no

---

TABLE 3.—VAP Diagnosis

Variable	Synbiotic	Placebo	P	Relative Risk (95% Confidence Interval)
Number of patients	130	129		
VAP (% of total)	12 (9)	17 (13)	0.42	0.70 (0.35–1.41)
Polymicrobial VAP	3	5		
Individual pathogens				
Enterobacteriaceae	6	7		
Pseudomonas aeruginosa		1		
MRSA		1		
Haemophilus influenzae		1		
Acinetobacter baumannii	3	1		
Stenotrophomonas maltophilia		1		
VAP episodes per 1,000 ventilator days	13	14.6	0.91	0.89 (0.42–1.87)
Number of ventilator days, median (IQR)	5 (2–9)	5 (3–11)	0.82	

TABLE 5.—Secondary Outcome Results

Variable	Synbiotic	Placebo	P	Relative Risk (95% CI)
Number of patients	130	129		
ICU length of stay in days, median (IQR)	6.0 (3–11)	7.0 (3–14)	0.45	
Hospital length of stay in days, median (IQR)	19 (8–36)	18 (7–32)	0.85	
Mortality				
ICU total (%)	28 (21.5)	34 (26.3)	0.44	0.82 (0.53–1.26)
Hospital total (%)	35 (26.9)	42 (32.5)	0.39	0.83 (0.57–1.20)

statistical difference was demonstrated between groups receiving synbiotic and placebo in the incidence of VAP (9 and 13%, $P = 0.42$), VAP rate per 1,000 ventilator days (13 and 14.6, $P = 0.91$) or hospital mortality (27 and 33%, $P = 0.39$), respectively.

Conclusions.—Enteral administration of Synbiotic 2000 FORTE® has no statistically significant impact on the incidence of VAP in critically ill patients (Tables 3 and 5).

▶ Ventilator-associated pneumonia (VAP) is associated with increased morbidity, mortality, length of stay, and cost of care. There are a number of strategies used to reduce the development of VAP. These strategies range from simplistic and economical (elevating the head of the bed) to elaborate and expensive (selective digestive decontamination). The use of enterally administered probiotics to protect the critically ill patient from infection with more severe pathogens is an intriguing concept and one certainly worth exploring. This study was well conducted, using prospectively defined definitions for VAP and blinded adjudicators to make the diagnosis. Unfortunately, the study was powered for a control VAP rate of 28% and only 13% of the control patients developed VAP. Hence, we are uncertain if there is no benefit from probiotics in the prevention of VAP, or if the study was underpowered and we are dealing with a type II error. At least we know the administration of probiotics appears to be safe in the critically ill ventilated patient.

R. A. Balk, MD

Decontamination of the Digestive Tract and Oropharynx in ICU Patients

de Smet AMGA, Kluytmans JAJW, Cooper BS, et al (Univ Med Ctr, Utrecht, the Netherlands; Amphia Hosp, Breda, the Netherlands; Centre for Infections Health Protection Agency Statistics, London)
N Engl J Med 360:20-31, 2009

Background.—Selective digestive tract decontamination (SDD) and selective oropharyngeal decontamination (SOD) are infection-prevention measures used in the treatment of some patients in intensive care, but reported effects on patient outcome are conflicting.

Methods.—We evaluated the effectiveness of SDD and SOD in a crossover study using cluster randomization in 13 intensive care units (ICUs), all in the Netherlands. Patients with an expected duration of intubation of more than 48 hours or an expected ICU stay of more than 72 hours were eligible. In each ICU, three regimens (SDD, SOD, and standard care) were applied in random order over the course of 6 months. Mortality at day 28 was the primary end point. SDD consisted of 4 days of intravenous cefotaxime and topical application of tobramycin, colistin, and amphotericin B in the oropharynx and stomach. SOD consisted of oropharyngeal application only of the same antibiotics. Monthly point-prevalence studies were performed to analyze antibiotic resistance.

Results.—A total of 5939 patients were enrolled in the study, with 1990 assigned to standard care, 1904 to SOD, and 2045 to SDD; crude mortality in the groups at day 28 was 27.5%, 26.6%, and 26.9%, respectively. In a random-effects logistic-regression model with age, sex, Acute Physiology and Chronic Health Evaluation (APACHE II) score, intubation status, and medical specialty used as covariates, odds ratios for death at day 28 in the SOD and SDD groups, as compared with the standard-care group, were 0.86 (95% confidence interval [CI], 0.74 to 0.99) and 0.83 (95% CI, 0.72 to 0.97), respectively.

Conclusions.—In an ICU population in which the mortality rate associated with standard care was 27.5% at day 28, the rate was reduced by an estimated 3.5 percentage points with SDD and by 2.9 percentage points with SOD. (Controlled Clinical Trials number, ISRCTN35176830.)

▶ This trial is the largest conducted to date on the use of selective digestive tract decontamination (SDD) or selective oropharyngeal decontamination (SOD) has been discussed for years as a method of reducing the rate of nosocomial infections in the ICU. The study is important in that it answers several key questions about SD and SOD. First, this was a highly cost-effective strategy with the regime costing $12 per day for protocol, and $1 per day for the SOD group. Second, the rate of resistant organisms or the rate of *Clostridium difficile* were no different between the groups. This trial demonstrates that SDD and SOD are safe, efficacious, and cost-effective. Intensivists should question why this approach has not been adopted to a significant extent in North America while seeing widespread use in Europe.

A. Kumar, MD
D. Funk, MD, FRCP(C)

Impact of a Monitored Program of Care on Incidence of Ventilator-Associated Pneumonia: Results of a Longterm Performance-Improvement Project

Weireter LJ Jr, Collins JN, Britt RC, et al (Eastern Virginia Med School, Norfolk)
J Am Coll Surg 208:700-705, 2009

Background.—Ventilator-associated pneumonia (VAP) remains a major source of morbidity, mortality, and expense in the ICU despite therapies directed against it.

Study Design.—A retrospective review of a prospectively developed performance-improvement project monitoring the incidence of VAP in two adjacent ICUs was conducted. In response to an excessive VAP rate, weekly multidisciplinary team meetings were instituted to review data, develop care protocols, and modify care routines. Protocol compliance was monitored daily and feedback provided weekly to the care teams. VAP rates were determined by the institutional Infection Control Committee and reviewed monthly with the ICU multidisciplinary team. Duration of the investigational period was 10 years.

Results.—A standardized ventilator-weaning protocol was instituted with confirmed 95% use. Additional modifications of care, such as patient positioning, use of specific endotracheal tubes to minimize aspiration of supraglottic secretions, an oral-care regimen, and aggressive antibiotic stewardship were standardized, with a compliance rate >90%. VAP rates dropped from 12.8 per 1,000 patient-days in 1998 to 1.1 in 2007 in the burn trauma ICU and from 21.2 to <1 in the neurotrauma ICU in the same time frame. Also, mean ventilator length of stay decreased from 6 days to 4.2 and from 5.8 days to 4.75 simultaneously in the respective ICUs. Such performance improvement has been sustained since implementation of the program.

Conclusion.—A systematic, monitored program of standardized care protocols can markedly reduce VAP rate in the ICU.

▶ The authors provide impressive results but provide a limited data set to explain them. For example, ventilator management protocols are not provided. It is unclear whether a new weaning strategy led to the reduction in ventilator length of stay. The authors appear to use rigorous infection control and pneumonia definitions but details of microbiology are also absent.

Three interventions are emphasized in this report. First, is the development of a therapist- and nurse-driven weaning protocol. The authors indicate that compliance with this protocol is high. Second, the authors have switched to endotracheal tubes incorporating aspiration of pharyngeal secretions to reduce this component of endotracheal tube-associated pneumonia. Finally, the authors have provided increased emphasis on oral care in their various critical care units.[1-3]

All of these interventions are important, but I am concerned that this report provides insufficient detail to explain the differing outcomes in patients described as opposed to other reports which indicate persisting, problematic respiratory infections in the trauma and burn populations.[4,5] In summary, I have no doubt that performance improvement projects as we see applied in industry may also be relevant in a problem such as ventilator-associated pneumonia. However, there is too little data provided here for a definitive decision to be made on the merits of this success story.

D. J. Dries, MSE, MD

References

1. Girard TD, Kress JP, Fuchs BD, et al. Efficacy and safety of a paired sedation and ventilator weaning protocol for mechanically ventilated patients in intensive care (Awaking and Breathing Controlled trial): a randomized controlled trial. *Lancet*. 2008;371:126-134.
2. Koeman M, van der Ven AJ, Hak E, et al. Oral decontamination with chlorhexidine reduces the incident of ventilator-associated pneumonia. *Am J Respir Crit Care Med*. 2006;173:1348-1355.
3. Lorente C, Del Castillo Y, Rello J. Prevention of infection in the intensive care unit: Current advances and opportunities for the future. *Curr Opin Crit Care*. 2002;8: 461-464.
4. Hedrick TL, Smith RL, McElearney ST, et al. Differences in early-and late-onset ventilator-associated pneumonia between surgical and trauma patients in a combined surgical or trauma intensive care unit. *J Trauma*. 2008;64:714-720.
5. Rangel EL, Butler KL, Johannigman JA, Tsuei BJ, Solomkin JS. Risk factors for relapse of ventilator-associated pneumonia in trauma patients. *J Trauma*. 2009; 67:91-96.

Mortality and time to extubation in severe hospital-acquired pneumonia

Connelly SM, Trinh JV, Johnson MD, et al (Duke Univ Med Ctr, Durham, NC; et al)

Am J Infect Control 37:143-149, 2009

Background.—This study examined predictors of in-hospital mortality and time to extubation among patients with acute, severe hospital-acquired pneumonia (HAP) managed in the intensive care unit (ICU).

Methods.—Patients with HAP prospectively identified between June 2001 and May 2003 were included in the study if they (1) met the Centers for Disease Control and Prevention's definition for HAP, (2) were treated in the ICU within 1 day of the HAP diagnosis, and (3) required intubation acutely or had a bloodstream infection within 48 hours of the HAP diagnosis.

Results.—The cohort included 219 patients, 83 of whom died (37.9%). Independent predictors of mortality included cancer (odds ratio [OR] = 4.2; 95% confidence interval [CI] = 1.7 to 10.5), age over 60 years (OR = 2.7; 95% CI = 1.3 to 5.6), APACHE-II score > 15 (OR = 2.0; 95% CI = 1.0 to 4.1), and receiving care in the medical ICU (OR = 3.0; 95% CI = 1.1 to 8.2). The following predictors were associated with an increased time to extubation: receipt of vancomycin (1.81-fold increase; $P = .001$), immunocompromised status (1.92-fold increase; $P = .07$), and treatment in the surgical or neurosurgical ICU (1.95-fold increase, $P = .01$; 1.83-fold increase, $P = .03$).

Conclusion.—Vancomycin was associated with increased time to extubation. Alternatives to vancomycin for treating patients with acute, severe HAP should be studied.

▶ Hospital-acquired pneumonia (HAP) is an important nosocomial infection that is associated with increased patient morbidity, mortality, hospital length of stay, and cost of care. Hospital-acquired infections are also on the radar screen of the reimbursement groups as "never events" that may be denied payment. Therefore, it is important for all of us to understand the risk factors for HAP and those parameters that impact outcome. This study evaluated patients at a large tertiary care, university hospital and uncovered risk factors associated with mortality and prolonged mechanical ventilatory support. Their conclusion regarding the need to find an alternative gram-positive antibiotic for vancomycin in hopes of shortening the duration of mechanical ventilation is of interest, but needs to be prospectively tested and proven. Fortunately, there are a few new gram-positive antibiotics in the pipeline for approval, the key to their success will be if they produce more favorable results than vancomycin in the setting of HAP.

R. A. Balk, MD

Gram-Negative Bacteremia upon Hospital Admission: When Should *Pseudomonas aeruginosa* Be Suspected?

Schechner V, Nobre V, Kaye KS, et al (Tel Aviv Univ, Israel; Univ of Geneva Hosps and Med School, Switzerland; Duke Univ Med Ctr, Durham, NC; et al)
Clin Infect Dis 48:580-586, 2009

Background.—*Pseudomonas aeruginosa* is an uncommon cause of community-acquired bacteremia among patients without severe immunodeficiency. Because tension exists between the need to limit unnecessary use of anti-pseudomonal agents and the need to avoid a delay in appropriate therapy, clinicians require better guidance regarding when to cover empirically for *P. aeruginosa*. We sought to determine the occurrence of and construct a model to predict *P. aeruginosa* bacteremia upon hospital admission.

Methods.—A retrospective study was conducted in 4 tertiary care hospitals. Microbiology databases were searched to find all episodes of bacteremia caused by gram-negative rods (GNRs) ≤48 h after hospital admission. Patient data were extracted from the medical records of 151 patients with *P. aeruginosa* bacteremia and of 152 randomly selected patients with bacteremia due to Enterobacteriaceae. Discriminative parameters were identified using logistic regression, and the probabilities of having *P. aeruginosa* bacteremia were calculated.

Results.—*P. aeruginosa* caused 6.8% of 4114 unique patient episodes of GNR bacteremia upon hospital admission (incidence ratio, 5 cases per 10,000 hospital admissions). Independent predictors of *P. aeruginosa* bacteremia were severe immunodeficiency, age >90 years, receipt of antimicrobial therapy within past 30 days, and presence of a central venous catheter or a urinary device. Among 250 patients without severe immunodeficiency, if no predictor variables existed, the likelihood of having *P. aeruginosa* bacteremia was 1:42. If ≥2 predictors existed, the risk increased to nearly 1:3.

Conclusions.—*P. aeruginosa* bacteremia upon hospital admission in patients without severe immunodeficiency is rare. Among immunocompetent patients with suspected GNR bacteremia who have ≥2 predictors, empirical anti-pseudomonal treatment is warranted.

▶ The timely administration of appropriate antimicrobial therapy is key to the survival of patients with severe sepsis and septic shock.[1,2] The administration of broad spectrum antibiotics to these patients has become part of the ABCs of sepsis therapy. There are competing concerns to this management strategy. Administering antibiotics that are not effective against the offending organism will increase the patient's mortality, even if appropriate antimicrobials are started after culture results become available. From a global perspective, however, the indiscriminate use of broad-spectrum antibiotics has led to increased rates of resistance, especially in *Pseudomonas* subspecies. Clinicians err on the side of broadly covering patients with antibiotics in case they harbor a drug-resistant organism. It would be advantageous to have a way of predicting which patients were at risk of these drug resistant organisms in order to tailor therapy appropriately.

The salient features of this article are the low incidence of *Pseudomonas* bacteremia in patients without severe immunodeficiency and the simple predictive rule that can be applied at the bedside. This article should help clinicians tailor their antimicrobial therapy in patients presenting with gram-negative bacteremia and decrease the selection pressure for *Pseudomonas* to develop drug resistance.

A. Kumar, MD

D. Funk, MD, FRCP(C)

References

1. Kumar A, Ellis P, Arabi Y, et al. Cooperative Antimicrobial Therapy of Septic Shock Database Research Group. Initiation of inappropriate antimicrobial therapy results in a five-fold reduction of survival in human septic shock. *Chest.* 2009;136:1237-1248.
2. Ibrahim EH, Sherman G, Ward S, Fraser VJ, Kollef MH. The influence of inadequate antimicrobial treatment of bloodstream infections on patient outcomes in the ICU setting. *Chest.* 2000;118:146-155.

Miscellaneous

Outcomes of Patients Hospitalized With Community-Acquired, Health Care–Associated, and Hospital-Acquired Pneumonia

Venditti M, the Study Group of the Italian Society of Internal Medicine (Univ of Rome, Italy; et al)
Ann Intern Med 150:19-26, 2009

Background.—Traditionally, pneumonia has been classified as either community- or hospital-acquired. Although only limited data are available, health care–associated pneumonia has been recently proposed as a new category of respiratory infection. "Health care–associated pneumonia" refers to pneumonia in patients who have recently been hospitalized, had hemodialysis, or received intravenous chemotherapy or reside in a nursing home or long-term care facility.

Objective.—To ascertain the epidemiology and outcome of community-acquired, health care–associated, and hospital-acquired pneumonia in adults hospitalized in internal medicine wards.

Design.—Multicenter, prospective observational study.

Setting.—55 hospitals in Italy comprising 1941 beds.

Patients.—362 patients hospitalized with pneumonia during two 1-week surveillance periods.

Measurements.—Cases of radiologically and clinically assessed pneumonia were classified as community-acquired, health care–associated, or hospital-acquired and rates were compared.

Results.—Of the 362 patients, 61.6% had community-acquired pneumonia, 24.9% had health care–associated pneumonia, and 13.5% had hospital-acquired pneumonia. Patients with health care–associated pneumonia had higher mean Sequential Organ Failure Assessment scores than did those with community-acquired pneumonia (3.0 vs. 2.0), were more frequently malnourished (11.1% vs. 4.5%, and had more frequent bilateral (34.4% vs. 19.7%) and multilobar (27.8% vs. 21.5%) involvement on a chest radiograph. Patients with health care–associated pneumonia also had higher fatality rates (17.8% [CI, 10.6% to 24.9%] vs. 6.7% [CI, 2.9% to 10.5%]) and longer mean hospital stay (18.7 days [CI, 15.9 to 21.5 days] vs. 14.7 days [CI, 13.4 to 15.9 days]). Logistic regression analysis revealed that depression of consciousness (odds ratio [OR], 3.2 [CI, 1.06 to 9.8]), leukopenia (OR, 6.2 [CI, 1.01 to 37.6]), and receipt of empirical antibiotic therapy not recommended by international guidelines (OR, 6.4 [CI, 2.3 to 17.6]) were independently associated with increased intrahospital mortality.

Limitations.—The number of patients with health care–associated pneumonia was relatively small. Microbiological investigations were not always homogeneous. The study included only patients with pneumonia that required hospitalization; results may not apply to patients treated as outpatients.

Conclusion.—Health care–associated pneumonia should be considered a distinct subset of pneumonia associated with more severe disease, longer hospital stay, and higher mortality rates. Physicians should differentiate between patients with health care–associated pneumonia and those with community-acquired pneumonia and provide more appropriate initial antibiotic therapy.

▶ Health care-associated pneumonia is a relatively recent distinct clinical entity defined in the American Thoracic Society/Infectious Disease Society guidelines.[1] It is estimated that the patient population residing in long-term care facilities and, thus having some contact with health care, will reach more than 5 million by 2030.[2] In response to this ever-enlarging patient population, investigators have recently begun defining the epidemiology of infections in this group.

Adding to the epidemiologic characteristics of health care-associated pneumonia (HCAP) initially put forward by Kollef et al, Venditti and colleagues conducted a prospective multicenter observational study to delineate differences between the various categories of pneumonia patients.[3] Intensivists should be aware of the major epidemiologic points highlighted in this study. Many patients with HCAP are at increased risk for colonization and infection with multidrug resistant pathogens and have a crude mortality higher than patients with community-acquired pneumonia. Targeted antimicrobial therapy with activity against resistant pathogens needs to be considered early in this group of patients and especially so for patients presenting with signs of severe sepsis or septic shock. The findings in this study add to the growing body of literature that HCAP is a unique entity differing from community-acquired pneumonia both bacteriologically and in outcome.

A. Kumar, MD

References

1. American Thoracic Society; Infectious Diseases Society of America. Guidelines for the management of adults with hospital acquired, ventilator-associated, and healthcare-associated pneumonia. *Am J Respir Crit Care Med.* 2005;171:388-416.
2. Hiramatsu K, Niederman MS. Health-care-associated pneumonia: a new therapeutic paradigm. *Chest.* 2005;128:3784-3787.
3. Micek ST, Kollef KE, Reichley RM, Roubinian N, Kollef MH. Health care-associated pneumonia and community-acquired pneumonia: a single-center experience. *Antimicrob Agents Chemother.* 2007;51:3568-3573.

PIRO score for community-acquired pneumonia: A new prediction rule for assessment of severity in intensive care unit patients with community-acquired pneumonia

Rello J, Rodriguez A, Lisboa T, et al (Univ Rovira and Virgili, CIBER Enfermedades Respiratorias, Tarragona, Spain; et al)
Crit Care Med 37:456-462, 2009

Objective.—To develop a severity assessment tool to predict mortality in community-acquired pneumonia (CAP) patients in intensive care unit (ICU), comparing its performance with Acute Physiology and Chronic Health Evaluation (APACHE) II score and American Thoracic Society/Infectious Disease Society of America (ATS/IDSA) criteria as a prognostic index in CAP patients requiring ICU admission.

Design.—Secondary analysis of prospective observational cohort study.

Setting.—Thirty-three ICUs.

Patients.—Five hundred and twenty-nine adult patients with CAP requiring ICU admission.

Measurements and Main Results.—A severity assessment score was developed based on the PIRO (predisposition, insult, response, and organ dysfunction) concept including the presence of the following variables: Comorbidities (chronic obstructive pulmonary disease, immunocompromise); age > 70 years; multilobar opacities in chest radiograph; shock, severe hypoxemia; acute renal failure; bacteremia and acute respiratory distress syndrome. PIRO score was obtained at ICU within 24 hours from admission, and one point was given for each present feature (range, 0–8 points). The mean PIRO score was significantly higher in nonsurvivors than in survivors (4.6 ± 1.2 vs. 2.3 ± 1.4). Considering the observed mortality for each PIRO score, the patients were stratified in four levels of risk: a) Low, 0–2 points; b) Mild, 3 points; c) high, 4 points; and d) Very high, 5–8 points. Mild-risk (hazard ratio [HR] 1.8; 95% confidence interval [CI] 1.1–2.9; $p < 0.05$), high-risk (HR 3.1; 95% CI = 2.0–4.7; $p < 0.001$), and very high risk levels (HR 6.3; 95% CI = 4.2–9.4; $p < 0.001$) were significantly associated with higher risk of death in Cox proportional hazards regression analysis. Furthermore, analysis of variance showed that higher levels of PIRO score were significantly associated with higher mortality ($p < 0.001$), prolonged length of stay in the ICU ($p < 0.001$), and days of mechanical ventilation ($p < 0.001$). Receiver operating characteristic curves showed that PIRO score (area under the curve [AUC] = 0.88) performed better than APACHE II (AUC = 0.75, $p < 0.001$) and ATS/IDSA criteria (AUC = 0.80, $p < 0.001$) to predict 28-day mortality.

Conclusions.—The PIRO score performed well as 28-day mortality prediction tool in CAP patients requiring ICU admission with a better performance than APACHE II and ATS/IDSA criteria in this subset of patients. Furthermore, PIRO score also is associated with increased healthcare resource utilization in CAP patients admitted in the ICU.

▶ There have been many strategies used to identify those patients with severe community-acquired pneumonia (CAP). Some are quite complex, such as the pneumonia severity index from the PORT database.[1] While others may be relatively simple such as the British Thoracic Society criteria (elevated respiratory rate, elevated BUN, and low blood pressure).[2] Many acronyms depict the criteria used in the scoring system such as CURB-65 and CUROX-85.[3,4] The American Thoracic Society (IDSA) and Infectious Disease Society of America (ATS) have also provided guidance using major and minor criteria.[5] This study used the predisposition, insult, response, organ dysfunction (PIRO) concept from the sepsis consensus conference to derive a scoring system that performed very well for this group of CAP patients cared for in the ICU. As shown in the graphs in the original article, there was good correlation with mortality, days of ventilatory support, and better performance than other predictors of mortality. The assessment was also quite easy to use in addition to performing quite well. Further studies are needed to confirm the predictive value of the PIRO method for severe CAP, but this initial data are quite impressive.

R. A. Balk, MD

References

1. Fine MJ, Auble TE, Yealy DM, et al. A prediction rule to identify low-risk patients with community-acquired pneumonia. *N Engl J Med*. 1997;336:243-250.
2. British Thoracic Society Research Committee. Community-acquired pneumonia in adults in British hospitals in 1982–1983: a survey of aetiology, mortality, prognostic factors, and outcome. *Q J Med*. 1987;62:195-220.
3. Lim WS, van der Eerden MM, Laing R, et al. Defining community acquired pneumonia severity on presentation to hospital. An international derivation and validation study. *Thorax*. 2003;58:377-382.
4. Espana PP, Capelastegui A, Gorordo I, et al. Development and validation of a clinical prediction rule for severe community-acquired pneumonia. *Am J Rspir Crit Care Med*. 2006;174:1249-1256.
5. Mandell LA, Wunderink RG, Anzueto A, et al. Infectious Disease Society of America/American Thoracic Society Consensus Guidelines on the management of community-acquired pneumonia in adults. *Clin Infect Dis*. 2007;44:S27-S72.

Usefulness of the "*Candida* score" for discriminating between *Candida* colonization and invasive candidiasis in non-neutropenic critically ill patients: A prospective multicenter study
León C, on behalf of the Cava Study Group (Hosp Universitario de Valme, Sevilla, Spain; et al)
Crit Care Med 37:1624-1633, 2009

Objective.—To assess the usefulness of the "*Candida* score" (CS) for discriminating between *Candida* species colonization and invasive candidiasis (IC) in non-neutropenic critically ill patients. A rate of IC <5% in patients with CS <3 was the primary end point.

Design.—Prospective, cohort, observational study.

Setting.—Thirty-six medical-surgical intensive care units of Spain, Argentina, and France.

Patients.—A total of 1,107 non-neutropenic adult intensive care unit patients admitted for at least 7 days between April 2006 and June 2007.

Measurements and Main Results.—Clinical data, surveillance cultures for fungal growth, and serum levels of (1–3)-beta-D-glucan and anti-*Candida* antibodies (in a subset of patients) were recorded. The CS was calculated as follows (variables coded as absent $= 0$, present $= 1$): total parenteral nutrition $\times 1$, plus surgery $\times 1$, plus multifocal *Candida* colonization $\times 1$, plus severe sepsis $\times 2$. A CS ≥ 3 accurately selected patients at high risk for IC. The colonization index was registered if ≥ 0.5. The rate of IC was 2.3% (95% confidence interval [CI] 1.06–3.54) among patients with CS <3, with a linear association between increasing values of CS and IC rate ($p \leq 0.001$). The area under the receiver operating characteristic curve for CS was 0.774 (95% CI 0.715–0.832) compared with 0.633 (95% CI 0.557–0.709) for CI. (1–3)-Beta-D-glucan was also an independent predictor of IC (odds ratio 1.004, 95% CI 1.0–1.007). The relative risk for developing IC in colonized patients without antifungal treatment was 6.83 (95% CI 3.81–12.45).

Conclusions.—In this cohort of colonized patients staying >7 days, with a CS <3 and not receiving antifungal treatment, the rate of IC was <5%. Therefore, IC is highly improbable if a *Candida*-colonized non-neutropenic critically ill patient has a CS <3.

▶ Invasive fungal infections in the non-neutropenic ICU patient remain a concern to practicing intensivists. These infections are difficult to detect and occur in patients with complex underlying disease processes. Furthermore, the incidence of these infections including nonalbicans candidal infections is on the rise (up to 10%), and there is evidence to suggest that the delayed treatment of candidemia has a negative effect on mortality.[1-3] The development of a predictive score to determine who is at high risk for invasive candidiasis (IC) would allow clinicians to treat this high-risk group of patients earlier.

Previous models to predict the risk of IC have been cumbersome and not vetted with prospective validation studies. In previous work, the authors of this study have developed a *Candida* score, that in a retrospective study accurately predicted who was at risk for IC. This work is a prospective evaluation of their *Candida* score.

This study confirms the usefulness of the *Candida* score as an accurate discriminator of those patients who are at risk of IC. It is simple to use and has immediate bedside applicability. A *Candida* score < 3 will accurately predict those patients at low risk for IC. Increasing values of the CS and a recent history of abdominal surgery are strong predictors of IC.

A. Kumar, MD

D. Funk, MD, FRCP(C)

References

1. Wisplinghoff H, Bischoff T, Tallent SM, Seifert H, Wenzel RP, Edmond MB. Nosocomial bloodstream infections in US hospitals: analysis of 24,179 cases from a prospective nationwide surveillance study. *Clin Infect Dis.* 2004;39:309-317.
2. Garey KW, Rege M, Pai MP, et al. Time to initiation of fluconazole therapy impacts mortality in patients with candidemia: a multi-institutional study. *Clin Infect Dis.* 2006;43:25-31.
3. Kumar A, Roberts D, Wood KE, et al. Duration of hypotension before initiation of effective antimicrobial therapy is the critical determinant of survival in human septic shock. *Crit Care Med.* 2006;34:1589-1596.

Epidemiology, management, and risk factors for death of invasive *Candida* infections in critical care: A multicenter, prospective, observational study in France (2005–2006)
Leroy O, for the AmarCand Study Group (Centre Hospitalier Gustave Dron, Tourcoing, France; et al)
Crit Care Med 37:1612-1618, 2009

Objective.—To describe the evolving epidemiology, management, and risk factors for death of invasive *Candida* infections in intensive care units (ICUs).

Design.—Prospective, observational, national, multicenter study.

Setting.—One hundred eighty ICUs in France.

Patients.—Between October 2005 and May 2006, 300 adult patients with proven invasive *Candida* infection who received systemic antifungal therapy were included.

Interventions.—None.

Measurements and Main Results.—One hundred seven patients (39.5%) with isolated candidemia, 87 (32.1%) with invasive candidiasis without documented candidemia, and 77 (28.4%) with invasive candidiasis and candidemia were eligible. In 37% of the cases, candidemia occurred within the first 5 days after ICU admission. *C. albicans* accounted for 57.0% of the isolates, followed by *C. glabrata* (16.7%), *C. parapsilosis* (7.5%), *C. krusei* (5.2%), and *C. tropicalis* (4.9%). In 17.1% of the isolates, the causative *Candida* was less susceptible or resistant to fluconazole. Fluconazole was the empirical treatment most commonly introduced (65.7%), followed by caspofungin (18.1%), voriconazole (5.5%), and amphotericin B (3.7%). After identification of the causative species and susceptibility testing results, treatment was modified in 86 patients (31.7%). The case fatality ratio in ICU was 45.9% and did not differ significantly according to the type of episode. Multivariate analysis showed that factors independently associated with death in ICU were type 1 diabetes mellitus (odds ratio [OR] 4.51; 95% confidence interval [CI] 1.72–11.79; $p = 0.002$), immunosuppression (OR 2.63; 95% CI 1.35–5.11; $p = 0.0045$), mechanical ventilation (OR 2.54; 95% CI

1.33–4.82; $p = 0.0045$), and body temperature >38.2°C (reference, 36.5–38.2°C; OR 0.36; 95% CI 0.17–0.77; $p = 0.008$).

Conclusions.—More than two thirds of patients with invasive candidiasis in ICU present with candidemia. Non-*albicans Candida* species reach almost half of the *Candida* isolates. Reduced susceptibility to fluconazole is observed in 17.1% of *Candida* isolates. Mortality of invasive candidiasis in ICU remains high.

▶ Mortality from invasive candidiasis remains exceedingly high. Although several matched cohort studies have described varying attributable mortality rates (5-71%), it remains clear that timely and appropriate antifungal therapy significantly reduces mortality.[1,2] Risk stratifying patients according to risk profiles can aid clinicians in determining both the probability of invasive candidemia and the choice of appropriate antifungal agent.

The study by Leroy and colleagues adds to the growing literature that invasive candidemia in intensive care units results in high case fatality rates. While this study identifies risk factors for invasive disease in mixed populations (ie, immunocompetent and immunocompromised), several uniform conclusions are applicable to the practicing intensivist. Clinicians should recognize that immunocompetent patients who have undergone gastrointestinal surgery, have long-term central venous catheters, and/or receiving total parenteral nutrition are at increased risk for candidemia. Despite the findings by Leroy et al of high mortalities despite central venous catheter removal, several studies have clearly shown benefit in fungal reduction and survival in removal of catheters in these patients.[3,4] Further, physicians should be aware that immunocompromised patients, while at high risk of invasive candidiasis, have higher risk of fluconazole resistant candidemia if recently exposed to fluconazole. Thus, if patients are at risk for candidemia based on the discussed risk factors, empiric therapy should be instituted based on host immune status, requirement of central venous catheter (CVC) removal, and previous receipt of antifungal agents.

A. Kumar, MD

S. Kethireddy, MD

References

1. Falagas ME, Apostolou KE, Pappas VD. Attributable mortality of candidemia: a systematic review of matched cohort and case control studies. *Eur J clin Microbiol Infect Dis.* 2006;25:419-425.
2. Morrel M, Fraser VJ, Kollef MH. Delaying the empiric treatment of candida bloodstream infection until positive blood culture results are obtained: a potential risk factor for hospital mortality. *Antimicrob Agents Chemother.* 2005;49: 3640-3645.
3. Anaissie EJ, Rex JH, Uzun O, Vartivarian S. Predictors of adverse outcome in cancer patients with candidemia. *Am J Med.* 1998;104:238-245.
4. Rex JH, Bennett JE, Sugar AM, et al. Intravascular catheter exchanges and the duration of candidemia. NIAID Mycoses Study Group and the Candidemia Study Group. *Clin Infect Dis.* 1995;21:994-996.

Contamination of Portable Radiograph Equipment With Resistant Bacteria in the ICU

Levin PD, Shatz O, Sviri S, et al (Hebrew Univ-Hadassah Med School, Jerusalem, Israel; et al)
Chest 136:426-432, 2009

Background.—Approximately 15% of nosocomial infections in the ICU result from spread of bacteria on caregivers' hands. The routine chest radiograph provides an unexamined opportunity for bacterial spread: close contact with each patient and sequential examination of ICU patients. This study examined infection control procedures performed during routine chest radiographs, assessed whether resistant bacteria were transferred to the radiograph machine, and determined whether improved infection control practices by radiograph technicians could reduce bacterial transfer.

Methods.—Radiograph technicians were observed performing chest radiographs on all ICU patients. Culture specimens were taken from the radiograph machine. An educational intervention directed at technicians was instituted, and its effect on infection control and machine contamination was measured.

Results.—Surveillance of 173, 113, and 120 chest radiographs during observation, intervention, and follow-up periods was performed. Adequate infection control was practiced during the performance of 2 of 173 observation period radiographs (1%), 48 of 113 intervention period radiographs (42%; $p < 0.001$), and 12 of 120 follow-up period radiographs (10%; ($p < 0.001$) [follow-up vs intervention and observation

TABLE 3.—Bacteriologic Results of Radiograph Machine Culture Samples Obtained at the End of the Daily Radiograph Round

Variables	Observation (Phases 1 and 2)	Intervention (Phase 3)	Follow-up (Phase 4)	p Value* 1	2	3
Culture samples, No.	30	29	14			
Culture result						
Resistant organisms						
A baumannii	5 (17)	0 (0)	4 (29)		2b	
K pneumoniae	6 (20)	0 (0)	4 (29)	1a	2b	
Pseudomonas aeruginosa	1 (3)	0 (0)	0 (0)			
Stenotrophomonas maltophilia	1 (3)	0 (0)	0 (0)			
Resistant Gram negatives†	12 (39)	0 (0)	6 (43)	1c	2c	
VRE	1 (3)	0 (0)	1 (7)			
Nonresistant organisms						
Gram positives	6 (19)	6 (21)	11 (79)		2c	3c
Gram negatives	6 (19)	5 (17)	8 (57)		2c	3b
Culture negative	11 (37)	22 (67)	1 (7)	1b	2c	

Data are presented as No. of isolates cultured (%) unless otherwise indicated.
*Observation vs intervention: 1a, $p < 0.05$; 1b, $p < 0.01$; 1c, $p < 0.001$. Intervention vs follow-up: 2a, $p < 0.05$; 2b, $p < 0.01$; 2c, $p < 0.001$. Observation vs follow-up: 3a, $p < 0.05$; 3b, $p < 0.01$; 3c, $p < 0.001$.
†Total No. of cultures with resistant Gram-negative organism; exceeds number of individual cultures as multiple bacteria grew in single cultures.

periods]. Radiograph machine surface culture samples yielded resistant Gram-negative bacteria on 12 of 30 occasions (39%), 0 of 29 occasions, and 7 of 14 occasions (50%), respectively, for the observation, intervention, and follow-up periods (p < 0.001).

Conclusion.—Multiresistant bacteria are frequently transferred from patients to the radiograph machine in the presence of poor infection control practices, and may be a source of cross-infection/colonization. Improved infection control practices decrease the occurrence of resistant organisms on the radiograph equipment. Radiograph technicians should be included in efforts to improve infection control measures (Table 3).

▶ To have effective infection control measures in the ICU it must be a 24-7-365 operation, and you must understand the full range of potential opportunities for the system to fail. This study has brought forward 2 very important lessons. Most of us have adopted the use of bundles of care to help ensure achievement of desired outcomes. These bundles often focus on the common aspects of management that we are responsible for and often omit the interaction of others, such as the X-ray technician and their equipment, in the infection control strategy. The investigators nicely identified the potential problem during a covert observation period and then confirmed the issue during an overt study period. Armed with the data, the investigators could then educate the X-ray technicians about their potential to contribute to infection spread in the ICU, and this education was successful in reducing the numbers and types of resistant bacteria. Unfortunately, lesson 2 reveals how rapidly humans forget, especially when they are busy trying to accomplish their work and move on to the next area. All of the success from the education phase was lost as the technicians went back to their usual way of business.

In the battle to control infections in the ICU we must adopt a relentless strategy that encompasses all aspects of patient care. Frequent education and surveillance are definitely a requirement for maintenance of successful outcomes.

R. A. Balk, MD

Polymorphisms in innate immunity genes predispose to bacteremia and death in the medical intensive care unit

Henckaerts L, Nielsen KR, Steffensen R, et al (Catholic Univ of Leuven, Belgium; Aalborg Hosp, Denmark; et al)
Crit Care Med 37:192-201, 2009

Objective.—Critically ill patients are at risk of sepsis, organ failure, and death. Studying the impact of genetic determinant may improve our understanding of the pathophysiology and allow identification of patients who would benefit from specific treatments. Our aim was to study the influence of single nucleotide polymorphisms in selected genes involved in innate immunity on the development of bacteremia or risk of death in patients admitted to a medical intensive care unit.

Design, Setting, and Patients.—DNA was available from 774 medical intensive care unit patients. We selected 31 single nucleotide polymorphisms in 14 genes involved in host innate immune defense. Serum levels of MASP2 and chemotactic capacity, phagocytosis, and killing capacity of monocytes at admission were quantified. Univariate Kaplan–Meier estimates with log-rank analysis and multivariate logistic regression were performed. Bootstrap resampling technique and ten-fold cross-validation were used to assess replication stability, prognostic importance of the variables, and repeatability of the final regression model.

Main Results.—Patients with at least one *NOD2* variant were shown to have a reduced phagocytosis by monocytes ($p = 0.03$) and a higher risk of bacteremia than wild-type patients ($p = 0.02$). The *NOD2/TLR4* combination was associated with bacteremia using survival analyses (time to bacteremia development, log-rank $p < 0.0001$), univariate regression ($p = 0.0003$), and multivariate regression analysis (odds ratio [OR] 4.26, 95% confidence interval [CI] 1.85–9.81; $p = 0.0006$). Similarly, the same combination was associated with hospital mortality using survival analysis (log-rank $p = 0.03$), univariate regression ($p = 0.02$), and multivariate regression analysis (OR 2.27, 95% CI 1.09–4.74; $p = 0.03$). Also variants in the *MASP2* gene were significantly associated with hospital mortality (survival analysis log-rank-$p = 0.003$; univariate regression $p = 0.02$; multivariate regression analysis OR 2.35, 95% CI 1.38–3.99; $p = 0.002$).

Conclusions.—Functional polymorphisms in genes involved in innate immunity predispose to severe infections and death, and may become part of a risk model, allowing identification of patients at risk, who could benefit from early introduction of specific preventive or therapeutic interventions.

▶ For years, clinicians and scientists were unable to explain why similar infections in outwardly similar patients could result in disparate outcomes. Adoption and twin studies have demonstrated a strong genetic link to the susceptibility to infection.[1] More recent work has suggested that in some cases, susceptibility to infection can be related to single nucleotide changes in the individual's genetic code. Such single nucleotide polymorphisms (or SNPs) can be associated with variations in genes responsible for the inflammatory response.

Several SNPs have already been identified in genes that code for expression of cytokines such as tumor necrosis factor α (TNFα), interleukin 6 and interleukin 10, and for the toll like receptors.[2] This article by Henckaerts et al is one of the most recent to look at the association of SNPs with the risk of infection. In 774 ICU patients they studied the effects of 31 different SNPs for 14 genes involved in the innate immune response. A combination of an SNP in the *NOD1* gene (nucleotide binding oligomerization domain) and in the toll like receptor 4 (*TLR4*) gene was associated with an increased risk of death.

Numerous studies have been published in recent years looking at these genetic associations. With time, an individual's risk of death from sepsis might be predicted based on their SNP profile, which might also help to tailor therapy.

A. Kumar, MD

D. Funk, MD, FRCP(C)

References

1. Sorensen TI, Nielsen GG, Andersen PK, Teasdale TW. Genetic and environmental influences on premature death in adult adoptees. *N Engl J Med*. 1988;318: 727-732.
2. Lin MT, Albertson TE. Genomic polymorphisms in sepsis. *Crit Care Med*. 2004; 32:569-579.

Severity of Meningococcal Disease Associated with Genomic Bacterial Load
Darton T, Guiver M, Naylor S, et al (Univ of Sheffield, UK; Health Protection Agency, Manchester, UK; et al)
Clin Infect Dis 48:587-594, 2009

Background.—Diagnostic polymerase chain reaction (PCR) detection of *Neisseria meningitidis* has enabled accurate quantification of the bacterial load in patients with meningococcal disease.

Methods.—Quantification of the *N. meningitidis* DNA level by real time-PCR was conducted on whole-blood samples obtained from patients presenting with meningococcal disease to hospitals throughout England and Wales over a 3-year period. Levels were correlated with clinical outcome, infecting serogroup, and host factors including, interleukin-1 genotype (*IL-1*).

Results.—Bacterial loads were available for 1045 patients and were not associated with the age of the patient, delay in sample submission, or administration of antibiotics prior to admission. The median log bacterial load was higher in 95 patients who died (5.29 $\log_{10}$copies/mL; interquartile range, 4.41–6.30 $\log_{10}$copies/mL) than in 950 patients who survived (3.79 $\log_{10}$copies/mL; interquartile range, 2.87–4.71 $\log_{10}$copies/mL). Logistic regression revealed that age (odds ratio, 1.04 per 1-year increase in age) and bacterial load (odds ratio, 2.04 per $\log_{10}$-copies/mL increase) had a statistically significant effect on the risk of death. Infection with *N. meningitidis* serogroup C was associated with increased risk of death and an increased bacterial load. Also associated with a higher bacterial load were prolonged hospitalization (duration, >10 days); digit, limb, or soft-tissue loss; and requirement of hemodialysis. Carriage of *IL-1RN*(+2018) was associated with increased mortality (odds ratio, 2.14; *P* =.07) but not with a higher bacterial load.

Conclusions.—In meningococcal disease, bacterial load is associated with likelihood of death, development of permanent disease sequelae, and prolonged hospitalization. The bacterial load was relatively higher in patients infected with *N. meningitidis* serogroup C than in those infected with other serogroups. The effects of age and *IL-1* genotype on mortality are independent of a high genomic bacterial load.

▶ Meningococcal disease remains a major worldwide health problem. Recent epidemics in Africa, New Zealand, Singapore as well as the international outbreak of *Neisseria meningitidis* W135 following the Hajj pilgrimage in 2000 and 2001 highlight the ongoing threat of disease.[1] The sensitivity of detection for meningococcal disease has markedly improved with the use of polymerase chain reaction (PCR). With sensitivity and specificity rates greater than 90%, this technique has proven to be particularly useful for confirmation of diagnosis in situations of previous antibiotic administration.[2]

Darton and colleagues studied the association between quantitative bacterial loads of *N meningitidis* in clinical samples with outcome. As previously shown by Hackett et al, this study confirmed the prognostic value of high bacterial loads in predicting poor outcome.[3] While bacterial DNA identification and elimination was unaffected by previous antibiotic administration, appropriate therapy and time to presentation, the data illustrate that untreated infection can result in rapid doubling times (within hours) and increased severity of illness. PCR testing while highly sensitive is not readily available at most centers. Given the rapidity of organism expansion with *N meningitidis* and data showing poor outcomes with delayed therapy (measured in hours) in septic shock,[4] early clinical suspicion and early appropriate empiric therapy remain the cornerstones to effective treatment.

A. Kumar, MD

S. Kethireddy, MD

References

1. Mandell G, Bennett JE, Dolin R, eds. *Principles and Practices of Infectious Diseases*. 6th ed. Philadelphia, PA: Elsevier; 2006.
2. Cummings KC, Louie J, Probert WS, et al. Increased detection of meningococcalinfections in California using a polymerase chain reaction assay. *Clin Infect Dis*. 2008;46:1124-1126.
3. Hackett SJ, Guiver M, Marsh J, et al. Meningococcal bacterial DNA load at presentation correlates with disease severity. *Arch Dis Child*. 2002;86:44-46.
4. Kumar A, Roberts D, Wood K, et al. Duration of hypotension before initiation of effective antimicrobial therapy is the critical determinant of survival in human septic shock. *Crit Care Med*. 2006;34:1589-1596.

Chlorhexidine-Impregnated Sponges and Less Frequent Dressing Changes for Prevention of Catheter-Related Infections in Critically Ill Adults: A Randomized Controlled Trial

Timsit J-F, Schwebel C, Bouadma L, et al (Univ Joseph Fourier, Grenoble CEDEX, France; Albert Michallon Univ Hosp, Grenoble, France; Bichat-Claude Bernard Univ Hosp, Paris, France; et al)
JAMA 301:1231-1241, 2009

Context.—Use of a chlorhexidine gluconate–impregnated sponge (CHGIS) in intravascular catheter dressings may reduce catheter-related infections (CRIs). Changing catheter dressings every 3 days may be more frequent than necessary.

Objective.—To assess superiority of CHGIS dressings regarding the rate of major CRIs (clinical sepsis with or without bloodstream infection) and noninferiority (less than 3% colonization-rate increase) of 7-day vs 3-day dressing changes.

Design, Setting, and Patients.—Assessor-blind, 2 × 2 factorial, randomized controlled trial conducted from December 2006 through June 2008 and recruiting patients from 7 intensive care units in 3 university and 2 general hospitals in France. Patients were adults (>18 years) expected to require an arterial catheter, central-vein catheter, or both inserted for 48 hours or longer.

Interventions.—Use of CHGIS vs standard dressings (controls). Scheduled change of unsoiled adherent dressings every 3 vs every 7 days, with immediate change of any soiled or leaking dressings.

Main Outcome Measures.—Major CRIs for comparison of CHGIS vs control dressings; colonization rate for comparison of 3- vs 7-day dressing changes.

Results.—Of 2095 eligible patients, 1636 (3778 catheters, 28 931 catheter-days) could be evaluated. The median duration of catheter insertion was 6 (interquartile range [IQR], 4-10) days. There was no interaction between the interventions. Use of CHGIS dressings decreased the rates of major CRIs (10/1953 [0.5%], 0.6 per 1000 catheter-days vs 19/1825 [1.1%], 1.4 per 1000 catheter-days; hazard ratio [HR], 0.39 [95% confidence interval {CI}, 0.17-0.93]; $P = .03$) and catheter-related bloodstream infections (6/1953 catheters, 0.40 per 1000 catheter-days vs 17/1825 catheters, 1.3 per 1000 catheter-days; HR, 0.24 [95% CI, 0.09-0.65]). Use of CHGIS dressings was not associated with greater resistance of bacteria in skin samples at catheter removal. Severe CHGIS-associated contact dermatitis occurred in 8 patients (5.3 per 1000 catheters). Use of CHGIS dressings prevented 1 major CRI per 117 catheters. Catheter colonization rates were 142 of 1657 catheters (7.8%) in the 3-day group (10.4 per 1000 catheter-days) and 168 of 1828 catheters (8.6%) in the 7-day group (11.0 per 1000 catheter-days), a mean absolute difference of 0.8%(95% CI, −1.78% to 2.15%) (HR, 0.99; 95% CI, 0.77-1.28), indicating noninferiority of 7-day changes. The median number of dressing changes per catheter was 4(IQR, 3-6) in the 3-day group and 3 (IQR, 2-5) in the 7-day group ($P < .001$).

Conclusions.—Use of CHGIS dressings with intravascular catheters in the intensive care unit reduced risk of infection even when background infection rates were low. Reducing the frequency of changing unsoiled adherent dressings from every 3 days to every 7 days modestly reduces the total number of dressing changes and appears safe.

▶ What intervention will take us to the pinnacle step to free our ICUs of catheter-related blood stream infections (CRBSIs)? Education, barrier precautions, chlorhexidine for skin antisepsis, use of the subclavian site, removal of unnecessary catheters, surveillance, and feedback have done wonders in decreasing the rate of infection in our institution. Decreasing the rate of CRBSIs even in centers with a rate that appears to be low can be of benefit in reducing the rate further.

This randomized controlled trial was conducted in France to evaluate the superiority of a chlorhexidine gluconate-impregnated sponge (CHGIS) in reducing intravascular infections and an assessment of noninferiority of 7-day versus 3-day dressing changes. The authors concluded that CHGIS dressings decreased the rate of major catheter-related infections (CRIs) when the baseline is already low. Additionally, reducing the frequency of dressing changes from every 3 days to 7 days appears to be safe as long as the dressings are monitored and changed if soiled or if a separation occurs. This study included more than 2000 subjects from 7 ICUs in 5 different hospitals demonstrating a combination of patients and staff.

There are several limitations in this study, which may impact how the results may be transferred to other centers. The authors did not have 2% chlorhexidine available for skin antisepsis, which may have further reduced the CRI rate in this study. Compliance with bundled care in prevention of infection was not measured in this study. Venkatram and colleagues report that the application of bundled care to prevent infection was shown to decrease their CRBSI rates from 10.77 to 1.67 per 1000 central line days.[1] We practice infection prevention bundled care and integrate central venous catheter insertion simulation education in my institution to help prevent CRBSI. In a study by Barsuk et al, using a simulation based central venous insertion training course has been effective in decreasing the rate of CRBSI.[2]

New therapies and devices continue to be studied in an attempt to bring the CRI rate to zero. The cost effectiveness and significant decrease in CRI using impregnated central venous catheters, use of special central catheter caps, or the use of special composite dressings continues to be evaluated. A review by Hockenhull et al points toward future studies needing to place more emphasis in determining if the clinical effectiveness of these new therapies are at all impacted by the centers where infection prevention bundles of care are incorporated as routine practice.[3] Additional studies using a standardized the definition of CRBSI along with monitoring of the effective use of the bundles, while studying new devices and dressing techniques requires further research.

C. A. Schorr, RN, MSN

References

1. Barsuk JH, Cohen ER, Feinglass J, McGaghie WC, Wayne DB. Use of simulation-based education to reduce catheter-related bloodstream infections. *Arch Intern Med.* 2009;169:1420-1423.
2. Venkatram S, Rachmale S, Kanna B. Study of device use adjusted rates in health care-associated infections after implementation of "bundles" in a closed-model medical intensive care unit. *J Crit Care.* 2009 Aug 12; [Epub ahead of print].
3. Hockenhull JC, Dwan KM, Smith GW, et al. The clinical effectiveness of central venous catheters treated with anti-infective agents in preventing catheter-related bloodstream infections: a systematic review. *Crit Care Med.* 2009;37:702-712.

Chlorhexidine-Impregnated Sponges and Less Frequent Dressing Changes for Prevention of Catheter-Related Infections in Critically III Adults: A Randomized Controlled Trial

Timsit J-F, for the Dressing Study Group (Univ Joseph Fourier, France; et al)
JAMA 301:1231-1241, 2009

Context.—Use of a chlorhexidine gluconate–impregnated sponge (CHGIS) in intravascular catheter dressings may reduce catheter-related infections (CRIs). Changing catheter dressings every 3 days may be more frequent than necessary.

Objective.—To assess superiority of CHGIS dressings regarding the rate of major CRIs (clinical sepsis with or without bloodstream infection) and noninferiority (less than 3% colonization-rate increase) of 7-day vs 3-day dressing changes.

Design, Setting, and Patients.—Assessor-blind, 2 × 2 factorial, randomized controlled trial conducted from December 2006 through June 2008 and recruiting patients from 7 intensive care units in 3 university and 2 general hospitals in France. Patients were adults (>18 years) expected to require an arterial catheter, central-vein catheter, or both inserted for 48 hours or longer.

Interventions.—Use of CHGIS vs standard dressings (controls). Scheduled change of unsoiled adherent dressings every 3 vs every 7 days, with immediate change of any soiled or leaking dressings.

Main Outcome Measures.—Major CRIs for comparison of CHGIS vs control dressings; colonization rate for comparison of 3- vs 7-day dressing changes.

Results.—Of 2095 eligible patients, 1636 (3778 catheters, 28 931 catheter-days) could be evaluated. The median duration of catheter insertion was 6 (interquartile range [IQR], 4-10) days. There was no interaction between the interventions. Use of CHGIS dressings decreased the rates of major CRIs (10/1953 [0.5%], 0.6 per 1000 catheter-days vs 19/1825

[1.1%], 1.4 per 1000 catheter-days; hazard ratio [HR], 0.39 [95% confidence interval {CI}, 0.17-0.93]; $P = .03$) and catheter-related bloodstream infections (6/1953 catheters, 0.40 per 1000 catheter-days vs 17/1825 catheters, 1.3 per 1000 catheter-days; HR, 0.24 [95% CI, 0.09-0.65]). Use of CHGIS dressings was not associated with greater resistance of bacteria in skin samples at catheter removal. Severe CHGIS-associated contact dermatitis occurred in 8 patients (5.3 per 1000 catheters). Use of CHGIS dressings prevented 1 major CRI per 117catheters.Catheter colonization rates were 142 of 1657 catheters (7.8%) in the 3-day group (10.4 per 1000 catheter-days) and 168 of 1828 catheters (8.6%) in the 7-day group (11.0 per 1000 catheter-days), a mean absolute difference of 0.8%(95% CI, −1.78% to 2.15%) (HR, 0.99; 95% CI, 0.77-1.28), indicating noninferiority of 7-day changes. The median number of dressing changes per catheter was 4(IQR, 3-6) in the 3-day group and 3 (IQR, 2-5) in the 7-day group ($P<.001$).

TABLE 1.—Patient Characteristics

Characteristic	All Patients, ITT Analysis (N = 1636)	Dressing Control (n = 819)	Dressing CHGIS (n = 817)	Dressing Change Interval 3 d (n = 818)	Dressing Change Interval 7 d (n = 818)
Age, median (IQR), y	62 (50-74)	63 (50-74)	62 (50-73)	62 (50-74)	62 (50-73)
Men	1052 (64.3)	518 (63.2)	534 (65.4)	542 (66.3)	510 (62.3)
≥1 Chronic disease	536 (32.8)	288 (35.2)	248 (30.4)	269 (32.9)	267 (32.6)
Immune deficiency	93 (5.7)	48 (5.9)	45 (5.6)	50 (6.2)	43 (5.3)
Hematologic malignancy	52 (3.2)	28 (3.4)	24 (3)	28 (3.5)	24 (2.9)
Metastatic cancer	64 (3.9)	33 (4)	31 (3.8)	28 (3.5)	36 (4.4)
AIDS	54 (3.3)	30 (3.7)	24 (3)	24 (3)	30 (3.7)
SAPS II, median (IQR)[a]	53 (40-65)	53 (40-67)	52 (40-65)	52 (40-67)	53 (40-65)
SOFA, median (IQR)[b]	12 (9-15)	12 (9-15)	12 (9-15)	12 (9-15)	12 (9-15)
Admission category					
Medical	1143 (69.9)	568 (69.4)	575 (70.4)	578 (70.7)	565 (69)
Scheduled surgery	107 (6.5)	66 (8.1)	41 (5.0)	50 (6.1)	57 (7)
Emergency surgery	386 (23.6)	185 (22.5)	201 (24.6)	190 (23.2)	196 (24)
Main reason for ICU admission					
Septic shock	349 (21.3)	163 (19.9)	186 (22.8)	180 (22)	169 (20.7)
Cardiogenic shock	155 (9.5)	66 (8.1)	89 (10.9)	80 (9.8)	75 (9.2)
De novo respiratory failure	326 (19.9)	167 (20.4)	159 (19.5)	160 (19.6)	166 (20.3)
Coma	225 (13.8)	115 (14)	110 (13.5)	107 (13.1)	118 (14.4)
Trauma	178 (10.9)	84 (10.3)	94 (11.5)	83 (10.1)	95 (11.6)
Mechanical ventilation	1411 (86.9)	693 (85.1)	718 (88.8)	689 (85.3)	722 (88.6)
Length of ICU stay, median (IQR), d	11 (5-22)	10 (5-21)	12 (5-25)	10 (5-22)	11 (5-23)
ICU death	549 (33.6)	280 (34.2)	269 (32.9)	261 (31.9)	288 (35.2)
Hospital death	645 (39.4)	333 (40.7)	312 (38.2)	314 (38.4)	331 (40.5)

Abbreviations: AIDS, acquired immunodeficiency syndrome; CHGIS, chlorhexidine gluconate–impregnated sponge; ICU, intensive care unit; IQR, interquartile range; ITT, intention-to-treat; SAPS II, Simplified Acute Physiology Score II; SOFA, Sequential Organ Failure Assessment.
[a]Range of possible scores, 0-162.
[b]Range of possible scores, 0-24.

TABLE 3.—Hazard Ratios in the Intention-To-Treat and Per-Protocol Analyses

	Dressing						Dressing Change Interval					
	Incidence, No./1000 Catheter-Days		ITT Analysis		Per-Protocol Analysis[a]		Incidence, No./1000 Catheter-Days		ITT Analysis		Per-Protocol Analysis[a]	
Variable	Control (n = 1825)	CHGIS (n = 1953)	HR (95% CI)	P Value	HR (95% CI)	P Value	3 d (n = 1815)	7 d (n = 1963)	HR (95% CI)	P Value	HR (95% CI)	P Value
Catheter colonization >10 CFUs/plate	15.8	6.3	0.36 (0.28-0.46)	<.001	0.35 (0.27-0.45)	<.001	10.4	11.0	0.99 (0.77-1.28)	.95	0.99 (0.77-1.28)	.95
Catheter-related bloodstream infection	1.3	0.4	0.24 (0.09-0.65)	.005	0.24 (0.09-0.63)	.004	0.7	0.9	1.26 (0.47-3.34)	.65	1.28 (0.48-3.40)	.62
Major catheter-related infection	1.4	0.6	0.39 (0.16-0.93)	.03	0.38 (0.16-0.92)	.03	0.9	1.1	1.16 (0.50-2.69)	.74	1.18 (0.51-2.73)	.70

Abbreviations: CFU, colony-forming unit; CHGIS, chlorhexidine gluconate–impregnated sponge; CI, confidence interval; HR, hazard ratio; ITT, intention-to-treat.
[a]Analysis adjusted on imbalanced parameters (ie, presence of ≥1 chronic disease for comparison of control and CHGIS groups).

TABLE 5.—Relationship Between Semiquantitative Skin Culture and Study Groups[a]

Culture	All Catheters (n = 2903)	Dressing Control (n = 1358)	CHGIS (n = 1545)	Dressing Change Interval 3 d (n = 1386)	7 d (n = 1517)
Sterile	1887 (65.0)	786 (57.8)	1101 (71.3)	935 (67.5)	952 (62.7)
1-9 CFUs/plate	326 (11.2)	148 (10.9)	178 (11.5)	168 (12.1)	158 (10.4)
10-99 CFUs/ plate	462 (15.9)	261 (19.2)	201 (13)	183 (13.2)	279 (18.4)
≥100 CFUs/ plate	228 (7.90)	163 (12)	65 (4.2)	100 (7.2)	128 (8.4)

Abbreviations: CFU, colony-forming unit; CHGIS, chlorhexidine gluconate–impregnated sponge.
[a]Missing data: all catheters, 875; control dressings, 467; CHGIS dressings, 408; 3-day dressing change interval, 429; 7-day dressing change interval, 446. $P<.01$ for comparisons between CHGIS and control dressings (χ^2 for trends); $P<.01$ for comparisons between 3-day and 7-day dressing changes (χ^2 for trends).

Conclusions.—Use of CHGIS dressings with intravascular catheters in the intensive care unit reduced risk of infection even when background infection rates were low. Reducing the frequency of changing unsoiled adherent dressings from every 3 days to every 7 days modestly reduces the total number of dressing changes and appears safe.

Trial Registration.—clinicaltrials.gov Identifier: NCT00417235

▶ This is an important study investigating the benefits of a chlorhexidine-impregnated sponge for the prevention of catheter-related infections. The data showed a benefit to the sponges for catheter colonization and catheter-related bloodstream infections (Table 3). The authors found no statistical difference if the dressing was changed on a 7-day cycle as compared with a 3-day cycle supporting the need for less often changes. Caution however is warranted before change in practice as there are some important potential limitations to the study. Approximately 45% of dressing changes actually occurred before the planned interval. The intention to treat analysis assumed that any catheter not cultured was not colonized, and I would have liked for the authors to have stacked the deck against their hypothesis and assumed that uncultured catheters were actually positive. Assessment of the induction of resistance to chlorhexidine was not possible under these study conditions, but could be an extremely important long-term impact that could prove devastating for infection control in general. Table 3 shows that the rates of catheter colonization and catheter-related bloodstream infections were higher, and although not statistically different, this may have clinical importance. Table 5 supports the concern that longer intervals between dressing changes is associated with higher colonization counts, and the higher mortality seen in the group (Table 1) is also concerning. Thus, although these findings are clearly important and may lead to practice change in the future, it would seem prudent to await further data.

T. Dorman, MD

Fulminant *Clostridium difficile* Colitis: Patterns of Care and Predictors of Mortality

Sailhamer EA, Carson K, Chang Y, et al (Massachusetts General Hosp, Boston)
Arch Surg 144:433-439, 2009

Hypothesis.—There exist predictors of mortality and the need for colectomy among patients with fulminant *Clostridium difficile* colitis.

Design.—Retrospective study.

Setting.—Academic tertiary referral center.

Patients.—We reviewed the records of 4796 inpatients diagnosed as having *C difficile* colitis from January 1, 1996, to December 31, 2007, and identified 199 (4.1%) with fulminant *C difficile* colitis, as defined by the need for colectomy or admission to the intensive care unit for *C difficile* colitis.

Main Outcome Measures.—Risk of inpatient mortality was determined by multivariate analysis according to clinical predictors, colectomy, and medical team.

Results.—The inhospital mortality rate for fulminant *C difficile* colitis was 34.7%. Independent predictors of mortality included the following: (1) age of 70 years or older, (2) severe leukocytosis or leukopenia (white blood cell count, $\geq 35\,000/\mu L$ or $<4000/\mu L$) or bandemia (neutrophil bands, $\geq 10\%$), and (3) cardiorespiratory failure (intubation or vasopressors). When all 3 factors were present, the mortality rate was 57.1%; when all 3 were absent, the mortality rate was 0%. Patients who underwent colectomy had a trend toward decreased mortality rates (odds ratio, 0.49; 95% confidence interval, 0.21-1.1; $P = .08$). Among patients admitted primarily for fulminant *C difficile* colitis, care in the surgical department compared with the nonsurgical department resulted in a higher rate of operation (85.1% vs 11.2%; $P < .001$) and lower mortality rates (12.8% vs 39.3%; $P = .001$). Patients admitted directly to the surgical department had a shorter mean (SD) interval from admission to operation (0 vs 1.7 [2.8] days; $P = .001$).

Conclusions.—Despite awareness and treatment, fulminant *C difficile* colitis remains a highly lethal disease. Reliable predictors of mortality exist and should be used to prompt aggressive surgical intervention. Survival rates are higher in patients who were cared for by surgical vs nonsurgical departments, possibly because of more frequent and earlier operations.

▶ *Clostridium difficile* infection (CDI) is now considered to be one of the most important causes of health care associated morbidity. An estimated 15 000 to 20 000 patients die from CDI every year.[1] The alarming increase in fulminant CDI initially described at the University of Pittsburgh in 2002 was the first in a series of reports describing the continuous rise and severity of CDI.[2]

The retrospective review conducted by Sailhamer et al confirms the high rate of mortality associated with fulminant CDI. The predictors of severity (age greater than 70, brisk leukocytosis/leucopenia, cardiorespiratory compromise) are important to note for the practicing intensivist. While the rapidity of progression was not discussed in this article, the data suggest that an elevated clinical suspicion of a surgical abdomen resulted in admission to a surgical unit, earlier time to colectomy, and improved survival. The increased mortality among patients who had a delayed time to colectomy compels us to use these clinical predictors of fulminant CDI. Early identification of severe illness mandates that physicians advocate for early surgical management along with prompt administration of oral vancomycin in these patients.

A. Kumar, MD

S. Kethireddy, MD

References

1. Rupnik M, Wilcox MH, Gerding DN. *Clostridium difficile* infection: new developments in epidemiology and pathogenesis. *Nat Rev Microbiol.* 2009;7:526-536.
2. Dallal RM, Harbrecht BG, Boujoukas AJ, et al. Fuliminant *Clostridium difficile*: an underappreciated and increasing cause of death and complications. *Ann Surg.* 2002;235:363-372.

Analysis of an outbreak of *Clostridium difficile* infection controlled with enhanced infection control measures
Salgado CD, Mauldin PD, Fogle PJ, et al (Med Univ of South Carolina, Charleston)
Am J Infect Control 37:458-464, 2009

Background.—In October 2004, our *Clostridium difficile* infection (CDI) rate increased (relative risk, 3.51; 95% confidence interval: 2.96-4.16) from a baseline rate of 1.35 per 1000 patient-days. We describe the outbreak, the relationship between antibiotic use and CDI, and the effect of enhanced infection control measures (EICM) on CDI.

Methods.—Rates were calculated as positive *C difficile* toxin A or B tests among patients with nosocomial diarrhea per 1000 patient-days (duplicates removed). Antibiotic use was calculated as defined daily dose per 1000 patient-days. EICM consisted of (1) placing patients with diarrhea into empiric Contact Precautions, (2) cleaning with a bleach product in areas with CDI patients, and (3) requiring soap and water hand hygiene when caring for CDI patients. CDI rates were analyzed by χ^2 for trend. Time series methodology was used to examine the association between CDI and antibiotic use.

Results.—During the outbreak (October 2004-May 2005), we observed 144 excess cases of CDI. The CDI rate decreased after EICM were implemented ($P < .0001$) and has been maintained for 36 months beyond the outbreak. Multivariate analysis revealed positive associations between CDI rates and cefazolin use ($P = .008$) and levofloxacin/gatifloxacin use ($P = .015$).

Conclusion.—Despite an association between some antibiotic use and CDI rates, we achieved sustained control of an outbreak using EICM

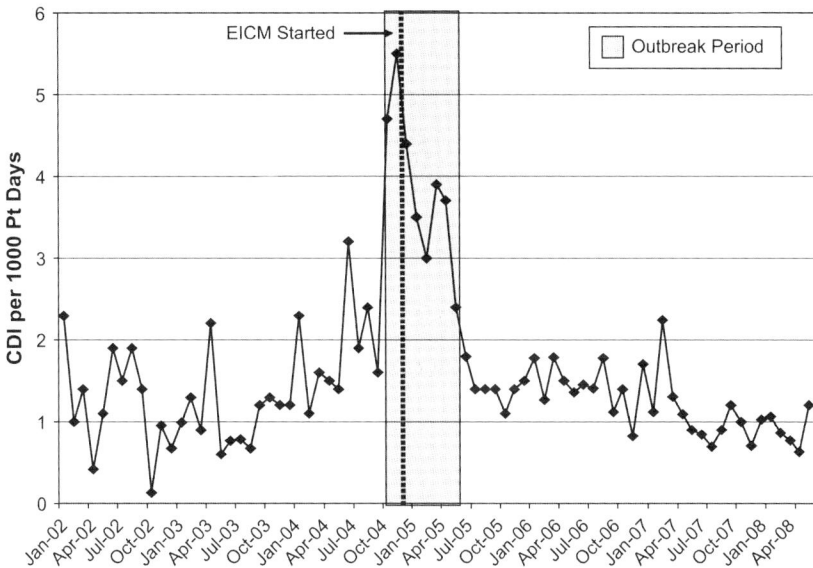

FIGURE 1.—Monthly CDI rates before, during, and after the outbreak period. CDI rates decreased significantly after EICM were implemented, χ^2 for trend $P < .0001$. (Reprinted from Salgado CD, Mauldin PD, Fogle PJ, et al. Analysis of an outbreak of *Clostridium difficile* infection controlled with enhanced infection control measures. *Am J Infect Control*. 2009;37:458-464.)

without formulary changes or new antibiotic control policies. This suggests that patient-to-patient spread may be a more important cause of increased CDI rates (Fig 1).

▶ *Clostridium difficile* infection (CDI) affects millions of hospitalized patients every year in the United States. Estimates indicate that as many as 10% of patients hospitalized for more than 2 days are affected by CDI. CDI has also been associated with significant morbidity, increased costs of care, and increased mortality. More recently, the incidence of CDI has been increasing, and a new strain of *C difficile* with increased virulence has caused multiple outbreaks in North America. CDI has also become an increasing problem in critically ill patients in the intensive care unit. In this study, Salgado and collaborators analyzed an outbreak of *C difficile* infection in their hospital and evaluated the impact of enhanced infection control measures (EICM) on controlling this outbreak. The investigators report an outbreak with an increase in cases from 1.35 per 1000 patient-days to 4.74 cases per 1000 patient-days. During this time, EICM were implemented and all cases were followed. EICM implemented during the outbreak consisted of (1) placing patients with diarrhea into empiric Contact Precautions until CDI was ruled out as a cause of diarrhea, (2) cleaning equipment and the environment with a bleach product in areas occupied by CDI patients, and (3) requiring soap and water for hand hygiene among health care providers when caring for patients with CDI (rather than alcohol hand gel). All the elements of the EICM were fully implemented at once. The investigators found that there was significant decrease immediately after the implementation of EICM and that this decrease persisted for a 33-month period follow-up (Fig 1). The investigators also evaluated antibiotic use in correlation with the increase in the CDI rate. They concluded that the use of cefazolin and fluoroquinolones (gatifloxacin-levofloxacin) were independently associated with an increased rate of CDI. Of interest, no modifications were done to antibiotic practices. This article adds important information to our understanding of CDI. CDI has become an increasingly common problem in intensive care units; it becomes very important for intensivists to understand what are the measures that can have impact in controlling the rate of *C difficile* infection. This study suggests that enhanced intervention control measures are sufficient to control outbreaks and more importantly have a long sustained effect on keeping the incidence of CDI low. Whether further benefit is obtained from antibiotic stewardship, along with a more controlled prescription pattern, is not determined by this study.

S. L. Zanotti-Cavazzoni, MD

Active cytomegalovirus infection is common in mechanically ventilated medical intensive care unit patients
Chiche L, Forel J-M, Roch A, et al (Université de la Méditerranée, Marseille, France)
Crit Care Med 37:1850-1857, 2009

Objective.—To assess the incidence, risk factors, and outcome of active cytomegalovirus (CMV) infection in nonimmunosuppressed intensive care unit (ICU) patients.

Design.—Prospective epidemiologic study.

Setting.—A medical ICU in a university hospital.

Patients.—Two hundred forty-two nonimmunosuppressed ICU patients mechanically ventilated for ≥ 2 days.

Interventions.—Routine pp65 antigenemia and serology for CMV were performed at admission, and then weekly. Bronchoalveolar lavage viral cultures were done when pneumonia was suspected.

Measurements and Main Results.—Thirty-nine of the 242 ICU patients (16.1%, confidence interval 11.5% to 20.7%) developed an active CMV infection, as diagnosed by positive antigenemia (85%) and/or positive rapid viral culture in bronchoalveolar lavage (26%). Antiviral treatment was initiated in 21 (54%) patients. ICU mortality (54% vs. 37%, $p = 0.082$) and in-hospital mortality (59% vs. 41%, $p = 0.058$) were increased in patients with active CMV infection, as compared with those without active CMV infection. Active CMV infection and Simplified Acute Physiology Score II at admission were associated with ICU death on multivariate analysis. The patients with active CMV infection had longer mechanical ventilation and longer ICU stay and were significantly more prone to developing bacterial nosocomial infections ($p < 0.001$). Logistic regression analysis showed that prior admission to other wards

TABLE 5.—ICU Patient Outcomes

	CMV Infection		
	Yes (n = 39)	No (n = 203)	*p*
ICU mortality, n (%)	21 (54)	76 (37)	0.082
In-hospital mortality, n (%)	23 (59)	84 (41)	0.058
ICU length of stay (d) median (IQR)	32 (18–47)	12 (7–21)	<0.001
Ventilator-free days and alive at day 28, median (IQR)	0 (0–0)	2 (0–19)	<0.001
Ventilator-free days and alive at day 60, median (IQR)	0 (0–23.25)	34 (0–51)	<0.001
Length of mechanical ventilation in survivors (d), median (IQR)	27 (19–44)	10 (5–19)	<0.001
At least one bacterial VAP, n(%)[a]	22 (56)	47 (23)	<0.001
At least one bacteremia, n (%)[a]	10 (26)	23 (11)	0.033
At least one urinary tract infection, n (%)[a]	4 (10)	13 (6)	0.61
At least one catheter-related infection, n (%)[a]	4 (10)	7 (3)	0.14
At least one bacterial nosocomial infection, n (%)[a]	27 (69)	68 (33)	<0.001
Shock, n (%)	27 (69)	126 (62)	0.50
ARDS, n (%)	17 (44)	59 (29)	0.11
Acute renal failure requiring renal replacement therapy, n (%)	15 (38)	44 (22)	0.042
Antiviral therapy directed against Herpesviridae, n (%)	21 (54)	9 (4)	<0.001
Aciclovir	0 (0)	7 (3)	0.52
Ganciclovir	20 (51)	1 (0.5)	<0.001
Foscarnet	1 (3)	0 (0)	0.36
Valaciclovir	0 (0)	1 (0.5)	0.35

ICU, intensive care unit; IQR, interquartile range; VAP, ventilator-associated pneumonia; ARDS, acute respiratory distress syndrome.
[a]Bacterial nosocomial infections diagnosed during ICU stay.

($p = 0.043$; odds ratio [OR], 2.49), blood transfusions ($p = 0.04$; OR, 3.31), enteral feeding ($p = 0.005$; OR, 3.00), recent corticosteroid use before ICU admission ($p = 0.08$; OR, 2.26), and age ($p = 0.07$; OR, 1.026) were associated with the occurrence of active CMV infection.

Conclusions.—Active CMV infection is common among previously healthy patients under mechanical ventilation in a medical ICU. Further studies are needed to evaluate the role of antiviral treatments to reduce both the incidence and the outcome impact of active CMV infection.

▶ While the observation of cytomegalovirus (CMV) in the airways of immuno-compromised patients is not new, the findings of this study do cause intensivists to change their usual thoughts concerning the types of organisms and the treatment of critically ill mechanically ventilated patients. Finding evidence of CMV in 16% of the patients involved in this observational cohort is indeed surprising. Additionally, as seen in Table 5, the impact of the CMV is also impressive. Keep in mind that not all of the CMV was treated by the attending physicians, so the true impact of the isolation of CMV in a ventilated patient remains to be seen, but suffice to say the preliminary observations from this report give us a healthy respect for acquisition of this virus in immunocompetent ventilated patients.

R. A. Balk, MD

Prevalence and mortality associated with cytomegalovirus infection in nonimmunosuppressed patients in the intensive care unit
Kalil AC, Florescu DF (Univ of Nebraska Med Ctr, Omaha)
Crit Care Med 37:2350-2358, 2009

Introduction.—Cytomegalovirus is the most common viral opportunistic infection in immunocompromised patients. However, recent studies have demonstrated active cytomegalovirus infection in nonimmunosuppressed intensive care unit patients.

Objective.—To define the frequency and mortality rate associated with cytomegalovirus infection in nonimmunosuppressed patients in the intensive care unit.

Methods.—A systematic review up to October 2008 was performed. Pooled results were analyzed by fixed- and random-effects models. Cochran Q and I^2 were performed for heterogeneity.

Results.—Thirteen studies (n = 1258) were selected. The overall rate of active cytomegalovirus infection was 17% (95% confidence interval [CI], 11% to 24%; $p < .0001$; $I^2 = 86\%$). When the patients were screened for ≥5 intensive care unit days, the overall rate of infection increased to 21% (95% CI, 15% to 29%; $p < .001$). The infection rate for studies that used cytomegalovirus DNA/antigen for diagnosis was 20% (95% CI, 13% to 31%; $p < .0001$) and for studies that used culture was 12% (95% CI, 6% to 22%; $p < .0001$). The cytomegalovirus rate for patients with unknown serology was 7% (95% CI, 3% to 14%; $p < .0001$), whereas the rate for patients with positive serology was 31% (95% CI, 22% to 42%; $p < .0001$). The rate of infection was higher in patients with severe sepsis: 32% (95% CI, 22% to 45%; $p < .0001$). And in patients with high disease severity: 32% (95% CI, 23% to 42%; $p < .0001$). The overall mortality rate associated with active cytomegalovirus infection was 1.93 times (95% CI, 1.29 to 2.88; $p = .001$) as high as that without cytomegalovirus infection.

Conclusions.—Active cytomegalovirus infection occurs frequently in nonimmunosuppressed patients in intensive care, especially in those with positive cytomegalovirus serology, intensive care unit stay ≥5 days, severe sepsis, and high disease severity, in whom the rate of cytomegalovirus infection is up to 36%. Mortality rate is significantly doubled with cytomegalovirus, but a cause-effect relationship cannot be established yet. A large prospective cohort study on the patient population identified by our findings is needed to define who is at the highest risk for developing active cytomegalovirus infection and to determine its effects on mortality.

▶ Cytomegalovirus (CMV) is the most common viral pathogen isolated from immunocompromised hosts. There is increasing evidence that CVM infection (either reactivation or de novo infection) may be common in nonimmunosuppressed ICU patients. The authors of this article conducted a systematic review of the literature and a meta-analysis to evaluate both the prevalence and the mortality of immunocompetent patients in the ICU who had active CMV infection (detected by either viral culture, CMV DNA, or the presence of the CMV antigen pp65). Thirteen studies that included a total of 1258 patients were included in the analysis.

This article amalgamates several articles that have described the presence of active CMV infection in nonimmunosuppressed ICU patients.[1-3] Interestingly, this infection appears to be present in a significant fraction (17%) only in patients who have been in the ICU for ≥5 days. In studies where patients were screened for <5 days, the rate of CMV infection was only 1%. This could be related to either the severity of disease in the patients in the ICU for ≥5 days, or the natural life cycle of the virus.

The almost 2-fold increase in mortality was also an interesting finding. Other studies have shown that CMV infection has resulted in higher numbers of nosocomial infections, and longer ICU and hospital stays. The study does not, however, answer the question as to whether or not CMV infection is a causative factor in the increased mortality, or if it is a marker of disease severity. To truly answer this question, a randomized controlled trial comparing treatment of active CMV infection with placebo must be conducted.

A. Kumar, MD

D. Funk, MD, FRCP(C)

References

1. Jaber S, Chanques G, Borry J, et al. Cytomegalovirus infection in critically ill patients: associated factors and consequences. *Chest.* 2005;127:233-241.
2. Limaye AP, Kirby KA, Rubenfeld GD, et al. Cytomegalovirus reactivation in critically ill immunocompetent patients. *JAMA.* 2008;300:413-422.
3. von Müller L, Klemm A, Weiss M, et al. Active cytomegalovirus infection in patients with septic shock. *Emerg Infect Dis.* 2006;12:1517-1522.

The effect of daily bathing with chlorhexidine on the acquisition of methicillin-resistant *Staphylococcus aureus*, vancomycin-resistant *Enterococcus*, and healthcare-associated bloodstream infections: Results of a quasi-experimental multicenter trial

Climo MW, Sepkowitz KA, Zuccotti G, et al (Hunter Holmes McGuire Veteran Affairs Med Ctr, Richmond, VA; Memorial Sloan-Kettering Cancer Ctr, NY; Brigham and Women's Hosp, Welksley, MA; et al)
Crit Care Med 37:1858-1865, 2009

Objective.—Spread of multidrug-resistant organisms within the intensive care unit (ICU) results in substantial morbidity and mortality. Novel strategies are needed to reduce transmission. This study sought to determine if the use of daily chlorhexidine bathing would decrease the incidence of colonization and bloodstream infections (BSI) because of methicillin-resistant *Staphylococcus aureus* (MRSA) and vancomycin-resistant *Enterococcus* (VRE) among ICU patients.

Design, Setting, and Patients.—Six ICUs at four academic centers measured the incidence of MRSA and VRE colonization and BSI during a period of bathing with routine soap for 6 months and then compared results with a 6-month period where all admitted patients received daily bathing with a chlorhexidine solution. Changes in incidence were evaluated by Poisson and segmented regression modeling.

Interventions.—Daily bathing with a chlorhexidine-containing solution.

Measurements and Main Results.—Acquisition of MRSA decreased 32% (5.04 vs. 3.44 cases/1000 patient days, $p = 0.046$) and acquisition of VRE decreased 50% (4.35 vs. 2.19 cases/1000 patient days, $p = 0.008$) following the introduction of daily chlorhexidine bathing. Segmented regression analysis demonstrated significant reductions in VRE bacteremia ($p = 0.02$) following the introduction of chlorhexidine bathing. VRE-colonized patients bathed with chlorhexidine had a lower risk of developing VRE bacteremia (relative risk 3.35; 95% confidence interval 1.13–9.87; $p = 0.035$), suggesting that reductions in the level of colonization led to the observed reductions in BSI.

Conclusion.—We conclude that daily chlorhexidine bathing among ICU patients may reduce the acquisition of MRSA and VRE. The approach is simple to implement and inexpensive and may be an important adjunctive intervention to barrier precautions to reduce acquisition of VRE and MRSA and the subsequent development of healthcare-associated BSI.

▶ Resistant organisms frequently colonize critically ill patients before causing infections. Multidrug resistant pathogens frequently cocolonize patients with a significant subset of patients subsequently developing infection with the colonizing species. While the introduction of alcohol-based hand sanitizers has resulted in dramatic reductions in acquisition of methicillin-resistant *Staphylococcus aureus* (MRSA) and vancomycin-resistant *Enterococcus* (VRE), further efforts to reduce nosocomial acquisition of organisms are needed.

Climo and colleagues studied the impact of chlorhexidine bathing on acquisition of multidrug resistant pathogens and subsequent infection. In this before and after study chlorhexidine bathing was superior to routine soap bathing in most assessed measures. These findings are supported by a study Weinstein and colleagues conducted in a long-term care facility where 2% chlorhexidine baths markedly reduced central venous catheter-associated bloodstream infections (9.5-3.8/1000 CVC days).[1] Simple and cheap to implement, chlorhexidine bathing appears an effective intervention in reducing rates of nosocomial acquisition of multidrug resistant pathogens. The ease of implementation in any ICU along with the mounting data in support of chlorhexidine bathing suggests that practicing intensivists should consider replacing daily soap bathing with daily chlorhexidine bathing.

A. Kumar, MD

S. Kethireddy, MD

Reference

1. Munoz-Price LS, Hota B, Stemer A, Weinstein RA. Prevention of bloodstream infections by use of daily chlorhexidine baths for patients at a long term acute care hospital. *Infect Control Hosp Epidemiol.* 2009;30:1031-1035.

Salvage Treatment for Persistent Methicillin-Resistant *Staphylococcus aureus* Bacteremia: Efficacy of Linezolid With or Without Carbapenem
Jang H-C, Kim S-H, Kim KH, et al (Seoul Natl Univ College of Medicine, Republic of Korea)
Clin Infect Dis 49:395-401, 2009

Background.—Persistent methicillin-resistant *Staphylococcus aureus* (MRSA) bacteremia is associated with high mortality rates, but no treatment strategy has yet been established. We performed this study to evaluate the efficacy of linezolid with or without carbapenem in salvage treatment for persistent MRSA bacteremia.

Methods.—All adult patients with persistent MRSA bacteremia for ≥7 days from January 2006 through March 2008 who were treated at Seoul National University Hospital were studied. The results of linezolid salvage therapy with or without carbapenem were compared with those of salvage therapy with vancomycin plus aminoglycosides or rifampicin.

Results.—Thirty-five patients with persistent MRSA bacteremia were studied. The early microbiological response (ie, negative results for follow-up blood culture within 72 hours) was significantly higher in the linezolid-based salvage therapy group than the comparison group (75% vs 17%; $P = .006$). Adding aminoglycosides or rifampicin to vancomycin was not successful in treating any of the patients, whereas linezolid-based therapy gave an 88% salvage success rate ($P < .001$). The *S. aureus*–related mortality rate was lower for patients treated with a linezolid salvage regimen than for patients continually treated with a vancomycin-based regimen (13% vs 53%; $P = .030$).

Conclusions.—Linezolid-based salvage therapy effectively eradicated *S. aureus* from the blood for patients with persistent MRSA bacteremia. The salvage success rate was higher for linezolid therapy than for vancomycin-based combination therapy.

▶ *Staphylococcus aureus* is an increasingly common cause of both community and nosocomial acquired bloodstream infections. Although high-level vancomycin resistance to methicillin resistant *S aureus* (MRSA) remains rare, problems of increased vancomycin tolerance raise concerns over how best to treat persistent MRSA infections.[1]

Jang and colleagues investigated the role of linezolid alone and in synergistic combination with carbapenem for the treatment of persistent MRSA bacteremia. Despite the inherent limitations of this retrospective study, the data support the concept of Sakoulas et al[1] of decreased susceptibility of MRSA to vancomycin after prolonged repeated administration. The investigators did not identify increasing minimum inhibitory concentrations (MICs), heteroresistance, or source eradication as clear causes for therapeutic failure. While this study suggests linezolid to be a viable salvage regimen in persistent MRSA infections, several important pharmacodynamic issues should be highlighted before considering a therapeutic change to linezolid. Recent data strongly suggest that microbial eradication with vancomycin decreases dramatically as the MIC increases from 0.05 to 1 to 2 mg/L.[2] Practicing intensivists should inquire as to the MIC of the MRSA isolate ie, if the MIC is 1 mg/L, increasing the daily dose of vancomycin to 3 to 4 gm would result in a 90% probability of target pharmacokinetic index attainment.[2] Secondly the addition of linezolid to vancomycin should be avoided in cases of persistent bacteremia. In vitro time kill studies have identified the combination of linezolid and vancomycin to be antagonistic, reducing killing of MRSA 100 to 1000 fold.[3] Finally while in vitro synergy between linezolid and carbapenems has been described, this study failed to show any increased benefit of combination therapy over isolated therapy with linezolid. In summary clinicians should be aware that while, source eradication remains the most important curative intervention, pharmacodynamic optimization needs to be strongly considered at the initiation of therapy. If these measures fail, switching to linezolid is a reasonable alternative.

A. Kumar, MD

S. Kethireddy, MD

References

1. Sakoulas G, Gold HS, Cohen RA, Venkataraman L, Moellering RC, Eliopoulos GM. Effects of prolonged vancomycin administration on methicillin resistant *Staphylococcus aureus* (MRSA) in a patient with recurrent bacteremia. *J Antimicrob Chemother.* 2006;57:699-704.
2. Rybak M, Lomaestro BM, Rotschafer JC, et al. Therapeutic monitoring of vancomycin in adults: summary of consensus recommendations from the American society of health-system pharmacists, the infectious disease society of America,

and the society of infectious diseases pharmacists. *Pharmacotherapy.* 2009;29: 1275-1279.
3. Deresinski S. Vancomycin in combination with other antibiotics for the treatment of serious methicillin-resistant *Staphylococcus aureus* infection. *Clin Infect Dis.* 2009;49:1072-1079.

Methicillin-Resistant *Staphylococcus aureus* Central Line–Associated Bloodstream Infections in US Intensive Care Units, 1997-2007
Burton DC, Edwards JR, Horan TC, et al (Ctrs for Disease Control and Prevention, Atlanta, GA)
JAMA 301:727-736, 2009

Context.—Concerns about rates of methicillin-resistant *Staphylococcus aureus* (MRSA) health care–associated infections have prompted calls for mandatory screening or reporting in efforts to reduce MRSA infections.

Objective.—To examine trends in the incidence of MRSA central line–associated bloodstream infections (BSIs) in US intensive care units (ICUs).

Design, Setting, and Participants.—Data reported by hospitals to the Centers for Disease Control and Prevention (CDC) from 1997-2007 were used to calculate pooled mean annual central line–associated BSI incidence rates for 7 types of adult and nonneonatal pediatric ICUs. Percent MRSA was defined as the proportion of *S aureus* central line–associated BSIs that were MRSA. We used regression modeling to estimate percent changes in central line–associated BSI metrics over the analysis period.

Main Outcome Measures.—Incidence rate of central line–associated BSIs per 1000 central line days; percent MRSA among *S aureus* central line–associated BSIs.

Results.—Overall, 33 587 central line–associated BSIs were reported from 1684 ICUs representing 16 225 498 patient-days of surveillance; 2498 reported central line–associated BSIs (7.4%) were MRSA and 1590 (4.7%) were methicillin-susceptible *S aureus* (MSSA). Of evaluated ICU types, surgical, nonteaching-affiliated medical surgical, cardiothoracic, and coronary units experienced increases in MRSA central line–associated BSI incidence in the 1997-2001 period; however, medical, teaching-affiliated medical-surgical, and pediatric units experienced no significant changes. From 2001 through 2007, MRSA central line–associated BSI incidence declined significantly in all ICU types except in pediatric units, for which incidence rates remained static. Declines in MRSA central line–associated BSI incidence ranged from −51.5% (95% CI, −33.7% to −64.6%; *P* < .001) in nonteaching-affiliated medical-surgical ICUs (0.31 vs 0.15 per 1000 central line days) to −69.2% (95% CI, −57.9% to −77.7%; *P* < .001) in surgical ICUs (0.58 vs 0.18 per 1000 central line days). In all ICU types, MSSA central line–associated BSI incidence declined from 1997 through 2007, with changes in incidence ranging from −60.1% (95% CI, −41.2% to −73.1%; *P* < .001) in surgical

ICUs (0.24 vs 0.10 per 1000 central line days) to -77.7% (95% CI, -68.2% to -84.4%; $P < .001$) in medical ICUs (0.40 vs 0.09 per 1000 central line days). Although the overall proportion of *S aureus* central line–associated BSIs due to MRSA increased 25.8% ($P = .02$) in the 1997-2007 period, overall MRSA central line–associated BSI incidence decreased 49.6% ($P < .001$) over this period.

Conclusions.—The incidence of MRSA central line–associated BSI has been decreasing in recent years in most ICU types reporting to the CDC. These trends are not apparent when only percent MRSA is monitored.

▶ Invasive MRSA infections remain a significant public health problem. Point estimates of MRSA infections, while helpful in estimating burden of disease, do not describe changes in epidemiology or the impact that infection control efforts have made in decreasing infections.[1]

Burton and colleagues defined an 11 year decreasing trend of catheter-associated bloodstream infection rate due to MRSA. The data are proof that effective infection control practices have had a significant impact on reducing MRSA infections from vascular catheters. However, clinicians should be aware that, while catheter-related infections due to MRSA have decreased over the years, other multicenter longitudinal surveillance studies suggest that nosocomial bloodstream infections from multidrug resistant pathogens are increasing.[2] Although the results of this study by Burton et al are reassuring, it is important to note that the demographics of invasive MRSA infection are no longer only confined to intensive care units or acute care settings.[1]

A. Kumar, MD

S. Kethireddy, MD

References

1. Klevens RM, Morrison MA, Nadle J, et al. Invasive methicillin-resistant Staphylococcus aureus infections in the United States. *JAMA*. 2007;298:1763-1771.
2. Wisplinghoff H, Bischoff T, Tallent SM, Siefert H, Wenzel RP, Edmond MB. Nosocomial bloodstream infections in US Hospitals: analysis of 24,179 cases from a prospective nationwide surveillance study. *Clin Infect Dis*. 2004;39: 309-317.

The usefulness of the semiquantitative procalcitonin test kit as a guideline for starting antibiotic administration
Oh JS, Kim SU, Oh YM, et al (The Catholic Univ of Korea, Seoul)
Am J Emerg Med 27:859-863, 2009

Objectives.—The Surviving Sepsis Campaign has recommended that antibiotic therapy should be started within the first hour of recognizing severe sepsis. Procalcitonin has recently been proposed as a biomarker of bacterial infection, although the quantitative procalcitonin assay is often time consuming, and it is not always available in many emergency departments (EDs). Our aim is to evaluate usefulness of the semiquantitative procalcitonin fast kit as a guideline for starting antibiotic administration for patients with severe sepsis or septic shock that requires prompt antibiotic therapy in the ED.

Methods.—We include those patients who were admitted to the ED and who were suspected of having infection. The procalcitonin concentration was determined by semiquantitative PCT-Q strips, and the points of the severity scoring system were calculated. The receiver operating characteristic curve was used to assess the diagnostic value of the PCT-Q strips to predict severe sepsis or septic shock.

Results.—Of the 80 recruited patients, 33 patients were categorized as having severe sepsis or septic shock according to the definition. At a procalcitonin cutoff level of 2 ng/mL or greater, the sensitivity of the PCT-Q for detecting severe sepsis or septic shock was 93.94% and the specificity was 87.23. The receiver operating characteristic curve for PCT-Q to predict severe sepsis or septic shock had an area under the curve of 0.916.

Conclusion.—PCT-Q is probably a fast, useful method for detecting severe sepsis in the ED, and it can be used as a guideline for antibiotic treatment.

▶ Early adequate antibiotic therapy paralleled with hemodynamic support (early-directed therapy [EGDT]) remains a cornerstone in the management of severe sepsis and septic shock. Despite the recommendations of the Surviving Sepsis Campaign of instituting antibiotic therapy within the first hour of recognition of severe sepsis, specific antibiotic treatment is often delayed. This delay has been in part attributed to the limitations on presentation to establish the diagnosis of infection versus systemic inflammatory response syndrome (SIRS) based on the common clinical manifestations of fever, tachycardia, tachypenea, and leukocytosis. More often, and especially true in the emergency department (ED), a microbiologic pathogen is often unidentified. To bridge this gap, biomedical markers of sepsis, such as C-reactive protein (CRP) and procalcitonin (PCT), were studied extensively, and their use to establish diagnosis of SIRS versus sepsis was tested in multiple clinical trials. Bell et al[1] reported that the measurement of PCT alone or in combination with CRP can be useful in discrimination of septicemia/bacteremia with associated SIRS versus noninfectious SIRS in an ICU setting. Moreover, Christ-Crain et al[2] showed that in patients with suspected respiratory tract infections, the use of PCT was helpful in deciding whether the patients should be treated with antibiotics.

In this article, Joo Suk Oh et al raised a very novel question about the usefulness of the semiquantitative PCT fast kit as a guideline to establish the diagnosis of SIRS versus sepsis. If achieved, the test can be used as a future reference to guide antibiotic administration in the emergency room. Extending the role of PCT to the ED seems very interesting. Overall, the test was proven easy, reliable, fast, and correlated well with the diagnosis of SIRS/sepsis spectrum. The early diagnosis of severe sepsis and septic shock in the ED would prompt early administration of antibiotics and could lead to better outcome in this category of patients.

However, the study has some limitations. The rapid semiquantitative PCT test was not compared with the regular PCT test to verify sensitivity and specificity, knowing already that the regular PCT test has its own limitations, in particular when used in conditions with localized infections and systemic effects but without bacteremia. Other limitations in the study include the small sample. The absence of the demographic data and comorbidities among patients paralleled with significant discrepancy in mortality (very low in severe sepsis 0%, very high in septic shock 68%) raises a compelling question about the heterogeneity of the different groups of patients and whether the PCT levels are well correlated. In addition, although secondary, this study showed that Acute Physiology and Chronic Health Evaluation II (APACHE II) and Sequential Organ Failure Assessment (SOFA) scores does not predict severe sepsis and septic shock. This is not in concordance with multiple other studies that showed strong correlation of PCT CRP, APACHE II, and SOFA with the presence of severe sepsis. If any, this emphasizes more the need for reporting the different physiologic parameters on which such conclusions were based.

Despite these limitations, the question raised in this article deserves adequate attention, as it holds the promise to provide a very important tool for diagnosis and management of severe sepsis in the ED.

S. L. Zanotti-Cavazzoni, MD

References

1. Bell K, Wattie M, Byth K, et al. Procalcitonin: a marker of bacteraemia in SIRS. *Anaesth Intensive Care.* 2003;31:629-636.
2. Christ-Crain M, Stolz D, Bingisser R, et al. Procalcitonin guidance of antibiotic therapy in community-acquired pneumonia: a randomized trial. *Am J Respir Crit Care Med.* 2006;174:84-93.

Emergence of a Novel Swine-Origin Influenza A (H1N1) Virus in Humans
Novel Swine-Origin Influenza A (H1N1) Virus Investigation Team (Ctrs for Disease Control and Prevention, Atlanta, GA)
N Engl J Med 360:2605-2615, 2009

Background.—On April 15 and April 17, 2009, novel swine-origin influenza A (H1N1) virus (S-OIV) was identified in specimens obtained from two epidemiologically unlinked patients in the United States. The same strain of the virus was identified in Mexico, Canada, and elsewhere. We describe 642 confirmed cases of human S-OIV infection identified from the rapidly evolving U.S. outbreak.

Methods.—Enhanced surveillance was implemented in the United States for human infection with influenza A viruses that could not be subtyped. Specimens were sent to the Centers for Disease Control and Prevention for real-time reverse-transcriptase–polymerase-chain-reaction confirmatory testing for S-OIV.

Results.—From April 15 through May 5, a total of 642 confirmed cases of S-OIV infection were identified in 41 states. The ages of patients ranged from 3 months to 81 years; 60% of patients were 18 years of age or younger. Of patients with available data, 18% had recently traveled to Mexico, and 16% were identified from school outbreaks of S-OIV infection. The most common presenting symptoms were fever (94% of patients), cough (92%), and sore throat (66%); 25% of patients had diarrhea, and 25% had vomiting. Of the 399 patients for whom hospitalization status was known, 36 (9%) required hospitalization. Of 22 hospitalized patients with available data, 12 had characteristics that conferred an increased risk of severe seasonal influenza, 11 had pneumonia, 8 required admission to an intensive care unit, 4 had respiratory failure, and 2 died. The S-OIV was determined to have a unique genome composition that had not been identified previously.

Conclusions.—A novel swine-origin influenza A virus was identified as the cause of outbreaks of febrile respiratory infection ranging from self-limited to severe illness. It is likely that the number of confirmed cases underestimates the number of cases that have occurred.

▶ Influenza viruses have the ability to reassort their genomes. They may also jump from animals to humans. These events can be associated with the occurrence of major antigenic "shifts" in human influenza virus infections and the emergency of pandemic strains 2 or 3 times a century. In early April, the first reported cases of a novel influenza A (H1N1) virus that contained genes from humans, swine, and birds were discovered. This marked the start of the first influenza pandemic of the 21st century.

The virus rapidly spread across the country, and this sentinel article describes the clinical characteristics of the first 642 cases in the United States. Further studies have been published describing the cases that occurred in Mexico and in Canadian intensive care units.[1,2] Atypically, this novel virus seemed to have a predilection to causing death for those under the age of 50, a pattern not seen in any influenza pandemic since 1918.

This virus is responsible for over 12 000 hospital admissions and over 500 deaths.[3] Ongoing studies will delineate the global epidemiology and pathogenesis of this virus, and aid in surge planning for future pandemics.

A. Kumar, MD

D. Funk, MD, FRCP(C)

References

1. Dominguez-Cherit G, Lapinsky SE, Macias AE, et al. Critically ill patients with 2009 influenza A (H1N1) in Mexico. *JAMA.* 2009;302:1880-1887.
2. Kumar A, Zarychanski R, Pinto R, et al. Critically ill patients with 2009 influenza A (H1N1) infection in Canada. *JAMA.* 2009;302:1872-1879.
3. Centers for Disease Control and Prevention. FluView: a weekly influenza surveillance report prepared by the Influenza Division. 2009-2010 influenza season week 43 ending October 31, 2009. http://cdc.gov/flu/weekly/. Accessed on November 3, 2009.

Influence of surgical treatment timing on mortality from necrotizing soft tissue infections requiring intensive care management

Boyer A, Vargas F, Coste F, et al (Hôpital Pellegrin-Tripode, Bordeaux cedex, France; et al)
Intensive Care Med 35:847-853, 2009

Purpose.—Surgical treatment is crucial in the management of necrotizing soft tissue infections (NSTIs). The aim of this study was to determine the influence of surgical procedure timing on hospital mortality in severe NSTI.

Methods.—A retrospective study including 106 patients was conducted in a medical intensive care unit equipped with a hyperbaric chamber. Data regarding pre-existing conditions, intensive care and surgical management were included in a logistic regression model to determine independent factors associated with hospital mortality.

Results.—Overall hospital mortality was 40.6%. In multivariate analysis, underlying cardiovascular disease, SAPS II, abdominoperineal compared to limb localization, time from the first signs to diagnosis <72 h, and time from diagnosis to surgical treatment >14 h in patients with septic shock were independently associated with hospital mortality.

Conclusion.—In patients with NSTI and septic shock, hospital mortality is influenced by the timing of surgical treatment.

▶ Necrotizing fasciitis is an uncommon and usually acute severe infection involving the subcutaneous soft tissues, superficial and often deep fascia. Two distinct bacteriologic entities are described in the literature ie, combination anaerobic infection and hemolytic streptococcal/staphylococcal gangrene; mortality for both types remains disturbingly high.[1]

While it is clear to most intensive care physicians that early goal directed therapy and source control is imperative to successfully treat severe infections, the impact of delays in diagnosis and surgical intervention on outcome of necrotizing fasciitis are poorly defined. The study by Boyer et al, shows marked mortality reductions follow early diagnosis,[2] and offers treating intensivists with distinct time parameters to consider when advocating for potentially disfiguring surgical debridement. Clinicians should be aware that the diagnosis of necrotizing fasciitis relies heavily on clinical decision-making and only partly on imaging results. This study should highlight the fact that patients clinically in septic shock presenting with a soft tissue infection should strongly be considered for surgical debridement preferably before or at the time of admission to the ICU.

A. Kumar, MD

S. Kethireddy, MD

References

1. Green RJ, Dafoe DC, Raffin TA. Necrotizing fasciitis. *Chest.* 1996;110:219-229.
2. Stamenkovic I. Early recognition of potentially fatal necrotizing fasciitis: use of frozen section biopsy. *N Engl Med.* 1984;310:1689-1693.

The impact of time on the systemic inflammatory response in pneumococcal pneumonia

Calbo E, Alsina M, Rodríguez-Carballeira M, et al (Universitat Autonoma de Barcelona, Spain)
Eur Respir J July 16, 2009 [Epub ahead of print]

Objective.—To analyze the impact of time from onset of symptoms on the systemic cytokine concentrations in patients with pneumococcal pneumonia.

Methods.—Adults with severe pneumococcal pneumonia were prospectively included. At admission, vital signs, time from onset of pneumonia symptoms and circulating levels of CRP, serum amyloid A (SAA), TNFα, IL1β, IL6, IL8, IL10, and IL1ra were recorded.

Results.—32 patients were included; 13 patients had <48h of evolution and 19 patients had been sick for >48h. The group with a longer time of evolution presented higher plasmatic levels of TNF-α (19.1(SD8.5) vs. 35.5(SD26) pg/mL; p=0.035), fibrinogen (6(SD1.8) vs. 9(SD2); p=0.001); CRP (130 (SD 85) vs. 327(SD 131; p=0.000) and SAA (678 (SD 509) vs. 984 (SD 391); p=0.025). Concentrations of TNFα were associated with the presence of bacteraemia (p=0.008), initial blood pressure < 90 mm Hg (p=0.050), and with a lower oxygen saturation at admission (p=0.047). Likewise, TNFα levels were correlated with concentrations of IL1β (r=0.49, p=0.008), IL6 (r=0.41, p=0.03), and IL8 (r=0.40, p=0.03)

Conclusions.—In pneumococcal pneumonia, patients with a longer time of evolution presented with higher levels of pro-inflammatory cytokines and a higher expression of acute phase proteins, suggesting a sustained release of pneumococcal antigens over time.

▶ The balance between pro and anti-inflammatory responses to severe infection is an area of research being continually refined by investigators. While differing opinions on the role of pro-inflammation versus anti-inflammation on mortality exist,[1] research has convincingly shown that delayed receipt of antimicrobials in setting of septic shock results in increased mortality.[2]

Calbo and colleagues studied the relationship of duration of pneumococcal infection and cytokine response. While methodologically supported largely on patient/family recall and thus subject to significant recall bias, the data presented in this study suggest that a longer duration of untreated infection results in increased pro-inflammatory cytokine release. The practicing intensivist should be aware of the growing body of literature in support of the concept that delayed anti-infective therapy in setting of severe infection is associated with progressive cytokine release, increasing bacterial loads, and ultimately higher mortality rates.[3]

A. Kumar, MD

S. Kethireddy, MD

References

1. Ashare A, Powers L, Butler NS, Doerschug KC, Monick MM, Hunninghake GW. Anti inflammatory response is associated with mortality and severity of infection in sepsis. *Am J Physiol Lung Cell Mol Physiol.* 2005;288:L633-L640.
2. Kumar A, Roberts D, Wood K, et al. Duration of hypotension before initiation of effective antimicrobial therapy is the critical determinant of survival in human septic shock. *Crit Care Med.* 2006;34:1589-1596.
3. Rello J, Lisboa T, Lujan M, et al. DNA-Neumococo Study Group. Severity of pneumococcal pneumonia associated with genomic bacterial load. *Chest.* 2009; 136:832-840.

Herpes simplex virus load in bronchoalveolar lavage fluid is related to poor outcome in critically ill patients
Linssen CFM, Jacobs JA, Stelma FF, et al (Univ Hosp Maastricht, The Netherlands)
Intensive Care Med 34:2202-2209, 2008

Objective.—To evaluate the relationship between the HSV-1 and -2 loads in BAL fluid (BALF) and clinical outcome.

Design.—Retrospective study.

Setting.—The general intensive care unit of the University Hospital Maastricht.

Patients.—Five hundred and twenty-one BALF samples from 462 patients were included. Patients were divided into three groups; (1) patients admitted to the hospital < 48 h before lavage (Community), (2) patients admitted to the ICU > 48 h before lavage (ICU) and (3) the remaining patients (non-ICU group).

Interventions.—No additional interventions were conducted.

Measurements and Results.—HSV-1 and HSV-2 loads were determined by real-time polymerase chain reaction (PCR). HSV-1 DNA was detected in 4.3% (4/92) of samples in the community group, 15% (18/121) in the non-ICU group and in 32% (99/308) of the ICU group. In the age group < 50 years HSV-1 DNA was less frequently isolated compared to the age group $\geq$ 50 years (16/129 (12%) versus 187/376 (25%), respectively, OR = 2.6; P < 0.001). HSV-1 loads of > 10^5 genome equivalents (ge)/ml were associated with an increased 14-day in-hospital mortality compared to patients with a HSV-1 load $\leq 10^5$ ge/ml in BALF (41 vs. 20%, respectively, $P = 0.001$). HSV-1 pneumonia was histologically proven in two patients with a HSV-1 load exceeding 10^5 ge/ml.

Conclusions.—HSV-1 occurred more in critically ill patients and high loads in BALF were associated with an increased mortality. The higher mortality observed in patients with HSV-1 load > 10^5 ge/ml enforces its clinical relevance and necessitates to start randomized medical intervention studies.

▶ Herpes simplex virus 1 (HSV-1) has been increasingly associated with pulmonary disease in critically ill patients. While observed associations between the qualitative presence of HSV-1, acute respiratory distress syndrome, and other severe respiratory disease have been reported in several series, the true pathogenic role of HSV-1 in severe respiratory disease is unknown.[1,2]

Linssen and colleagues studied the quantitative association between HSV-1 DNA load in lower respiratory samples and outcomes. The difference in viral DNA identification between the ICU (32%) and non-ICU groups (4-15%) suggested that increased severity or duration of illness results in higher viral expression. Berrington and colleagues have shown recently that the presence of HSV viremia among hospitalized patients was associated with higher mortality rates in both immunocompetent and immunocompromised hosts.[3] Interestingly, this study also found that 25% of patients with HSV viremia without an alternative explanation of acute illness had respiratory failure.[3]

These findings have implications for the practicing intensivist. The association of HSV viral load and severity of disease while compelling does not imply causality. Further studies are needed to distinguish between causality and reactivation of viral shedding as well as to determine whether antiviral treatment, if warranted, improves outcomes. At this time however the data are insufficient to recommend either diagnostic testing for HSV or targeted treatment in critically ill patients.

A. Kumar, MD

S. Kethireddy, MD

References

1. Simoons-Smit AM, Kraan EM, Beishuizen A, Strack van Schijndel RJ, Vandenbroucke-Grauls CM. Herpes simplex virus type 1 and respiratory disease in critically ill patients: real pathogen or innocent bystander? *Clin Microbiol Infect.* 2006;12:1050-1059.
2. Verheij J, Groeneveld AB, Beishuizen A, van Lingen A, Simoons-Smit AM, van Schijndel RJ. Herpes simplex virus type 1 and normal protein permeability in the lungs of critically ill patients: a case for low pathogenicity. *Crit Care.* 2004; 8:R139.
3. Berrington WR, Jerome KR, Cook L, Wald A, Corey L, Casper C. Clinical correlates of herpes simplex virus viremia among hospitalized adults. *Clin Infect Dis.* 2009;49:1295-1301.

6 Postoperative Management

Cardiovascular Surgery

In situ simulation-based team training for post-cardiac surgical emergency chest reopen in the intensive care unit
Nunnink L, Welsh A-M, Abbey M, et al (Princess Alexandra Hosp, Woolloongabba, Australia)
Anaesth Intensive Care 37:74-78, 2009

Emergency chest reopen of the post cardiac surgical patient in the intensive care unit is a high-stakes but infrequent procedure which requires a high-level team response and a unique skill set. We evaluated the impact on knowledge and confidence of team-based chest reopen training using a patient simulator compared with standard video-based training. We evaluated 49 medical and nursing participants before and after training using a multiple choice questions test and a questionnaire of self-reported confidence in performing or assisting with emergency reopen.

Both video- and simulation-based training significantly improved results in objective and subjective domains. Although the post-test scores did not differ between the groups for either the objective (P = 0.28) or the subjective measures (P = 0.92), the simulation-based training produced a numerically larger improvement in both domains. In a multiple choice question out of 10, participants improved by a mean of 1.9 marks with manikin-based training compared to 0.9 with video training (P = 0.03). On a questionnaire out of 20 assessing subjective levels of confidence, scores improved by 3.9 with manikin training compared to 1.2 with video training (P = 0.002).

Simulation-based training appeared to be at least as effective as video-based training in improving both knowledge and confidence in post cardiac surgical emergency resternotomy.

▶ The landscape of cardiac surgical care continues to change with decreasing resident training hours and a decline in the overall volume of cardiac surgical procedures but with increasing complexity of these patients. The first 2 factors may translate to a decreased overall number of experiences per caregiver, especially with regard to emergency chest reopening. Furthermore, there are data that support that resternotomy within 10 minutes is associated with improved outcomes[1] and is part of the recently published European Resuscitation Council guidelines for resuscitation in cardiac arrest after cardiac surgery.[2] Therefore, resternotomy may need to occur before a senior level surgical fellow or attending arrive. In order to address these goals of resuscitation and limitations in work force, the authors sought to assess the impact of 2 different training methods for emergent resternotomy in postcardiac surgical patients. They performed a prospective trial comparing in-situ simulation (in a standard bed space in the ICU) versus an instructional video. While they showed that both methods improved the knowledge and confidence in postcardiac surgical emergency resternotomy, they were unable to show how this impacted performance because they did not include an assessment of the speed and quality of performing such a task, which is as equally important as the operator's confidence and knowledge. To accomplish this, simulation may be a key tool. Dunning and colleagues[3] previously reported the use of a 3-day simulation course for training the management of postcardiac surgical patients. They were able to show a difference in the speed and quality of the care for cardiac surgical patients who suffered from a cardiac arrest. However, while they also assessed skill, as in this study they only assessed the immediate acquisition of knowledge and skill. Because of the infrequency of such events, it is important to also assess the retention of such knowledge and skills, and because of the cost associated with simulation projects, to assess whether such training sessions impact outcomes.

One of the potentially important characteristics of this study was the use of in-situ simulation. This methodology has the potential to not only teach important skills but also offers the unique opportunity to identify local problems with equipment and other potential system issues.[4] Future studies should not only compare simulation with other more traditional modalities of teaching, but also to compare in-situ versus off-site simulation programs in both the acquisition and retention of knowledge and skills and for the training of potentially new guidelines, such as those for resuscitation in cardiac arrest after cardiac surgery.[2]

E. A. Martinez, MD, MHS

References

1. Mackay JH, Powell SJ, Osgathorp J, Rozario CJ. Six-year prospective audit of chest reopening after cardiac arrest. *Eur J Cardiothorac Surg.* 2002;22:421-425.
2. Dunning J, Fabbri A, Kolh PH, et al, EACTS Clinical Guidelines Committee. Guideline for resuscitation in cardiac arrest after cardiac surgery. *Eur J Cardiothorac Surg.* 2009;36:3-28.
3. Dunning J, Nandi J, Ariffin S, Jerstice J, Danitsch D, Levine A. The Cardiac Surgery Advanced Life Support Course (CALS): delivering significant improvements in emergency cardiothoracic care. *Ann Thorac Surg.* 2006;81:1767-1772.
4. Rodriguez-Paz JM, Mark LJ, Herzer KR, et al. A novel process for introducing a new intraoperative program: a multidisciplinary paradigm for mitigating hazards and improving patient safety. *Anesth Analg.* 2009;108:202-210.

Cerebral Ischemic Lesions on Diffusion-Weighted Imaging Are Associated With Neurocognitive Decline After Cardiac Surgery
Barber PA, Hach S, Tippett LJ, et al (Auckland City Hosp, New Zealand; Univ of Auckland, New Zealand)
Stroke 39:1427-1433, 2008

Background and Purpose.—Improvements in cardiac surgery mortality and morbidity have focused interest on the neurological injury such as stroke and cognitive decline that may accompany an otherwise successful operation. We aimed to investigate (1) the rate of stroke, new ischemic change on MRI, and cognitive impairment after cardiac valve surgery; and (2) the controversial relationship between perioperative cerebral ischemia and cognitive decline.

Methods.—Forty patients (26 men; mean [SD] age 62.1 [13.7] years) undergoing intracardiac surgery (7 also with coronary artery bypass grafting) were studied. Neurological, neuropsychological, and MRI examinations were performed 24 hours before surgery and 5 days (MRI and neurology) and 6 weeks (neuropsychology and neurology) after surgery. Cognitive decline from baseline was determined using the Reliable Change Index.

Results.—Two of 40 (5%) patients had perioperative strokes and 22 of 35 (63%) tested had cognitive decline in at least one measure (range, 1 to 4). Sixteen of 37 participants (43%) with postoperative imaging had new ischemic lesions (range, 1 to 17 lesions) with appearances consistent with cerebral embolization. Cognitive decline was seen in all patients with, and 35% of those without, postoperative ischemic lesions ($P < 0.001$), and there was an association between the number of abnormal cognitive tests and ischemic burden ($P < 0.001$).

Conclusion.—We have provided a reliable estimate of the rate of stroke, postoperative ischemia, and cognitive impairment at 6 weeks after cardiac valve surgery. Cognitive impairment is associated with perioperative ischemia and is more severe with greater ischemic load.

▶ Brain injury following cardiac surgery remains a significant complication that leads to increased morbidity, mortality, and cost. Brain injury can include anything along the spectrum from encephalopathy to stroke to neurologic death. Furthermore, there are data to support that cognitive decline is a significant problem postcardiac surgery,[1] and more broadly, in patients with cardiovascular disease regardless of the treatment modality.[2] Despite significant efforts over the last 10 to 20 years to identify risk factors, develop risk-reduction strategies, and to improve diagnosis, the rate of perioperative strokes continues to be 1.1% to 6.6%, depending on the assessment methodology (ie, clinically evident vs a prospective systematic assessment). While long-term cognitive impairment or decline may not be directly, or solely, attributable to cardiac surgery,[2] perhaps early postoperative changes may be. Barber and colleagues hypothesized that those patients with postoperative findings of radiographic ischemia would be more likely to exhibit neurocognitive decline at 6 weeks after operation. They used the diffusion-weighted MRI (DWI) to assess for new lesions. DWI has been shown to be a more sensitive diagnostic test for new ischemic events following cardiac surgery.[3] The cohort of 40 patients included in this trial were undergoing an intracardiac procedure and were part of a larger clinical trial in which patients underwent pre and postoperative neurocognitive testing and DWI. While only 5% had a stroke, 43% of this small cohort had a new postoperative ischemic lesion. Of those with ischemia, a change in cognitive function was observed in 100%, compared with only 35% of the patients without a new ischemic focus ($P < .001$). Furthermore, they identified an association between the number of abnormal cognitive tests and the ischemic burden, supporting a "dose-like" response in deterioration of cognitive function.

The strengths of this study are that all of the cognitive tests were performed by the same neuropsychologist and patients were screened for mood disorders, which can have an effect on such testing. In addition, it offers more evidence that the DWI should be considered a key modality, or the best modality, for use as an outcome measure in cardiac surgery research where perioperative cerebral ischemia is the outcome of interest. One of the limitations of this study is that they only looked at relatively short-term outcomes (6 weeks), and it is unclear what the status of these individuals is long-term. Given that other trials have shown little difference between the trajectory of cognitive decline in patients with cardiovascular disease, regardless of their treatment,[2] the association with the ischemic burden found on DWI and long-term cognitive decline would be important to understand. While there are data supporting cognitive decline in the population of patients with cardiovascular disease, the association between early ischemic findings on DWI has not been assessed and would be an interesting follow-up study to this. Of course, the most important study to perform would be to answer the question what we can do to decrease the ischemic burden and whether that has any impact on decreasing both early and late cognitive decline.

E. A. Martinez, MD, MHS

References

1. Newman MF, Kirchner JL, Phillips-Bute B, et al. Longitudinal assessment of neurocognitive function after coronary-artery bypass surgery. N Engl J Med. 2001; 344:395-402.
2. Selnes OA, Grega MA, Bailey MM, et al. Do management strategies for coronary artery disease influence 6-year cognitive outcomes? Ann Thorac Surg. 2009;88: 445-454.
3. Gottesman RF, Sherman PM, Grega MA, et al. Watershed strokes after cardiac surgery: diagnosis, etiology, and outcome. Stroke. 2006;37:2306-2311.

Shop for Quality or Volume? Volume, Quality, and Outcomes of Coronary Artery Bypass Surgery

Auerbach AD, Hilton JF, Maselli J, et al (Univ of California, San Francisco; Tufts Univ School of Medicine, Springfield, MA)
Ann Intern Med 150:696-704, 2009

Background.—Care from high-volume centers or surgeons has been associated with lower mortality rates in coronary artery bypass surgery, but how volume and quality of care relate to each other is not well understood.

Objective.—To determine how volume and differences in quality of care influence outcomes after coronary artery bypass surgery.

Design.—Observational cohort.

Setting.—164 hospitals in the United States.

Patients.—81 289 patients 18 years or older who had coronary artery bypass grafting from 1 October 2003 to 1 September 2005.

Measurements.—Hospital and surgeon case volumes were estimated by using a data set. Quality measures were defined by whether patients received specific medications and by counting the number of measures missed. Hierarchical models were used to estimate effects of volume and quality on death and readmission up to 30 days.

Results.—After adjustment for clinical factors, lowest surgeon volume and highest hospital volume were associated with higher mortality rates and lower readmission risk, respectively. Patients who did not receive aspirin (odds ratio, 1.89 [95% CI, 1.65 to 2.16) or β-blockers (odds ratio, 1.29 [CI, 1.12 to 1.49]) had higher odds for death, after adjustment for clinical risk factors and case volume. Adjustment for individual quality measures did not alter associations between volume and readmission or death. However, if no quality measures were missed, mortality rates at the lowest-volume centers (adjusted mortality rate, 1.05% [CI, 0.81% to 1.29%]) and highest-volume centers (adjusted mortality rate, 0.98% [CI, 0.72% to 1.25%]) were similar.

Limitation.—Because administrative data were used, the quality measures may not replicate measures collected through chart abstraction.

Conclusion.—Maximizing adherence to quality measures is associated with improved mortality rates, independent of hospital or surgeon volume.

▶ The volume-outcome relationship in cardiac surgery remains a debate.[1] Early data suggested that higher-volume centers had better outcomes. These findings were the impetus for some insurers to push for evidence-based referrals to high-volume centers. Although recent literature refutes these findings with the use of different statistical analyses, data continue to show that there are variations in outcomes for cardiac surgery. In this retrospective study, the authors elegantly evaluate what factors may be contributing to these differences in outcomes. In a cohort of over 81 000 patients, Auerbach and colleagues set out to evaluate (1) whether there was a volume-outcome relationship in mortality and readmission following cardiac surgery, (2) whether overall quality explained this relationship, if it existed, and (3) the relationship between overall quality and mortality. Using billing data from a subset of premier hospitals, they captured hospital- and surgeon-specific volume, outcome variables (death, readmission), in addition to patient risk factors/comorbidities, and a measure of compliance with key quality indicators from the Surgical Care Improvement Project (SCIP). The SCIP measures included (Table 1) were abstracted retrospectively from the hospital billing data, and they appropriately note that this methodology had not been validated. In general there was variation (inconsistencies) in the associations between global volume and outcome (mortality and readmission) and between individual caregiver quality-of-care measures and outcomes. Furthermore, adjusting for individual quality-of-care measures did not change the association between volume and outcomes. Two quality indicators, "patients who did not receive aspirin or β-blockers," were associated with higher odds of death after adjustment for clinical risk factors and case volume. Importantly, they found that there was a relationship between the overall number of quality measures missed and the overall adjusted mortality (Table 5), with a statistically significantly increased mortality when a patient did not receive at least 3 of the indicated performance measures. This trend

TABLE 1.—Definitions and Descriptive Statistics for Quality Measures

Quality Measure	Definition	Exclusion Criteria	Total Patients, n (%)
No use of serial compression devices in the first 2 days	No charges for serial compression devices 2 days after surgery	None	62 231 (77)
No statins in the first 2 days after surgery	No charge for "statin" lipid-lowering drug 2 days after surgery (e.g., lovastatin, pravastatin, atorvastatin)	Principal or secondary diagnosis code for liver disease, cirrhosis, myopathy	45 579 (56)
Inappropriate choice of prophylactic antimicrobials	Use of antimicrobial not on approved list	Principal or secondary diagnosis code for preexisting infection, as defined by SCIP	29 486 (36)
No prophylactic antimicrobials	No charges for antimicrobials on approved list	Principal or secondary diagnosis code for preexisting infection, as defined by SCIP	5167 (6)
No aspirin in the first 2 days after surgery	No charge for aspirin 2 days after surgery	Principal or secondary diagnosis code for cerebrovascular hemorrhage, gastrointestinal bleeding, factor deficiencies, platelet disorders	28 183 (35)
No β-blockers in the first 2 days after surgery	No charges for adrenergic blocking agents 2 days after surgery	Principal or secondary diagnosis code for conduction system disorder, hypotension, sepsis, congestive heart failure, or bradycardia	15 998 (20)

SCIP = Surgical Care Improvement Project.

TABLE 5.—Quality Measures and Care Outcomes

Variable	30-Day Mortality Rate (n = 1825)			Readmission Rate (n = 8653)		
	Unadjusted OR (95% CI)	Adjusted OR (95% CI)* †	Adjusted OR (95% CI)† ‡	Unadjusted OR (95% CI)	Adjusted OR (95% CI)* §	Adjusted OR (95% CI)‡ §
Individual measures						
No aspirin	1.17 (1.06–1.29)	1.90 (1.66–2.16)	1.89 (1.65–2.16)	0.91 (0.87–0.95)	1.01 (0.94–1.08)	1.00 (0.94–1.06)
No β-blocker	0.82 (0.72–0.93)	1.29 (1.12–1.48)	1.29 (1.12–1.49)	0.83 (0.78–0.88)	0.95 (0.89–1.01)	0.96 (0.90–1.02)
No statin	1.23 (1.12–1.35)	1.07 (0.95–1.20)	1.07 (0.95–1.21)	0.95 (0.91–0.99)	0.97 (0.91–1.04)	0.96 (0.91–1.02)
No prophylactic antibiotics	1.12 (0.94–1.35)	1.25 (0.77–2.00)	1.25 (0.79–2.00)	0.82 (0.74–0.91)	0.87 (0.76–1.00)	0.90 (0.80–1.01)
Inappropriate antibiotics	2.05 (1.86–2.25)	0.66 (0.58–0.74)	0.66 (0.58–0.75)	1.26 (1.20–1.32)	1.10 (1.05–1.15)	1.12 (1.08–1.17)
No serial compression device	1.22 (1.09–1.37)	1.00 (0.82–1.22)	1.00 (0.83–1.22)	1.01 (0.95–1.06)	0.99 (0.90–1.09)	1.01 (0.93–1.09)
Missed measures||						
0	Reference	Reference	Reference	Reference	Reference	Reference
1	1.68 (1.35–2.10)	1.05 (0.79–1.37)	1.05 (0.80–1.38)	1.10 (1.01–1.20)	1.00 (0.92–1.10)	1.01 (0.92–1.10)
2	1.58 (1.28–1.95)	1.15 (0.87–1.53)	1.15 (0.87–1.53)	1.09 (1.01–1.18)	0.99 (0.91–1.08)	1.00 (0.92–1.09)
3	2.43 (1.99–2.98)	1.54 (1.20–1.98)	1.54 (1.20–1.98)	1.08 (0.99–1.17)	0.99 (0.90–1.10)	1.00 (0.91–1.10)
≥4	2.37 (1.92–2.92)	1.62 (1.23–2.14)	1.63 (1.24–2.15)	1.03 (0.95–1.13)	0.98 (0.88–1.10)	1.02 (0.93–1.13)

OR = odds ratio.
*Adjusted for confounders only.
†Confounders included in mortality rate models were age, sex, diagnosis-related group–predicted mortality, congestive heart failure, hypertension, neurologic disorders, diabetes with complications, renal failure, coagulopathy, deficiency anemia, and whether an internal mammary graft was used during the procedure.
‡Adjusted for volume measures and confounders.
§Confounders included in readmission models were age, sex, race, insurance type, admission status, diagnosis-related group–predicted mortality, chronic obstructive pulmonary disease, peripheral vascular disease, diabetes, diabetes with complications, renal failure, electrolyte disorders, deficiency anemia, psychoses, depression, and geographic region.
||9378 (12%) patients had 0 missed measures, 14 884 (18%) had 1 missed measure, 20 534 (25%) had 2 missed measures, 21 232 (26%) had 3 missed measures, and 15 261 (18%) had ≥4 missed measures.

held true for both surgeon and hospital volume. Equally as important with regard to health policy was that when adjusted for patient risk, if no quality measures were missed, mortality rates at high- and low-volume centers were not statistically different.

While there continues to be debate about the value of compliance with national quality measures and their association with improved outcomes, this study suggests that in fact there is a relationship. The question remains that if centers that perform poorly on these specific indicators improve their performance, will their outcomes be improved?

While this study has limitations inherent to its retrospective nature and use of administrative databases, it is strengthened by the quality and rigor of the statistical analysis. The insights into what might be contributing to variations in outcomes is compelling, and further studies evaluating the impact of improving performance on process measures on outcomes are needed. We need to continue to strive to identify what high performers are doing to get the results they do and broaden their implementation.

E. A. Martinez, MD, MHS

Reference

1. Birkmeyer JD, Dimick JB. Potential benefits of the new Leapfrog standards: effect of process and outcomes measures. *Surgery.* 2004;135:569-575.

Variation in perioperative vasoactive therapy in cardiovascular surgical care: Data from the Society of Thoracic Surgeons
Hernandez AF, Li S, Dokholyan RS, et al (Duke Univ School of Medicine, Durham, NC; e al)
Am Heart J 158:47-52, 2009

Background.—The appropriate use of vasoactive cardiovascular drugs in high-risk coronary artery bypass grafting (CABG) patients has not been well characterized.

Methods.—We performed a detailed chart analysis on 2,390 randomly selected patients undergoing CABG between January 2004 and June 2005 at 55 hospitals participating in the Society of Thoracic Surgeons' National Adult Cardiac Surgery Database. Patients were eligible if they had elective/urgent CABG with an ejection fraction (EF) <40%, or if they had an elective or urgent CABG at ≥65 years with diabetes, or a glomerular filtration rate <60 mL/min per 1.73 m². Logistic regression modeling was used to determine predictors of and provide risk-adjusted frequencies of postoperative vasoactive therapies.

Results.—Vasoactive therapy was used in 90% of patients. Inotropes/vasopressors were used in 28% (668), vasodilators in 18% (430), and the combination in 43% (1,037). Predictors of any inotrope use were preoperative atrial fibrillation (odds ratio [OR] 1.48), other arrhythmia (OR 2.09), EF (OR 1.09 per 5-unit decrease), severe mitral regurgitation

(OR 2.56), 3-vessel coronary artery disease (OR 1.35), New York Heart Association class IV (1.38), on-pump (OR 1.86), other procedure (OR 2.51), and peripheral vascular disease (OR 1.28) (all OR $P < .05$). Hospital-level risk-adjusted rates of any inotrope use varied significantly from 100% to 35% ($P < .01$) and vasodilator rates varied from 100% to 10% ($P < .01$).

Conclusions.—There is marked hospital variation in the use of vasoactive therapies in high-risk CABG patients in clinical practice, indicating an important area for further research to better clarify best practice.

▶ The use of vasoactive agents in cardiovascular surgery is ubiquitous. Patients are placed on inotropes, vasopressors, and vasodilators for multiple reasons, but the ultimate goals are to optimize myocardial function and end-organ perfusion and avoid increased risks in the perioperative setting (eg, ischemia or bleeding). Various combinations of vasoactive agents can achieve these goals. These authors describe the epidemiology of vasoactive drug use in cardiac surgical patients. In a subset of patients who are cared for in hospitals who report to the Society of Thoracic Surgeons' National Adult Cardiac Database (STS NCD), they sought to identify risk factors for and current use of vasoactive agents. As part of a larger project to assess current practices (Contemporary Analysis of Perioperative Cardiovascular Surgical Care), they performed an in-depth retrospective chart review of 2390 random, high-risk patients from 48 database participants (approximately 50 patients from each) who underwent a primary coronary artery bypass grafting (CABG) procedure. Eligible patients were ≥65 years old, had a preoperative ejection fraction (EF) of < 40%, and either history of diabetes or a preoperative estimated glomerular filtration rate < 60 mL/min per 1.73 m^2. For this analysis, they grouped patients by whether they received either an inotrope or vasopressor in contrast to a vasodilator. Not surprisingly, they found that 90% of patients were managed with a vasoactive agent within the first 12 hours postoperatively (Fig 1). Of these, the majority were on a combination of a vasopressor/inotrope plus

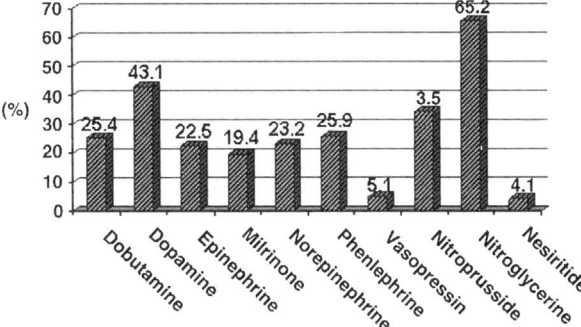

FIGURE 1.—Overall frequency of vasoactive medications during hospitalization (surgery through discharge). (Reprinted from Hernandez AF, Li S, Dokholyan RS, et al. Variation in perioperative vasoactive therapy in cardiovascular surgical care: data from the society of thoracic surgeons. *Am Heart J.* 2009;158:47-52, with permission from Elsevier.)

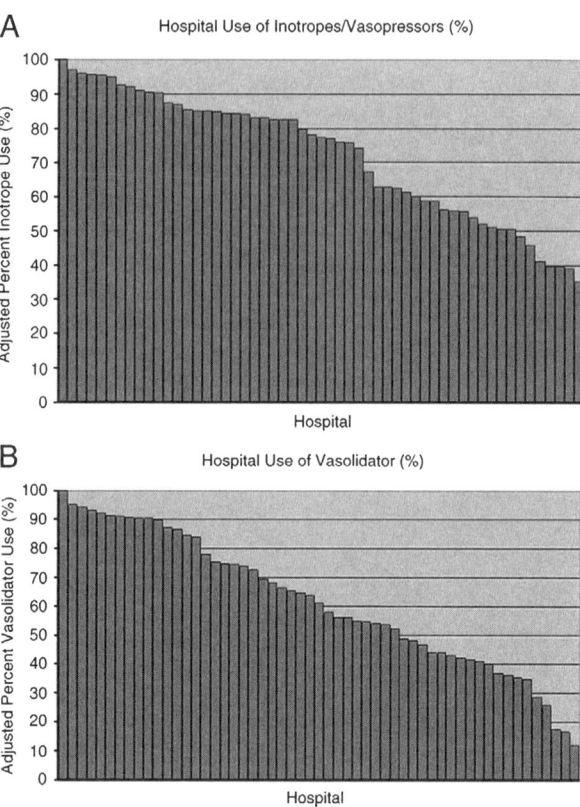

FIGURE 2.—A, Risk-adjusted hospital use of inotropes/vasopressors. B, Risk-adjusted hospital use of vasodilators (frequencies shown from highest to lowest and hospitals are not in the same order as A). (Reprinted from Hernandez AF, Li S, Dokholyan RS, et al. Variation in perioperative vasoactive therapy in cardiovascular surgical care: data from the society of thoracic surgeons. *Am Heart J*. 2009;158:47-52, with permission from Elsevier.)

a vasodilator, and over 90% of those were on these simultaneously. In the subset of patients who underwent an off-pump procedure, the use of vasoactive agents was approximately 80%. While the great majority in each population was on vasoactive agents, the hospital-level risk-adjusted rates of usage varied significantly (*P* < .01) for both inotropes/vasopressors and vasodilators (Fig 2), and these differences did not seem to be attributable to hospital-level characteristics. The findings in this article highlight the current variation and practices in use of vasoactive agents. It will be important to study this further as we must strive to not only identify these variations, but also rigorously evaluate how they impact outcomes so that we can identify best practices and better inform guidelines for care.

E. A. Martinez, MD, MHS

Risk of Assessing Mortality Risk in Elective Cardiac Operations: Age, Creatinine, Ejection Fraction, and the Law of Parsimony

Ranucci M, Castelvecchio S, Menicanti L, et al (IRCCS Policlinico S. Donato, Milan, Italy)
Circulation 119:3053-3061, 2009

Background.—Several mortality risk scores exist in cardiac surgery. All include a considerable number of independent risk factors. In elective cardiac surgery patients, the operative mortality is low, the number of events recorded per year is limited, and the risk model may be overfitted. The present study aims to develop and validate an operative mortality risk score for elective patients based on a limited number of factors.

Methods and Results.—The development series included 4557 adult patients who had undergone an elective cardiac operation at our institution from 2001 to 2003; the validation series includes the 4091 patients who subsequently underwent an operation. Three independent factors were included in the mortality risk model: age, creatinine, and left ventricular ejection fraction (ACEF). The ACEF score was computed as follows: age (years)/ejection fraction (%)+1 (if serum creatinine value was >2 mg/dL). The ACEF score was compared with 5 other risk scores in the validation series. Discriminatory power (accuracy) was defined with a receiver-operating characteristics analysis. The best accuracy was achieved by the Cleveland Clinic score (0.812), with ACEF score just below it (0.808). In coronary operations, the 2 scores performed equally well (0.815 versus 0.813), and in isolated coronary operations, the best accuracy was achieved by ACEF (0.826), with the Cleveland Clinic score at 0.806.

Conclusion.—A risk model limited to 3 independent predictors has similar or better accuracy and calibration compared with more complex risk scores if applied to elective cardiac operations.

▶ There has been a longstanding interest in developing an accurate mortality risk score in cardiac surgery. Currently, the Euro score and the Society of Thoracic Surgeons risk scores are probably the most commonly used in research. However, it is unclear how frequently providers use these in clinical practice or use these to discuss risks with an individual patient. One of the reasons for this is that both of these, and other historical risk scores, are relatively cumbersome to use in the everyday management of patients because they incorporate anywhere from 9 to 17 independent risk factors. The authors of this article sought to develop and validate a more parsimonious model of risk for patients presenting for elective cardiac surgery only. From 33 variables that are constituents of these more complex risk scores, they identified 3 independent variables—age, creatinine, and left ventricular ejection fraction (ACEF)—that were associated with, and had the best area under the curve association with, in-hospital or 30-day mortality. The ACEF score was based on data from the 4557 patients in the development cohort and was computed based on the respective regression coefficients of each variable and is: age (years)/ejection fraction (EF) (%) +1 (if baseline serum creatinine was

> 2 mg/dL). Interestingly, they found that the risk associated with a creatinine > 2 mg/dL versus ≥2 mg/dL was 5.3 (95% confidence interval [CI], 3.5 to 7.8), which was similar to the odds ratio for mortality for each point of the age/EF score. This finding led to the inclusion of the creatinine, potentially adding 1 additional point to the risk model. The association between the ACEF risk score and predicted mortality rate is shown in Fig 2 in the original article. They then compared this risk score with 5 widely used mortality scores in the validation cohort. The mortality scores, which were used for comparison, are the additive and logistic EuroSCORE, Parsonnet, Cleveland Clinic, and Northern New England scores. The predicted mortality rates using the ACEF score compared with various patient populations are shown in Figs 3 to 5 in the original article. The ACEF performed well in all subsets of patients. Each risk score performed differently for the different patient populations, and much of this reflected the patient population in whom they were originally intended. For example, most included emergency procedures in their development and validation while the ACEF score did not.

Perhaps the greatest strength of the ACEF score is its simplicity, with 3 easily obtained variables, and its reliance on relatively stable and nondisputable data points (age, serum creatinine). The third variable, EF, may be vulnerable to subjective interpretations, as we frequently will see various different EFs reported for a patient, especially when they are based on echocardiography versus angiography. The authors included in their model the most recent measure of EF or the lowest value—so this model incorporates both modalities and still performed well. Many of the other models incorporate other comorbidities such as chronic obstructive pulmonary disease and cerebrovascular disease, all of which are vulnerable to the vagaries of a patient's medical history unless clearly defined and confirmed with a diagnostic test.

The authors astutely point out that while the ACEF score compared favorably with more complex scores, none have the ability to accurately identify patients at risk of having a poor outcome (poor positive predictive value). While these scores do allow us to identify patients who are unlikely to die (good negative predictive value), we must continue to develop models that will improve our ability to give patients more accurate information about their individual mortality risk.

E. A. Martinez, MD, MHS

Safety and Efficacy of Recombinant Activated Factor VII: A Randomized Placebo-Controlled Trial in the Setting of Bleeding After Cardiac Surgery
Gill R, Herbertson M, Vuylsteke A, et al (Southampton Univ Hosps, UK; Papworth Hosp, Cambridge, UK; et al)
Circulation 120:21-27, 2009

Background.—Blood loss is a common complication of cardiac surgery. Evidence suggests that recombinant activated factor VII (rFVIIa) can decrease intractable bleeding in patients after cardiac surgery. Our objective was to investigate the safety and possible benefits of rFVIIa in patients who bleed after cardiac surgery.

Methods and Results.—In this phase II dose-escalation study, patients who had undergone cardiac surgery and were bleeding were randomized to receive placebo (n = 68), 40 μg/kg rFVIIa (n = 35), or 80 μg/kg rFVIIa (n = 69). The primary end points were the number of patients suffering critical serious adverse events. Secondary end points included rates of reoperation, amount of blood loss, and transfusion of allogeneic blood. There were more critical serious adverse events in the rFVIIa groups. These differences did not reach statistical significance (placebo, 7%; 40 μg/kg, 14%; $P = 0.25$; 80 μg/kg, 12%; $P = 0.43$). After randomization, significantly fewer patients in the rFVIIa group underwent a reoperation as a result of bleeding ($P = 0.03$) or required allogeneic transfusions ($P = 0.01$).

Conclusions.—On the basis of this preliminary evidence, rFVIIa may be beneficial for treating bleeding after cardiac surgery, but caution should be applied and further clinical trials are required because there is an increase in the number of critical serious adverse events, including stroke, in those patients randomized to receive rFVIIa.

▶ Blood loss following cardiac surgery is a serious complication, and transfusions are associated with increased morbidity and mortality.[1] Recombinant factor VIIa (rFVIIa; NovoSeven, Novo Nordisk A/S, Bagsvaerd, Denmark) is approved for management of patients with hemophilia and inhibitors to coagulation factors VIII or IX, FVII deficiency, and acquired hemophilia. There is, however, significant interest in using this product for patients without such underlying diseases, and many providers have explored its use in trauma. Many concerns have arisen that, although it has been associated with a decrease in transfusion requirements, its use has also been associated with an increased risk of thrombotic complications. Nonetheless, rFVIIa is being used off-label in cardiac surgical centers in patients with postoperative bleeding but with no history of hematologic diseases. These authors used a randomized, dose-escalation, placebo-controlled trial to evaluate the safety and efficacy of the use of rFVIIa for bleeding following cardiac surgery. They included adult cardiac surgical patients who had either ≥200 ml/hr for 1 hour or ≥2 ml/cc/kg for 2 consecutive hours after the first 30 minutes in the ICU and did not require urgent reoperation based on the provider's judgment. The primary endpoint was the incidence of critical significant adverse events (cSAE) out to 30 days postoperatively, which included death, myocardial infarction, cerebral infarction, clinically symptomatic pulmonary embolus, and other clinically symptomatic thrombotic events confirmed by follow-up investigation. They used a logistic regression to evaluate the risk of having a cSAE, which included prespecified variables (previous cardiac surgery, use of antifibrinolytic, and treatment allocation). Patients were consented preoperatively and randomized once they met inclusion criteria. A total of 172 patients were randomized. While those patients who received rFVIIa required fewer reoperations, received fewer allogeneic blood products, and had lower chest tube output, a trend toward more cSAEs was seen in the rFVIIa group. Although this finding did not reach statistical significance because of the small sample size, the potential harm is important. Based on the findings in this underpowered trial, the risk of having an adverse event may be decreased by 50% or, importantly, it might be increased by as much as 5 times (odds ratio 1.67 [0.5-5.47]). This is an extremely important finding and certainly warrants further study in an adequately powered trial so that we can better understand the risk-to-benefit ratio of blood transfusions compared with complications attributable to factor VIIa. This same understanding should be sought as we use other agents that are targeted to decrease perioperative bleeding in cardiac surgery.

E. A. Martinez, MD, MHS

Reference

1. Koch CG, Li L, Duncan AI, Loop FD, Starr NJ, Blackstone EH. Transfusion in coronary artery bypass grafting is associated with reduced long-term survival. *Ann Thorac surg.* 2006;81:1650-1657.

Impact of 24-Hour In-House Intensivists on a Dedicated Cardiac Surgery Intensive Care Unit
Kumar K, on behalf of the Cardiovascular Health Research in Manitoba Investigator Group (St. Boniface General Hosp/I.H. Asper Clinical Res Inst, Manitoba, Canada; et al)
Ann Thorac Surg 88:1153-1161, 2009

Background.—Intensive care unit (ICU) physician staffing models for cardiac surgery patients vary widely and correlate poorly with outcomes. Clinical outcomes associated with 24-hour, in-house intensivists working in a dedicated post–cardiac surgical unit have not been previously investigated. We sought to examine the safety and efficacy of such a model.

Methods.—A retrospective, propensity-matched, cohort study of all patients undergoing a cardiac surgical procedure at a single tertiary center was performed. The control cohort (n = 1,467) consisted of patients admitted to the traditional, mixed surgical intensive care unit (SICU) from January 2005 to January 2007. The intervention cohort (n = 1,089) consisted of patients admitted to a newly created "hybrid" cardiac surgery ICU (CICU) from January 2007 to January 2008, which was staffed by 24-hour in-house consultant intensivists and a daytime, fast track cardiac anesthesiologist. The primary outcomes were blood product utilization, requirement for ventilation, and ICU recidivism.

Results.—The proportion of patients in the CICU cohort who received transfused red blood cells was decreased compared with the SICU cohort (30.2% versus 42.3%, $p < 0.001$). Similar reductions in platelets and fresh frozen plasma were also observed. The CICU patients were less likely to arrive to the ICU intubated (43.7% versus 66.5%, $p < 0.001$). There were no differences in postoperative complications. Overall hospital length of stay was reduced in the CICU cohort by a median of 1 day (6 days [interquartile range, 5 to 8] versus 7 days [5 to 9], $p < 0.001$). Significant reductions in mortality and ICU recidivism were not observed.

Conclusions.—The current Manitoba CICU model of 24-hour intensive care physician/cardiac anesthesiologist staffing in postoperative cardiac surgery care is associated with reduced transfusion of blood components, decreased requirement for mechanical ventilation, and shorter hospital length of stay.

▶ Studies have shown that the presence of an intensivist is associated with decreased mortality and frequently decreased length of stay.[1] However, there are few data assessing this association in isolated cardiac surgery intensive care units (CICUs). The authors report on their experience with the introduction of a dedicated CICU and implementation of a 24-hour in-house coverage model. They performed a retrospective, propensity-matched, cohort study of over 2000 patients. They sought to evaluate the impact of the interventions on blood use, requirement for ventilation, and ICU readmission. The care model before this intervention consisted of admission of patients to a mixed surgical ICU. Daytime coverage consisted of a consultant intensivist and junior residents. The overnight coverage consisted of an in-house junior resident and an intensivist providing home-call backup. Following the ICU, patients were discharged to a step-down/intermediate care unit and then to the general cardiac surgical floor. The new unit and model were created in 2007 during which year the cardiac surgical volume increased from 700 to 1000 cases per year because of national (Canadian) referral mandates. The new model, a hybrid CICU, consisted of 8 to 10 beds, of which some were designated for fast-track and were managed during the day by a cardiac anesthesiologist who was free of all other duties. An intensivist managed the remainder of the beds. The night-time coverage was managed by a different intensivist who was dedicated to that CICU. Care was continued in the CICU until the patient was appropriate for transfer to the regular ward setting, because the step-down unit was eliminated with the new model. All patients were included in the analysis and matched by propensity scores (85.7% of entire cohort), which adds strength to the analysis given its prepost design and vulnerability to temporal bias. The authors report a significant reduction in the proportion of patients receiving blood products (Fig 2) and a shorter length of stay, although the interquartile ranges overlap. They also observed a trend toward a decrease in ICU and 30-day mortality. Interestingly, they report that fewer patients arrived in the ICU intubated; therefore a significant change in the intraoperative technique (a fast-track anesthetic plan) cannot be ruled out as a significant contributor to the difference in outcome, or at a minimum as a confounder.

While this is an interesting article and explores a very important question in how postoperative cardiac care can best be delivered, it doesn't quite give us the answer as to what component of this hybrid system contributed most to the improvements. We cannot rule out that it was the institution of a dedicated unit itself, a dedicated nursing staff with expertise in cardiac care, a different physician-to-patient ratio with the addition of the anesthesiologist who cared

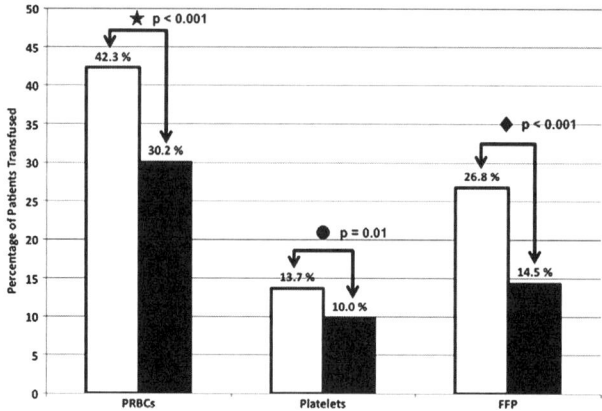

FIGURE 2.—A significant reduction in the proportion of patients receiving packed red blood cells (PRBCs), platelets, and fresh frozen plasma (FFP) was observed in the cardiac surgery intensive care unit cohort (solid bars) compared with the surgical intensive care unit cohort (open bars). (Reprinted from Kumar K, on behalf of the Cardiovascular Health Research in Manitoba Investigator Group. Impact of 24-hour in-house intensivists on a dedicated cardiac surgery intensive care unit. *Ann Thorac Surg.* 2009;88:1153-1161, with permission from The Society of Thoracic Surgeons.)

for a proportion of the patients, a possible change in the nurse-to-patient ratio staffing pattern, the avoidance of an additional transfer of care (a known vulnerable point in the care of patients) to the intermediate care unit, or a change in resident coverage (resident coverage not described for the hybrid unit). Further research is warranted to identify the best structures and processes of care in the postoperative care of cardiac surgical patients that are associated with improved outcomes. Teasing out the contribution of each of these would be very important as centers prioritize which components of such a model they might implement.

E. A. Martinez, MD, MHS

Reference

1. Pronovost PJ, Angus DC, Dorman T, Robinson KA, Dremsizov TT, Young TL. Physician staffing patterns and clinical outcomes in critically ill patients: a systematic review. *JAMA.* 2002;288:2151-2162.

Serum Myoglobin and Renal Morbidity and Mortality following Thoracic and Thoraco-Abdominal Aortic Repair: Does Rhabdomyolysis Play a Role?
Miller CC III, Villa MA, Sutton J, et al (Univ of Texas Med School at Houston)
Eur J Vasc Endovasc Surg 37:388-394, 2009

Objectives.—The intractability of renal dysfunction following thoracic and thoraco-abdominal aortic repair leads us to believe that the accepted mechanisms of renal injury – ischaemia and embolism – are incompletely explanatory. We studied postoperative myoglobinaemia and renal dysfunction following aortic surgery.

Methods.—Between September 2006 and February 2008, we studied serum myoglobin in 109 patients requiring thoracic/thoraco-abdominal repair for three postoperative days. Forty-two of the 109 (38%) patients were female. The median age was 67 years (range 23–84 years). As we have focussed more attention on renal function, our independent renal consultants have dialysed more aggressively. We divided dialysis into: (1) creatinine indication, (2) non-creatinine indication and (3) no dialysis.

Results.—Thirteen of the 109 (12%) patients met creatinine indication for dialysis (>4 mg dl^{-1}) and an additional 28 (26%) were dialysed for other reasons. Overall mortality was 12 out of 109 (11%) cases: 11 out of 41 (27%) in dialysed patients and one out of 68 (1.5%) in non-dialysed patients. Mortality did not differ between the indications for dialysis. Predictors of mortality were baseline glomerular filtration rate (GFR), postoperative myoglobin and dialysis. The only predictor of dialysis was postoperative myoglobin.

Conclusion.—A strong relationship between postoperative serum myoglobin and renal failure suggests a rhabdomyolysis-like contributing aetiology following thoraco-abdominal aortic repair. We postulate

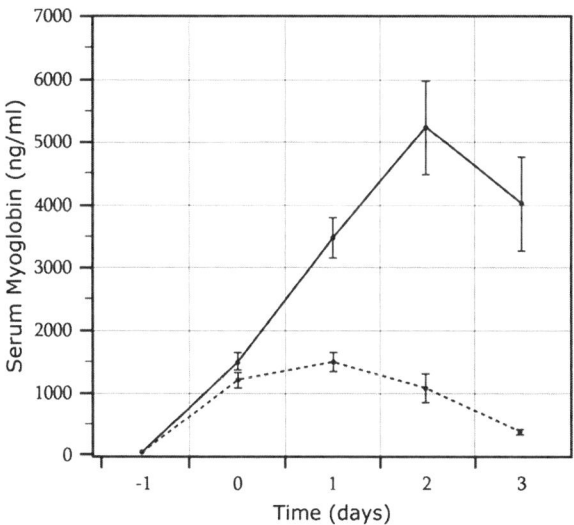

FIGURE 2.—Time course of serum myoglobin. Day 1 is the day before surgery. Day 0 is day of surgery, and days 1–3 are postoperative days 1–3. The solid line indicates patients with renal failure and dashed line indicates patients without. Rhabdomyolysis is described in the literature as occurring at myoglobin levels of 1000–5000 ng ml^{-1}. Upper limit of normal range for our laboratory is 85 ng ml^{-1}. (Reprinted from Miller III CC, Villa MA, Sutton J, et al. Serum myoglobin and renal morbidity and mortality following thoracic and thoraco-abdominal aortic repair: does rhabdomyolysis play a role? *Eur J Vasc Endovasc Surg.* 2009;37:388-394, with permission from the European Society for Vascular Surgery.)

a novel mechanism of renal injury for which mitigation strategies should be developed.

▶ Although these authors have identified an interesting association, this study has significant limitations that preclude its use for more than hypothesis generation. The dataset may not be standardized and thus may contain bias itself. The patients were not controlled for cardiac output, reperfusion, creatine kinases (CKs), or statin use. Initiation of dialysis was also not standardized, impacting outcome groups. As can be seen in Fig 2, those who went on to have myoglobin elevation went on to have higher rates of creatinine rise. Again, this association is interesting and offers a hypothesis that should be tested prospectively with adequate controls.

T. Dorman, MD

On-Pump versus Off-Pump Coronary-Artery Bypass Surgery
Shroyer AL, for the Veterans Affairs Randomized On/Off Bypass (ROOBY) Study Group (Northport Veterans Affairs (VA) Med Ctr; et al)
N Engl J Med 361:1827-1837, 2009

Background.—Coronary-artery bypass grafting (CABG) has traditionally been performed with the use of cardiopulmonary bypass (on-pump CABG). CABG without cardiopulmonary bypass (off-pump CABG) might reduce the number of complications related to the heart–lung machine.

Methods.—We randomly assigned 2203 patients scheduled for urgent or elective CABG to either on-pump or off-pump procedures. The primary short-term end point was a composite of death or complications (reoperation, new mechanical support, cardiac arrest, coma, stroke, or renal failure) before discharge or within 30 days after surgery. The primary long-term end point was a composite of death from any cause, a repeat revascularization procedure, or a nonfatal myocardial infarction within 1 year after surgery. Secondary end points included the completeness of revascularization, graft patency at 1 year, neuropsychological outcomes, and the use of major resources.

Results.—There was no significant difference between off-pump and on-pump CABG in the rate of the 30-day composite outcome (7.0% and 5.6%, respectively; P = 0.19). The rate of the 1-year composite outcome was higher for off-pump than for on-pump CABG (9.9% vs. 7.4%, P = 0.04). The proportion of patients with fewer grafts completed than originally planned was higher with off-pump CABG than with on-pump CABG (17.8% vs. 11.1%, P<0.001). Follow-up angiograms in 1371 patients who underwent 4093 grafts revealed that the overall rate of graft patency was lower in the off-pump group than in the on-pump group (82.6% vs. 87.8%, P<0.01). There were no treatment-based differences in neuropsychological outcomes or short-term use of major resources.

Conclusions.—At 1 year of follow-up, patients in the off-pump group had worse composite outcomes and poorer graft patency than did patients in the on-pump group. No significant differences between the techniques were found in neuropsychological outcomes or use of major resources. (ClinicalTrials.gov number, NCT00032630.)

▶ The advent of "off-pump" coronary artery bypass surgery was greeted with great enthusiasm, as many of the postoperative complications of cardiac bypass surgery were directly linked to cardiopulmonary artery bypass. This includes activation of complement and the proinflammatory cascade, and depletion of clotting factors and microembolic phenomenon to the brain. Early preliminary reports failed to demonstrate a decrease in postoperative complications and morbidities, which was unexpected. This is an important article because of the size (2203 patients) and the randomization. This trial once again shows not only no benefit from off-pump, but it shows worse outcomes with poorer graft patency than on-pump. Since there is no way one could say that bypass itself is of benefit, the only explanation for these results is that use of bypass allows better surgical technique to be deployed.

R. P. Dellinger, MD

Miscellaneous

Use of Helical CT Is Associated with an Increased Incidence of Postoperative Pulmonary Emboli in Cancer Patients with No Change in the Number of Fatal Pulmonary Emboli

Auer RC, Schulman AR, Tuorto S, et al (Univ of Ottawa, Ontario, Canada; Memorial Sloan-Kettering Cancer Center, NY)
J Am Coll Surg 208:871-878, 2009

Background.—Multidetector computed tomography (MDCT) scanning technology has increased the ease with which pulmonary emboli (PE) are evaluated. Our aim was to determine whether the incidence and severity of postoperative PE have changed since adoption of Multidetector computed tomography.

Study Design.—A prospective postoperative morbidity and mortality database from a single institution was used to identify all cancer patients who experienced a PE within 30 days of thoracic, abdominal, or pelvic operations. The incidence, type (central, segmental, and subsegmental), and severity of PE were examined.

Results.—A total of 295 PE were documented among 47,601 postoperative cancer patients. The incidence of PE increased yearly from 2.3 per 1,000 patients in 2000 to 9.3 per 1,000 patients in 2005 ($p < 0.0001$). This corresponded to an increasing number of CT scans of the chest performed (6.6 CT scans per 1,000 postoperative patients in 2000 versus 45 in 2005; $p < 0.0001$). The increased incidence was because of a 7.8%

(CI, 4.0 to 11.7) and 5.4% (CI, 4.1 to 6.7) average annual increase in segmental and subsegmental PE, respectively. There was no change in the number of central (0.1%; CI, −1.0 to 1.12) PE. Overall incidence of fatal PE was 0.4 and did not change during the time period (p = 0.3). A central PE was more commonly associated with hypoxia, ICU admission, and 30-day mortality (33% versus 5% for peripheral; p = 0.02).

Conclusions.—Chest CT scans are being performed more frequently on postoperative cancer patients and have resulted in an increased diagnosis of peripheral PE. The clinical significance of, and optimal treatment for, diagnosed subsegmental PE are incompletely defined.

▶ The authors document an observation that has also been made in the trauma patient population. The more you look for venous thromboembolic complications, the more frequently they appear.[1] Thus, to use the diagnosis of venous thromboembolic events (VTEs) as a quality marker, one must have a consistent surveillance policy.

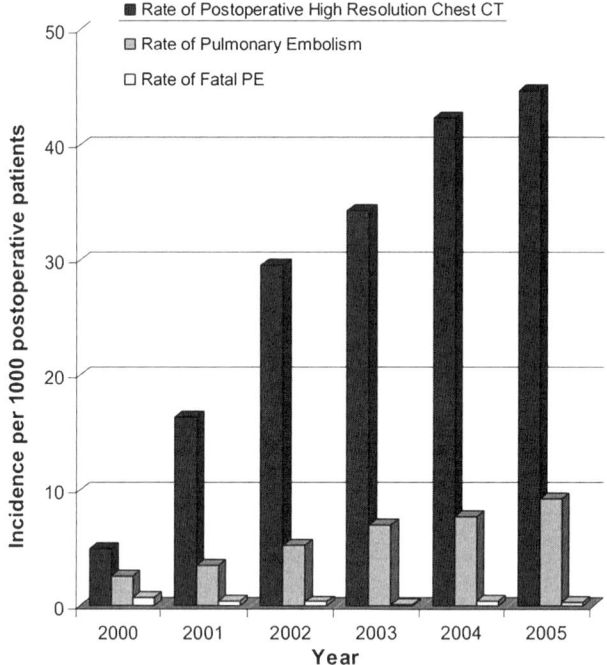

FIGURE 1.—Annual postoperative incidence of multidetector computed tomography (MDCT) scan of the chest, pulmonary embolism (PE), and fatal PE. The number (incidence per 1,000 postoperative patients) of MDCT of the chest performed to evaluate patients for a PE in the postoperative period (black bar) and the number of postoperative PEs (gray bar) detected have increased from 2000 to 2005, and the incidence of a fatal PE among surgical patients in the postoperative period has remained unchanged (white bar). (Reprinted from Auer RC, Schulman AR, Tuorto S, et al. Use of helical CT is associated with an increased incidence of postoperative pulmonary emboli in cancer patients with no change in the number of fatal pulmonary emboli. *J Am Coll Surg* 2009;208:871-878, with permission from the American College of Surgeons.)

I was surprised that pharmacologic VTE prophylaxis was administered in less than 60% of patients. As the authors clearly indicate, malignancy is a marker of increased risk for thromboembolic events. In addition, despite a fixed rate of fatal pulmonary emboli, there is no evolution in the approach to prophylactic use of heparins. I did note that patients who did not die of initial pulmonary emboli were noted to have a subsequent pulmonary embolus in 10% of cases. Early detection of patients with small pulmonary emboli may be a marker for patients at risk for a second, potentially more serious, event.

These data reinforce the importance of VTE prophylaxis, preferably with low molecular weight heparins, in oncologic patients undergoing major surgical procedures. While small pulmonary emboli are more likely to be identified with contemporary imaging modalities, these clots predict an increased risk for subsequent emboli and offer the opportunity for intervention (Fig 1).[2,3]

D. J. Dries, MSE, MD

References

1. Pierce CA, Haut ER, Kardooni S, et al. Surveillance bias and deep vein thrombosis in the national trauma data bank: the more we look, the more we find. *J Trauma.* 2008;64:932-937.
2. Carson JL, Kelley MA, Duff A, et al. The clinical course of pulmonary embolism. *N Engl J Med.* 1992;326:1240-1245.
3. Lazo-Langner A, Goss GD, Spaans JN, Rodger MA. The effect of low-molecular-weight heparin on cancer survival. a systematic review and meta-analysis of randomized trials. *J Thromb Haemost.* 2007;5:729-737.

Noninvasive ventilation for acute respiratory failure after lung resection: an observational study

Lefebvre A, Lorut C, Alifano M, et al (Université Paris 5, France)
Intensive Care Med 35:663-667, 2009

Background.—A single prospective randomized study found that, in selected patients with acute respiratory failure (ARF) following lung resection, noninvasive ventilation (NIV) decreases the need for endotracheal mechanical ventilation and improves clinical outcome.

Method.—We prospectively evaluated early NIV use for ARF after lung resection during a 4-year period in the setting of a medical and a surgical ICU of a university hospital. We documented demographics, initial clinical characteristics and clinical outcomes. NIV failure was defined as the need for tracheal intubation.

Results.—Among 690 patients at risk of severe complications following lung resection, 113 (16.3%) experienced ARF, which was initially supported by NIV in 89 (78.7%), including 59 with hypoxemic ARF (66.3%) and 30 with hypercapnic ARF (33.7%). The overall success rate of NIV was 85.3% (76/89). In-ICU mortality was 6.7% (6/89). The mortality rate following NIV failure was 46.1%. Predictive factors of NIV failure in univariate analysis were age ($P = 0.046$), previous cardiac comorbidities ($P = 0.0075$), postoperative pneumonia ($P = 0.0016$), admission in the surgical ICU ($P = 0.034$), no initial response to NIV ($P < 0.0001$) and occurrence of noninfectious complications ($P = 0.037$). Only two independent factors were significantly associated with NIV failure in multivariate analysis: cardiac comorbidities (odds ratio, 11.5; 95% confidence interval, 1.9–68.3; $P = 0.007$) and no initial response to NIV (odds ratio, 117.6; 95% confidence interval, 10.6–1305.8; $P = 0.0001$).

Conclusion.—This prospective survey confirms the feasibility and efficacy of NIV in ARF following lung resection.

▶ This important article studies a large number of patients at a single institution after pulmonary resection. Unfortunately, there is no randomization. Patients are assigned to invasive and noninvasive ventilation based on clinician judgment. Examination of the figure indicates a good selection of hypoxemic and hypercapnic respiratory failure treated with noninvasive ventilation (Fig 1). It appears that the practitioner using noninvasive ventilation after pulmonary resection

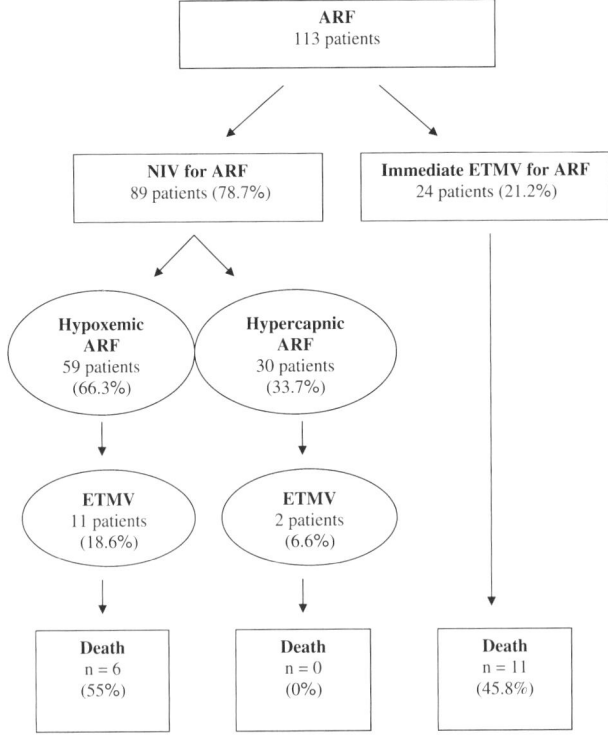

FIGURE 1.—Distribution and outcomes of mechanical ventilatory support for acute respiratory failure (*ARF*). (Reprinted from Lefebvre A, Lorut C, Alifano M, et al. Noninvasive ventilation for acute respiratory failure after lung resection: an observational study. *Intensive Care Med.* 2009;35:663-667, with kind permission from Springer-Verlag.)

TABLE 2.—Characteristics of Patients at NIV Initiation

Parameters	Overall Population $n = 89$	Hypoxemic ARF Group $n = 59$	Hypercapnic ARF Group $n = 30$	P value
Heart rate (beats/min)	99 ± 27.6	110 ± 29.6	85.3 ± 16.7	0.0003
Systolic pressure (mmHg)	125 ± 26.6	127 ± 25.8	122 ± 27.9	0.44
Respiratory rate (breaths/min)	25.9 ± 6.4	28.6 ± 4.5	20.7 ± 6.5	0.0001
SAPS II at ICU admission	28.9 ± 9	29.7 ± 7.7	27.4 ± 11.1	0.24
PaO_2/FiO_2	226 ± 10	189 ± 71	274 ± 112	0.008
$PaCO_2$ (mmHg)	46 ± 8.9	38.2 ± 5	54.1 ± 4.3	0.0001
pH	7.34 ± 0.06	7.38 ± 0.04	7.30 ± 0.05	<0.0001

Data are presented as mean values ± SD.
SAPS simplified acute physiologic score, PaO_2 arterial oxygen tension, $PaCO_2$ arterial carbon dioxide tension.

must be careful of cardiac complications in the patient with hypoxemic ARF. The patient with hypercapnic ARF did well in this study. Of concern, however, is the extremely high mortality rate (45% or more) in patients failing noninvasive ventilation or requiring immediate endotracheal mechanical ventilation. We are given no data regarding physiologic severity of illness in this population.

The patients studied included a variety of pulmonary procedures, including a small number of pneumonectomies (approximately 12%), lobectomy (64%), and lesser resections. Only one patient suffered a bronchial stump blowout. This patient also had bleeding complications and required a second thoracotomy. It is possible that the bronchial stump was compromised by hypoperfusion in this patient (Table 2).

A number of general observations can be made. First, bronchial stump blowout or gastrointestinal tract perforation is unlikely in patients receiving noninvasive ventilation after pulmonary resection. Gastrointestinal dysmotility, however, was noted frequently. The patient with hypoxemic respiratory failure in this trial was more severely ill and at increased risk to do poorly. Patients with hypercapnic respiratory failure appeared healthier than the hypoxemic group.[1-3]

D. J. Dries, MSE, MD

References

1. Brochard L, Mancebo J, Wysocki M, et al Noninvasive ventilation for acute exacerbations of chronic obstructive pulmonary disease. *N Engl J Med.* 1995; 333: 817-822.
2. Ferrer M, Esquinas A, Leon M, Gonzalez G, Alarcon A, Torres A. Noninvasive ventilation in severe hypoxemic respiratory failure: a randomized clinical trial. *Am J Respir Crit Care Med.* 2003;168:1438-1444.
3. Antonelli M, Conti G, Moro ML, et al. Predictors of failure of noninvasive positive pressure ventilation in patients with acute hypoxemic respiratory failure: a multi-center study. *Intensive Care Med.* 2001;27:1718-1728.

Going home to die from surgical intensive care units

Huang Y-C, Huang S-J, Ko W-J (Natl Taiwan Univ Hosp, Taipei)
Intensive Care Med 35:810-815, 2009

Purpose.—To better understand events related to going home to die (GHTD) from the intensive care unit (ICU), with the hope that this information might improve the palliative care of ICU patients.

Methods.—This retrospective observational study was performed at a tertiary medical center—the National Taiwan University Hospital. All surgical ICU mortality cases between 1 January 2003 and 31 December 2007 were included in this study.

Results.—The rate of GHTD from the ICU declined annually, but has reached a plateau of around 25% in recent years. Multivariate logistic regression analysis found independently significant factors associated with GHTD, including older age (OR: 1.013; $P = 0.001$), married status (OR: 2.128; $P < 0.001$), lower educational level (OR: 1.799; $P = 0.001$), and lack of DNR consent (OR: 1.499; $P = 0.006$). When treatment intensity was compared on the date of death, GHTD patients in general received more treatments and diagnostic procedures than those who died in the ICU. Univariate analysis showed that GHTD patients received significantly more advanced antibiotics, more chest radiography, greater use of sedatives, greater use of analgesics, and more transfusions, but less FiO_2 and mechanical circulatory support than patients who died in the ICU.

Conclusion.—GHTD from the ICU is a special phenomenon in the Chinese cultural area, representing a cultural tradition rather than a form of palliative care.

▶ Bioethicist Alexander Capron has argued:

There is no such thing as a "natural" death. Somewhere along the way for just about every patient, death is forestalled by human choice and human action, or death is allowed to occur because of human choice.

Life-support techniques make death a matter of human choice and hence a matter that provokes ethical concern.[1]

There are 4 medical actions that can lead to the death of a patient: withholding/withdrawing life-sustaining treatments, provision of palliative treatment that may hasten foreseeable death, euthanasia, and assisted suicide. These 4 actions can lead to a conflict in physicians, between their duty to relieve a patient's suffering and their duty to preserve life. For patients, their concern is not the physician's conflict, but their desire to die in a peaceful way in a place of their choosing, usually their home.

However, while a majority of the public desires to die in the comfort of their homes, many will die in inpatient settings such as hospitals. There are many factors that affect where people eventually die, including a person's financial means, access to health care resources such as hospices, and cultural beliefs. The assumption that states in America with higher home- and community-based services allow people to spend their last days at home has been shown to be incorrect.[2] In spite of growing hospice and palliative services, allowing patients to go home to die from hospitals has been constant challenge for health professionals in United States.

This study analyzed the events related to going home to die from the surgical intensive care unit (ICU) setting. They found that 25% of patients were discharged to home when death seemed imminent. Factors associated with going home to die included older age, married status, and religion. Patients going home to die also received more sedatives, analgesics, transfusions, and antibiotics to make the patients as comfortable as possible and increase the chances for the patient to arrive home to die.

The authors attributed a quarter of patients leaving the surgical ICU to die at home to the special cultural meaning of dying at home in Taiwan. This is in contrast to other countries where patients' transition from ICUs to hospices or nursing homes where palliative care can be given. In the United States, the percentage of Americans dying as hospital inpatients has dropped from 54% to 41% from 1980-1998.[2] During the end of that time period, African-Americans were more likely to die as inpatients when compared with Caucasians. This difference may be due to cultural differences and the lack of access for African-Americans to hospice and home health care services.

Going home to die from an ICU is a cultural phenomenon in Taiwan. While the percentage of Americans dying as hospital inpatients has decreased over the past 30 years, there need to be better resources to aid Americans who desire to die at home. Resources such as support for caregivers at home and the ability to provide health care in the home rather than a hospital will help in this regard. These resources will also need to be tailored for different cultures and ethnicities as well as different disease processes if they are to be used by the public. In conjunction, it needs to be determined what is the ethical responsibility of physicians when patients wish to die. There is constant conflict between the principle of patient autonomy and the obligation of physicians to respect patient's choices and the potential consequences of a policy that permits physicians to act in a way that would lead to a patient's death.

S. N. Patel, MD
V. Rajput, MD

References

1. Capron AM. Legal and ethical problems in decisions for death. *Law Med Health Care*. 1986;14:141-144.
2. Muramatsu N, Hoyem R, Yin H, Campbell RT. Place of death among older Americans: does state spending on home- and community-based services promote home death? *Med Care*. 2008;46:829-838.

Clinical Benefits After the Implementation of a Protocol of Restricted Perioperative Intravenous Crystalloid Fluids in Major Abdominal Operations

de Aguilar-Nascimento JE, Diniz BN, do Carmo AV, et al (The Federal Univ of Mato Grosso, Cuiaba, Brazil)
World J Surg 33:925-930, 2009

Background.—Perioperative fluid replacement is a challenging issue in surgical care. The purpose of the present study was to investigate the effect of two different perioperative hydration protocols on the outcome in patients undergoing major abdominal operations.

Methods.—This was a prospective study involving 61 patients (42 men/19 women; mean age: 52 years; age range: 18–81 years) who underwent major abdominal operations. The study had two distinct phases: before (conventional group; administered 30–50 ml/kg per day of crystalloid fluids; $n = 33$) and after the implementation of a protocol of restricted use of intravenous fluids (restricted group; administered less than 30 ml/kg per day of crystalloid fluids; $n = 28$). The total volume of intravenous crystalloid fluids infused was recorded until postoperative day (POD) 4. Morbidity, mortality, and the length of postoperative hospital stay were the main clinical variables.

Results.—Mortality was 4.9% ($p > 0.05$ between groups). Intravenous therapy in the restricted group was terminated earlier ($p < 0.001$) and the patients received 2.4 l less crystalloid fluid than did those in the conventional group from POD 1 through POD 4 ($p < 0.001$). The adoption of the restricted protocol shortened the postoperative hospital stay by 2 days ($p = 0.02$) and diminished the morbidity by 25% ($p = 0.04$).

Conclusions.—Restriction of perioperative intravenous crystalloid fluid is associated with reductions in morbidity and length of postoperative hospital stay after major abdominal operations.

▶ This important preliminary work argues that restriction of fluids in the perioperative period may be associated with early departure from hospital, reduction in complications, and earlier introduction of oral nutrition. There are several concerns that are relevant to this work. While the study is prospective, it is carried out over an extended period of time. Cases are not randomized. Control procedures are performed first followed by the study group receiving reduced postoperative fluid administration. When complications are examined in the conventional and restricted groups in this study, outcomes are similar with one exception. A greater number of pulmonary complications are noted in the patients receiving larger amounts of postoperative fluid. Unfortunately, pulmonary complications are not rigorously defined (Table 4).

Why is this preliminary work important? These results are similar to a recent study by the ARDSNet investigators, which compared 2 fluid management strategies in patients with acute lung injury.[1] As in this study, there was no difference in observed mortality. However, a conservative fluid management strategy was associated with improved lung function and reduced duration of

TABLE 4.—Distribution of Morbidities in the Two Groups

Complications	Conventional group ($n = 33$)	Restricted group ($n = 28$)	p Value
Surgical site infection	6	4	0.74
Anastomotic dehiscence	6	2	0.27
Pulmonary	9	2	0.05
Sepsis	2	2	1.00
Shock	2	1	1.00
Total number of complications[a]	25	11	<0.01
No. of patients with complications	14	9	0.04
No. of complications per patient with complication	1.7	1.2	0.14

[a]Some patients had more than one complication

mechanical ventilation and critical care stay. Nonpulmonary organ failures did not increase with reduced fluid administration. This more rigorous study corresponds to the pulmonary findings of the Brazilian group featured here.

Here is one more study which argues that we must think critically about fluid administration after operation.[1,2] To better study this question, we also have to standardize operating room fluid administration and critically assess the preoperative hydration status of investigated patients.

D. J. Dries, MSE, MD

References

1. National Heart, Lung, and Blood Institute Acute Respiratory Distress Syndrome (ARDS) Clinical Trials Network, Wiedemann HP, Wheeler AP, Bernard GR, et al. Comparison of two fluid-management strategies in acute lung injury. *N Engl J Med*. 2006;354:2564-2575.
2. Murphy CV, Schramm GE, Doherty JA, et al. The importance of fluid management in acute lung injury secondary to septic shock. *Chest*. 2009;136:102-109.

Intraoperative Transfusion of 1 U to 2 U Packed Red Blood Cells Is Associated with Increased 30-Day Mortality, Surgical-Site Infection, Pneumonia, and Sepsis in General Surgery Patients
Bernard AC, Davenport DL, Chang PK, et al (Univ of Kentucky, Lexington)
J Am Coll Surg 208:931-937, 2009

Background.—Transfusion of packed red blood cells (PRBCs) increases morbidity and mortality in select surgical specialty patients. The impact of low-volume, leukoreduced RBC transfusion on general surgery patients is less well understood.

Study Design.—The American College of Surgeons National Surgical Quality Improvement Program participant use file was queried for general surgery patients recorded in 2005 to 2006 (n = 125,223). Thirty-day morbidity (21 uniformly defined complications) and mortality, demographic, preoperative, and intraoperative risk variables were obtained. Infectious complications and composite morbidity and mortality were stratified across intraoperative PRBCs units received. Multivariable logistic regression was used to assess influence of transfusion on outcomes, while adjusting for transfusion propensity, procedure type, wound class, operative duration, and 30+ patient risk factors.

Results.—After adjustment for transfusion propensity, procedure group, wound class, operative duration, and all other important risk variables, 1 U PRBCs significantly ($p < 0.05$) increased risk of 30-day mortality (odds ratio [OR] = 1.32), composite morbidity (OR = 1.23), pneumonia (OR = 1.24), and sepsis/shock (OR = 1.29). Transfusion of 2 U additionally increased risk for these outcomes (OR = 1.38, 1.40, 1.25, 1.53, respectively; $p \leq 0.05$) plus surgical-site infection (OR = 1.25; $p < 0.05$). A risk index for calculating transfusion likelihood demonstrated very good discrimination (c-index = 0.844).

Conclusions.—Intraoperative transfusion of PRBCs increases risk for mortality and several morbidities in general surgery patients. These risks, substantial for even 1 U, remain after adjustment for transfusion propensity and numerous risk factors available in the American College of Surgeons National Surgical Quality Improvement Program. Transfusion

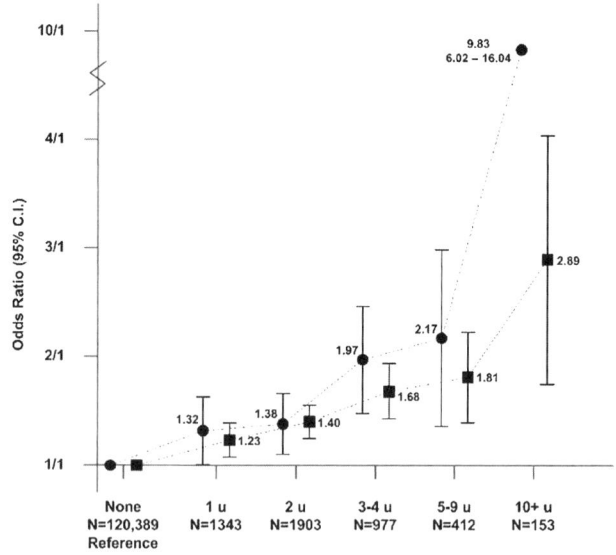

FIGURE 2.—Propensity and risk adjusted odds ratios (95% CI) for 30-day mortality and morbidity by level of intraoperative transfusion. Both morbidity and mortality risks were substantially increased after only 1 U RBC transfusion intraoperatively and continued to increase with increasing units. Circles, mortality; squares, morbidity. (Reprinted from Bernard AC, Davenport DL, Chang PK, et al. Intraoperative transfusion of 1 U to 2 U packed red blood cells is associated with increased 30-day mortality, surgical-site infection, pneumonia, and sepsis in general surgery patients. *J Am Coll Surg.* 2009;208:931-937, with permission from the American College of Surgeons.)

for mildly hypovolemic or anemic patients should be discouraged in light of these risks (Fig 2).

▶ Using the extensive National Surgical Quality Improvement Program of the American College of Surgeons, the authors document incremental morbidity and mortality associated with intraoperative red cell transfusion.[1] These data parallel observations made in the trauma community where adverse outcomes associated with the use of red blood cells have been documented for a decade and a half.[2]

There are several important limitations in this study. First, the most accurate data come from the intraoperative period. The database does not reflect carefully the amount of blood given during the time before operation and shortly thereafter. Thus, there is a significant risk that some transfusions are not included in this database. Second, platelet data are not incorporated. While the impact of platelets on transfusion-related morbidity remains unclear, we know nothing of their use in this patient group. Third is the list of limitations accompanying any large retrospective registry-based study.

Nonetheless, this work represents an important observation as the perioperative immune state in general surgery patients probably is dissimilar (in many cases) to multiply injured trauma patients having immune and metabolic stress added to the effects of transfusion. This article documents one more group of surgical patients in whom transfusion is a risk factor for adverse outcome.[3,4]

D. J. Dries, MSE, MD

References

1. Khuri SF, Henderson WG, Daley J, et al. The patient safety in surgery study: background, study design, and patient populations. *J Am Coll Surg.* 2007;204: 1089-1102.
2. Napolitano L. Cumulative risks of early red blood cell transfusion. *J Trauma.* 2006;60:S26-S34.
3. Scott BH, Seifert FC, Grimson R. Blood transfusion is associated with increased resource utilization, morbidity and mortality in cardiac surgery. *Ann Card Anaesth.* 2008;11:15-19.
4. Murphy GJ, Reeves BC, Rogers CA, Rizvi SI, Culliford L, Angelini GD. Increased mortality, postoperative morbidity, and cost after red blood cell transfusion in patients having cardiac surgery. *Circulation.* 2007;116:2544-2552.

7 Sepsis/Septic Shock

Outcome of patients receiving high dose vasopressor therapy: a retrospective cohort study

Jenkins CR, Gomersall CD, Leung P, et al (The Chinese Univ of Hong Kong, Shatin)

Anaesth Intensive Care 37:286-289, 2009

The aim of this study was to determine the hospital survival of patients receiving high doses of catecholamines.

A retrospective observational study was conducted in a 22-bed multidisciplinary adult intensive care unit of a tertiary referral university hospital. All patients (n = 64) receiving > 100 μg/min of adrenaline or noradrenaline or adrenaline and noradrenaline combined over a one-year period were studied to determine survival to intensive care unit and hospital discharge. Four patients survived to intensive care unit discharge and hospital discharge (6.25%, 95% CI 0.3 to 12.2%). Survival was 3.3% (95% CI 0 to 7.9%) in the subgroup of 60 patients who received > 100 μg/min noradrenaline and 3.6% (95% CI 0 to 8.6%) in the 55 patients who received > 2 μg/kg/min noradrenaline. None of the 32 patients who received > 200 μg/min noradrenaline survived.

We conclude that the survival of patients requiring high doses of catecholamines is poor, but the use of such doses is probably not futile. It remains for individual clinicians, patients and their surrogates to decide whether use of high doses of vasopressor is appropriate, given the low probability of survival.

▶ This is a retrospective review of outcomes from a single ICU for patients who received high-dose vasopressors. All clinicians find themselves with patients who seem to require these excessively high doses, and we all wonder if it's worth it. In the United States right now debate is raging regarding limitations of care given the high expenditures that exist at the terminus of life. These authors have shown that only a small percentage (5.7%) of their total patient population seems to require these very high doses of norepinephrine or epinephrine. Survival in the population that required more than 100 μg/min was only 3.3%. No patient that required this dose for more than 20 hours survived nor did any patient who received twice this dose. There are several obvious concerns in addition to the fact that only associations can be identified for future study from a project such as this. These additional concerns related to other aspects of care described within the article such as how the authors determined when to escalate pressor doses and the use of high-dose steroids

(100 mg every 8 hours) in patients with a diagnosis of septic shock. Importantly, the decision to limit support or even to withdraw support may have been impacted by the general belief that high doses are incompatible with life and thus could have served as a self-fulfilling prophecy.

T. Dorman, MD

Early Use of Polymyxin B Hemoperfusion in Abdominal Septic Shock: The EUPHAS Randomized Controlled Trial

Cruz DN, Antonelli M, Fumagalli R, et al (St Bortolo Hosp and International Renal Res Inst Vicenza, Italy; Catholic Univ of Sacred Heart, Rome, Italy; Milano Bicocca Univ, St Gerardo dei Tintori Hosp, Monza, Italy; et al)
JAMA 301:2445-2452, 2009

Context.—Polymyxin B fiber column is a medical device designed to reduce blood endotoxin levels in sepsis. Gram-negative–induced abdominal sepsis is likely associated with high circulating endotoxin. Reducing circulating endotoxin levels with polymyxin B hemoperfusion could potentially improve patient clinical outcomes.

Objective.—To determine whether polymyxin B hemoperfusion added to conventional medical therapy improves clinical outcomes (mean arterial pressure [MAP], vasopressor requirement, oxygenation, organ dysfunction) and mortality compared with conventional therapy alone.

Design, Setting, and Patients.—A prospective, multicenter, randomized controlled trial (Early Use of Polymyxin B Hemoperfusion in Abdominal Sepsis [EUPHAS]) conducted at 10 Italian tertiary care intensive care units between December 2004 and December 2007. Sixty-four patients were enrolled with severe sepsis or septic shock who underwent emergency surgery for intra-abdominal infection.

Intervention.—Patients were randomized to either conventional therapy (n=30) or conventional therapy plus 2 sessions of polymyxin B hemoperfusion (n=34).

Main Outcome Measures.—Primary outcome was change in MAP and vasopressor requirement, and secondary outcomes were PaO_2/FiO_2 (fraction of inspired oxygen) ratio, change in organ dysfunction measured using Sequential Organ Failure Assessment (SOFA) scores, and 28-day mortality.

Results.—MAP increased (76 to 84 mm Hg; $P = .001$) and vasopressor requirement decreased (inotropic score, 29.9 to 6.8; $P < .001$) at 72 hours in the polymyxin B group but not in the conventional therapy group (MAP, 74 to 77 mm Hg; $P = .37$; inotropic score, 28.6 to 22.4; $P = .14$). The PaO_2/FiO_2 ratio increased slightly (235 to 264; $P = .049$) in the polymyxin B group but not in the conventional therapy group (217 to 228; $P = .79$). SOFA scores improved in the polymyxin B group but not in the conventional therapy group (change in SOFA, -3.4 vs -0.1; $P < .001$), and 28-day mortality was 32% (11/34 patients) in the polymyxin B group and 53% (16/30 patients) in the conventional therapy group (unadjusted hazard ratio [HR], 0.43; 95% confidence interval [CI], 0.20-0.94; adjusted HR, 0.36; 95% CI, 0.16-0.80).

Conclusion.—In this preliminary study, polymyxin B hemoperfusion added to conventional therapy significantly improved hemodynamics and organ dysfunction and reduced 28-day mortality in a targeted population with severe sepsis and/or septic shock from intra-abdominal gram-negative infections.

Trial Registration.—clinicaltrials.gov Identifier: NCT00629382.

▶ Severe sepsis and septic shock are common problems in the ICU and are associated with a high morbidity and mortality. For many years, endotoxin, one of the principal components of the outer membrane of gram-negative bacteria, has been considered a relevant trigger to the host response in sepsis and an important component of the sepsis pathogenesis. High levels of endotoxin activity have been associated with worse clinical outcomes in patients with sepsis. However, several therapeutics strategies aimed at endotoxin have failed and the use of endotoxin-targeted treatment remains controversial. Polymyxin B, an antibiotic with high affinity for endotoxin, has been bound and immobilized to polystyrene fibers in a medical device for hemoperfusion. This device can effectively bind endotoxins both in vitro and in vivo. Based on this polymixin B hemoperfusion has been proposed as a therapy that could potentially interrupt the response triggered by endotoxin in sepsis. Polymyxin B hemoperfusion has been used principally in Asia for this purpose. A systemic review suggested that polymyxin B hemoperfusion may have favorable effects on mean arterial pressure, vasopressor use, oxygenation, and mortality.[1] However, the conclusion of this systemic review is limited due to the low methodological quality of the few studies available and the heterogeneous population of these studies. In a small European pilot study, polymyxin B was shown to improve cardiac and renal dysfunctions due to sepsis or septic shock, but had no effect on mortality.[2] With this context in mind, this group of Italian investigators conducted a prospective, multicenter, randomized controlled trial in patients with severe sepsis or septic shock who underwent emergency surgery for intraabdominal infection. Patients were randomized to either conventional therapy or conventional therapy plus 2 sessions of polymyxin B hemoperfusion. The authors argued that patients with abdominal sepsis were most likely to have gram-negative induced sepsis and, therefore, high circulating endotoxin levels. The primary outcome for this a study was a change in mean arterial pressure and vasopressor requirement, and secondary outcomes include PaO_2/FiO_2, change in organ dysfunction measured using sequential organ failure assessment (SOFA) scores, and 28-day mortality. In this preliminary study, polymyxin B hemoperfusion added to conventional therapy significantly improved hemodynamics and organ dysfunction and reduced 28-day mortality in a targeted population with severe sepsis and/or septic shock for intraabdominal gram-negative infections. Of interest, the authors state that the study was terminated early based on the surprising difference in the 28-day mortality (a secondary endpoint). Mortality in the polymyxin B group was 32% versus 53% with conventional therapy. It is unfortunate that this study was terminated early, thus precluding a larger patient enrollment with a higher chance of providing a more definitive trial regarding the true effects of polymyxin B hemoperfusion. We agree with the authors who state that further studies with polymyxin B hemoperfusion are warranted and needed to further define whether this should become a standard treatment in patients with gram-negative sepsis. Furthermore, questions regarding the wide applicability of polymixin B hemoperfusion to patients with gram-positive sepsis remain unanswered.

S. L. Zanotti-Cavazzoni, MD

References

1. Cruz DN, Perazella MA, Bellomo R, et al. Effectiveness of polymyxin B-immobolized fiber column in sepsis: a systematic review. *Crit Care.* 2007;11:R47.
2. Vincent JL, Laterre PF, Cohen J, et al. A pilot-controlled study of a polymyxin B-immobilized hemoperfusion catridge in patients with sever sepsis secondary to intra-abdominal infection. *Shock.* 2005;23:400-405.

Adverse outcomes associated with the use of drotrecogin alfa (activated) in patients with severe sepsis and baseline bleeding precautions
Gentry CA, Gross KB, Sud B, et al (Dept of Veterans Affairs Med Ctr, Oklahoma City; Univ of Oklahoma Health Sciences Ctr and Dept of Veterans Affairs Med Ctr)
Crit Care Med 37:19-25, 2009

Background.—Key clinical trials involving drotrecogin alfa (activated) (or recombinant human activated protein C) excluded patients with specific baseline bleeding precautions. However, not all such precautions are considered contraindications to treatment with recombinant human activated protein C in current product labeling.

Objective.—To compare outcomes of patients receiving recombinant human activated protein C with or without baseline bleeding precautions as defined by the Recombinant Human Activated Protein C Worldwide Evaluation in Severe Sepsis (PROWESS) trial.

Design.—Retrospective medical record review.

Setting.—Two tertiary care institutions: An academic medical center and an affiliated Veterans Affairs Medical Center.

Patients.—All patients receiving recombinant human activated protein C for treatment of sepsis.

Interventions.—Demographic information, characteristics associated with inclusion and exclusion criteria of the PROWESS trial, and 30-day postdischarge outcomes.

Measurements And Main Results.—Seventy-three patients received recombinant human activated protein C. Serious bleeding events occurred in 7 of 20 patients (35%) with any baseline bleeding precaution vs. only 2 of 53 patients (3.8%) without any bleeding precautions ($p < 0.0001$). More patients with a baseline bleeding precaution died compared with patients without any bleeding precautions (65% vs. 24.5%, $p = 0.0015$).

Patients with a baseline bleeding precaution had a higher mean Acute Physiology and Chronic Health Evaluation II score (27.5 vs. 22.7, $p = 0.015$). Multivariate analysis demonstrated that the presence of a baseline bleeding precaution was the only independent variable associated with occurrence of serious bleeding events. The presence of a baseline bleeding precaution, increased Acute Physiology and Chronic Health Evaluation II score, and the presence of bloodstream infection were independent variables associated with mortality.

Conclusions.—Patients with severe sepsis who received recombinant human activated protein C with baseline bleeding precautions as defined by product labeling had significantly higher rates of both serious bleeding events and deaths compared with those without bleeding precautions. These data suggest that strict adherence to PROWESS trial exclusion criteria would further limit serious bleeding events associated with the use of recombinant human activated protein C.

▶ Drotrecogin alfa (activated) or recombinant human activated protein C (rhAPC) received FDA approval for use in adult patients with severe sepsis and a high risk of death based on the results of the PROWESS trial. The PROWESS trial showed a significant reduction in mortality in patients receiving rhAPC compared with placebo (24.7 % vs 30.8%, $P = .005$).[1] Concerns with the potential for increased bleeding complications and results from follow-up studies that did not show a mortality benefit in lower-risk patient populations treated with rhAPC have raised questions regarding the proper role of rhAPC in treating patients with severe sepsis. Several conditions associated with increased risk of bleeding that were considered contraindications in the PROWESS trial have been placed as precautions or warnings on the current FDA labeling. This means that in clinical practice, outside the confines of a controlled clinical trial, it is more likely that patients with a higher risk of bleeding are being treated with rhAPC. With all the concerns raised regarding the risk/benefit ratio of rhAPC, understanding the impact of these precautions or warnings on outcomes in patients treated with rhAPC becomes critical. In this retrospective review of patients treated with rhAPC, the authors compared outcomes in patients with and without baseline bleeding precautions. The most important findings of this study are the increase in serious bleeding events, serious bleeding events involving the central nervous system, and increased mortality in patients with bleeding precautions that received rhAPC when compared with patients without baseline bleeding precautions. Furthermore, in a multivariate analysis, the only independent factor associated with increased risk of serious bleeding was the presence of a baseline bleeding precaution. Although further randomized trials with rhAPC are ongoing, clinicians still have to decide which patients are best suited to be treated with rhAPC based on the available data. The results from this study should be taken into account understanding that the size and design of the study present limitations. It is not possible to conclude that patients with a baseline bleeding precaution should not receive rhAPC. However, clinicians must recognize the increased risk of bleeding in this patient group and factor this into their risk/benefit assessment.

S. L. Zanotti-Cavazzoni, MD

A prospective, observational registry of patients with severe sepsis: The Canadian Sepsis Treatment and Response Registry
Martin CM, for the STAR Registry Investigators (Lawson Health Research Inst, London, Canada; Eli Lilly Canada Inc., Scarborough, Ontario, Canada; et al)
Crit Care Med 37:81-88, 2009

Objective.—To determine the location of acquisition, timing, and outcomes associated with severe sepsis in community and teaching hospital critical care units.

Design.—Prospective, observational study.

Setting.—Twelve Canadian community and teaching hospital critical care units.

Patients.—All patients admitted between March 17, 2003, and November 30, 2004 to the study critical care units with at least a 24-hr length of stay or severe sepsis identified during the first 24 hrs.

Interventions.—Daily monitoring for severe sepsis.

Measurements and Main Results.—We recorded data describing characteristics of patients, infections, systemic responses, and organ dysfunction. Severe sepsis occurred in 1238 patients (overall rate, 19.0%; range, 8.2%–35.3%). Hospital mortality was 38.1% (95% confidence interval [CI]: 35.4–40.8). Median intensive care unit length of stay was 10.3 days (interquartile range: 5.5, 17.9). Variables associated with mortality in multivariable analysis included age (odds ratio [OR] by decade 1.50; 95% CI: 1.36–1.65), acquisition location of severe sepsis (with community as the reference—hospital [OR: 1.69; CI: 1.16–2.46], early intensive care unit [OR: 2.15; CI: 1.42–3.25], late intensive care unit [OR: 2.65; CI: 1.82–3.87]), late intensive care unit (OR: 2.65; CI: 1.82–3.87), any comorbidity (OR: 1.42; CI: 1.04–1.93), chronic renal failure (OR: 2.03; CI: 1.10–3.76), oliguria (OR: 1.34; CI: 1.02–1.76), thrombocytopenia (OR: 2.12; CI: 1.43–3.13), metabolic acidosis (OR: 1.54; CI: 1.13–2.10), Multiple Organ Dysfunction Score (OR: 1.15; CI: 1.09–1.21) and Acute Physiology and Chronic Health Evaluation II predicted risk (OR: 3.75; CI: 2.08–6.76).

Conclusion.—These data confirm that sepsis is common and has high mortality in general intensive care unit populations. Our results can inform healthcare system planning and clinical study designs. Modifiable variables associated with worse outcomes, such as nosocomial infection (hospital acquisition), and metabolic acidosis indicate potential targets for quality improvement initiatives that could decrease mortality and morbidity.

▶ Sepsis is an important cause of morbidity and mortality in the intensive care unit. Several studies have shown increased hospital resource utilization and prolonged intensive care unit and hospital length of stays in patients with sepsis. Estimates on the annual economic burden of sepsis are in the billions of dollars for the United States alone. Over the last several years, initiatives such as the Surviving Sepsis Campaign have developed guidelines and bundles with the goal of improving patient outcomes in sepsis. However, despite increasing awareness and increased research in the field, the true incidence and epidemiology of sepsis remain undefined. The primary objective of this prospective cohort study conducted in several centers in Canada was to determine hospital mortality of patients in a combination of teaching and academic ICUs. Additional objectives were to determine the location and timing of acquisition of severe sepsis and variables present at the time of acquisition of severe sepsis that were associated with mortality and morbidity. Several findings in this study are valuable from a clinical perspective. First, the mortality of 38.1% illustrates the high severity of this disease and suggests that there is still much room for improvement. The incidence of severe sepsis in the ICU was reported to be almost 20%, reminding us that this is a common disease in critically ill patients. Of greater value perhaps are the findings related to factors associated with increased mortality. This study showed that factors such as age, comorbid diseases, presence of renal failure, and time between hospital and ICU admission were independently associated with increased mortality. Furthermore, a strong correlation was found between mortality and the acquisition location of severe sepsis, progressively increasing mortality if severe sepsis was acquired in the community (< 48 hours after admission), the hospital (> 48 hours after admission), early ICU (> 24 hours after ICU admission), or late ICU (> 4 days after ICU admission). This study provides important and valuable information regarding the epidemiology of sepsis. For the practicing clinician, the results of this study support greater efforts in preventing sepsis with improved infection control measures to decrease the incidences of nosocomial acquired sepsis.

S. L. Zanotti-Cavazzoni, MD

The Importance of Fluid Management in Acute Lung Injury Secondary to Septic Shock

Murphy CV, Schramm GE, Doherty JA, et al (Barnes-Jewish Hosp, St. Louis, MO; Hosp Pharmacy Services, Mayo Clinic, Rochester, MN; BJC Healthcare, St. Louis, MO; et al)
Chest 136:102-109, 2009

Background.—Recent studies have suggested that early goal-directed resuscitation of patients with septic shock and conservative fluid management of patients with acute lung injury (ALI) can improve outcomes. Because these may be seen as potentially conflicting practices, we set out to determine the influence of fluid management on the outcomes of patients with septic shock complicated by ALI.

Methods.—A retrospective analysis was performed at Barnes-Jewish Hospital (St. Louis, MO) and in the medical ICU of Mayo Medical Center (Rochester, MN). Patients hospitalized with septic shock were enrolled into the study if they met the American-European Consensus definition of ALI within 72 h of septic shock onset. Adequate initial fluid resuscitation (AIFR) was defined as the administration of an initial fluid bolus of ≥ 20 mL/kg prior to and achievement of a central venous pressure of ≥ 8 mm Hg within 6 h after the onset of therapy with vasopressors. Conservative late fluid management (CLFM) was defined as even-to-negative fluid balance measured on at least 2 consecutive days during the first 7 days after septic shock onset.

Results.—The study cohort was made up of 212 patients with ALI complicating septic shock. Hospital mortality was statistically lowest for those achieving both AIFR and CLFM and higher for those achieving only CLFM, those achieving only AIFR, and those achieving neither (17 of 93 patients [18.3%] vs 13 of 31 patients [41.9%] vs 30 of 53 patients [56.6%] vs 27 of 35 [77.1%], respectively; $p < 0.001$).

Conclusions.—Both early and late fluid management of septic shock complicated by ALI can influence patient outcomes.

▶ It is often confusing to the resident or medical student when integrating recent evidence-based medicine with regard to early resuscitation with management of the patient with septic shock when it continues into the ICU stay. The current emphasis is on aggressive resuscitation early to include increasing oxygen delivery based on high lactate or persistent hypotension, even to include red blood cell transfusion. As the patient transitions out of the early resuscitation phase into the subacute ICU, course strategy now shifts toward limiting red blood cell transfusion and limiting aggressiveness of resuscitation, both limiting intravascular volume in acute lung injury patients (including diuretic therapy) and recognizing that multiple studies targeting increasing oxygen delivery in the later ICU course failed to show benefit. Although this may be confusing to the resident and medical student, and perhaps even some practicing intensivists, it all makes sense when you look at the literature upon which this logic is based and the location of the patient at the time the research was done.

R. P. Dellinger, MD

Effectiveness of Treatments for Severe Sepsis: A Prospective, Multicenter, Observational Study

Ferrer R, Artigas A, Suarez D, et al (Hosp de Sabadell, Spain; Universidad Autónoma de Barcelona, Sabadell, Spain)

Am J Respir Crit Care Med 180:861-866, 2009

Rationale.—Several Surviving Sepsis Campaign Guidelines recommendations are reevaluated.

Objectives.—To analyze the effectiveness of treatments recommended in the sepsis guidelines.

Methods.—In a prospective observational study, we studied all adult patients with severe sepsis from 77 intensive care units. We recorded compliance with four therapeutic goals (central venous pressure 8 mm Hg or greater for persistent hypotension despite fluid resuscitation and/or lactate greater than 36 mg/dl, central venous oxygen saturation 70% or greater for persistent hypotension despite fluid resuscitation and/or lactate greater than 36 mg/dl, blood glucose greater than or equal to the lower limit of normal but less than 150 mg/dl, and inspiratory plateau pressure less than 30 cm H_2O for mechanically ventilated patients) and four treatments (early broad-spectrum antibiotics, fluid challenge in the event of hypotension and/or lactate greater than 36 mg/dl, low-dose steroids for septic shock, drotrecogin alfa [activated] for multiorgan failure). The primary outcome measure was hospital mortality. The effectiveness of each treatment was estimated using propensity scores.

Measurements and Main Results.—Of 2,796 patients, 41.6% died before hospital discharge. Treatments associated with lower hospital mortality were early broad-spectrum antibiotic treatment (treatment within 1 hour vs. no treatment within first 6 hours of diagnosis; odds ratio, 0.67; 95% confidence interval, 0.50–0.90; $P = 0.008$) and drotrecogin alfa (activated) (odds ratio, 0.59; 95% confidence interval, 0.41–0.84; $P = 0.004$). Fluid challenge and low-dose steroids showed no benefits.

Conclusions.—In severe sepsis, early administration of broad-spectrum antibiotics in all patients and administration of drotrecogin alfa (activated) in the most severe patients reduce mortality.

▶ Severe sepsis and septic shock are among the leading causes of morbidity and mortality in patients admitted to the ICU. Early appropriate antibiotic therapy, early goal-directed therapy (EGDT), corticosteroids, recombinant human-activated protein C (rhAPC), tight glucose control, and lung protective strategies have been associated with improved survival in sepsis. These therapeutic advances constitute the backbone of the evidence-based guidelines published by the Surviving Sepsis Campaign (SSC).[1] To have a greater impact at the bedside, the SCC and the Institute for Healthcare Improvement proposed the implementation of sepsis bundles. The 6-hour resuscitation bundle includes measuring a lactate, early cultures and antibiotics, and EGDT) and the 24-hour management bundle includes glycemic control, low tidal volume ventilation, and determination of appropriateness for corticosteroids and rhAPC. In a previous prospective before-and-after study (Edusepsis) it was shown that compliance with the sepsis bundles (introduced in multiple ICUs after a standardized educational program) can improve outcomes in patients with severe sepsis. Two recent studies, the CORTICUS study and the NICE-SUGAR study, have called into question the efficacy of some of the interventions included in the sepsis bundles,[2,3] therefore increasing the interest in a clear understanding of which individual components of the bundles are responsible for improving outcomes. The objective of this study was to analyze the impact of treatments for severe sepsis on hospital mortality in all patients included in the previous Edusepsis. In this large cohort of ICU patients with severe sepsis, the authors found that 2 of the 4 treatments recommended in the SSC care bundles (early administration of antibiotics and administration of rhAPC) were independently associated with lower hospital mortality after adjusting for multiple independent clinical predictors of death. The findings of this study should help clinicians understand the potential impact of individual components of the sepsis bundle. Furthermore, studies like this one will be needed in the future to better understand how bundles and protocols for severe sepsis can be improved.

For further reading on this subject I suggest an article by Ferrer et al.[4]

S. L. Zanotti-Cavazzoni, MD

References

1. Dellinger RP, Levy MM, Carlet JM, et al. Surviving Sepsis Campaign: international guidelines for management of severe sepsis and septic shock: 2008. *Crit Care Med.* 2008;26:296-327.
2. Sprung CL, Annane D, Keh D, et al. Hydrocortisone therapy for patients with septic shock. *N Engl J Med.* 2008;358:111-124.
3. Finfer S, Chittock DR, Su SY, et al. Intensive versus conventional glucose control in critically ill patients. *N Engl J Med.* 2009;360:1283-1297.
4. Ferrer R, Artigas A, Levy MM, et al. Improvement in process of care and outcome after a multicenter severe sepsis educational program in Spain. *JAMA.* 2008;299:2294-2303.

Acute kidney injury in septic shock: clinical outcomes and impact of duration of hypotension prior to initiation of antimicrobial therapy
Bagshaw SM, Lapinsky S, Dial S, et al (Univ of Alberta, Edmonton, Canada; Mount Sinai Hosp, Toronto, Canada; Davis Jewish General Hosp, Montreal, Canada; et al)
Intensive Care Med 35:871-881, 2009

Objective.—To describe the incidence and outcomes associated with early acute kidney injury (AKI) in septic shock and explore the association between duration from hypotension onset to effective antimicrobial therapy and AKI.

Design.—Retrospective cohort study.

Subjects.—A total of 4,532 adult patients with septic shock from 1989 to 2005.

Setting.—Intensive care units of 22 academic and community hospitals in Canada, the United States and Saudi Arabia.

Measurements and Main Results.—In total, 64.4% of patients with septic shock developed early AKI (i.e., within 24 h after onset of hypotension). By RIFLE criteria, 16.3% had risk, 29.4% had injury and 18.7% had failure. AKI patients were older, more likely female, with more co-morbid disease and greater severity of illness. Of 3,373 patients (74.4%) with hypotension prior to receiving effective antimicrobial therapy, the median (IQR) time from hypotension onset to antimicrobial therapy was 5.5 h (2.0–13.3). Patients with AKI were more likely to have longer delays to receiving antimicrobial therapy compared to those with no AKI [6.0 (2.3–15.3) h for AKI vs. 4.3 (1.5–10.8) h for no AKI, $P < 0.0001$). A longer duration to antimicrobial therapy was also associated an increase in odds of AKI [odds ratio (OR) 1.14, 95% CI 1.10–1.20, $P < 0.001$, per hour (log-transformed) delay]. AKI was associated with significantly higher odds of death in both ICU (OR 1.73, 95% CI 1.60–1.9, $P < 0.0001$) and hospital (OR 1.62, 95% CI, 1.5–1.7, $P < 0.0001$). By Cox proportional hazards analysis, including propensity score-adjustment, each RIFLE category was independently associated with a greater hazard ratio for death (risk 1.31; injury 1.45; failure 1.56).

Conclusion.—Early AKI is common in septic shock. Delays to appropriate antimicrobial therapy may contribute to significant increases in the incidence of AKI. Survival was considerably lower for septic shock associated with early AKI, with increasing severity of AKI, and with increasing delays to appropriate antimicrobial therapy.

▶ Acute kidney injury (AKI) is common in critically ill patients and is a predictor of increased morbidity and mortality. Estimates from recent studies suggest that more than a third of patients admitted to the ICU develop AKI. Although sepsis is often recognized as a predisposing factor for development of AKI, the incidence and outcomes of AKI in patients with sepsis are not fully described. In this large retrospective study (over 4000 patients with septic shock), Bagshaw et al evaluated the incidence of early AKI, the clinical characteristics and severity of early AKI, the association between duration from hypotension onset to effective antimicrobial therapy and the occurrence and severity of early AKI, and the survival relation to early AKI. The authors found that AKI is common and frequently occurs in septic shock. AKI was present in 64.4% of patients at 24 h after onset of hypotension. When classified according to the RIFLE criteria, 16.3% had risk, 29.4% had injury, and 18.7% had failure. Delays in initiating appropriate antibiotics after the onset of hypotension were associated with increased risk of developing AKI. Patients who developed AKI had higher mortality than those who did not. The impact on mortality of delays in starting appropriate antibiotics in patients with septic shock was demonstrated in a previous study from the same group.[1] The current study is the first to show that delays in starting appropriate antibiotics are also associated with organ dysfunction—more specifically acute kidney failure. This study in addition offers important information to clinicians regarding AKI in septic shock.

S. L. Zanotti-Cavazzoni, MD

Reference

1. Kumar A, Roberts D, Wood KE, et al. Duration of hypotension before initiation of effective antimicrobial therapy is the critical determinant of survival in human septic shock. *Crit Care Med.* 2006;34:1589-1596.

Influence of vasopressor agent in septic shock mortality. Results from the Portuguese Community-Acquired Sepsis Study (SACiUCI study)
Póvoa PR, on behalf of the Portuguese Community-Acquired Sepsis Study Group (São Francisco Xavier Hospital, Lisbon, Portugal; Santo António Hospital, Porto, Portugal; University of Porto, Portugal)
Crit Care Med 37:410-416, 2009

Objective.—Guidelines for the adrenergic support of septic shock are controversial. In patients with community-acquired septic shock, we assessed the impact of the choice of vasopressor support on mortality.

Design.—Cohort, multiple center, observational study.

Setting.—Seventeen Portuguese intensive care units (ICUs).

Patients.—All adult patients admitted to a participating ICU between December 2004 and November 2005.

Interventions.—None.

Measurements and Main Results.—Patients were followed up during the first five ICU days, the day of discharge or death, and hospital outcome. Eight hundred ninety-seven consecutive patients with community-acquired sepsis (median age, 63 years; 577 men; and hospital mortality, 38%) were studied. Of the 458 patients with septic shock, 73% received norepinephrine and 50.5% dopamine. The norepinephrine group had a higher hospital mortality (52% vs. 38.5%, $p = 0.002$). A Kaplan–Meier survival curve showed diminished 28-day survival in the norepinephrine group (log-rank $= 22.6$, $p < 0.001$). A Cox proportional hazard analysis revealed that the administration of norepinephrine was associated with an increased risk of death (adjusted hazard ratio, 2.501; 95% confidence interval, 1.413–4.425; $p = 0.002$). In a multivariate analysis with ICU mortality as the dependent factor, Simplified Acute Physiology Score II and norepinephrine administration were independent risk factors for ICU mortality in patients with septic shock.

Conclusions.—In patients with community-acquired septic shock, our data suggest that norepinephrine administration could be associated with worse outcome.

▶ Septic shock is one of the most challenging problems facing the critical care physician. Hemodynamic support for patients with septic shock has been based on the use of intravenous fluids and vasopressors. Recent evidence-based guidelines recommend the use of vasopressors in patients who do not respond to fluid resuscitation. Norepinephrine and dopamine are considered first-line vasopressors for septic shock. However, the discussion of which vasopressor is best has been going on for years and remains unresolved. The lack of conclusive randomized trials has perpetuated this discussion. In this study, Póvoa et al observed a large multicentered Portuguese population of septic shock patients, the various vasopressors used, and patients' outcomes. The authors report that the use of norepinephrine was associated with higher mortality when compared with the use of dopamine. This is contrary to findings in another large observational study, which reported a higher mortality in patients treated with dopamine when compared with norepinephrine.[1] Both of these studies are limited by their observational status, and it is not possible to attribute cause/effect or comment on which vasopressor is better. Recognizing that this study will not resolve the controversy of which vasopressor is superior, one should ask, "What can we learn from another observational study?" Of importance, this study also evaluated compliance with individual items of the sepsis resuscitation bundle. They found that although compliance with some elements of the 6-hour bundle was good, others were very low. If one used an all-or-none approach, >70% of the patients in this cohort failed the 6-hour resuscitation bundle. Perhaps the lesson for now should be to place less emphasis on vasopressor selection and more emphasis on compliance with proven bundles during the initial phases of resuscitation.

For further reading on this subject I suggest an article by Dellinger et al.[2]

S. L. Zanotti-Cavazzoni, MD

References

1. Sakr Y, Reinhart K, Vincent JL, et al. Does dopamine administration in shock influence outcome? Results of the Sepsis Occurrence in Acutely Ill Patients (SOAP) study. *Crit Care Med.* 2006;34:589-597.
2. Dellinger RP, Levy MM, Carlet JM, et al. Surviving Sepsis Campaign: international guidelines for management of severe sepsis and septic shock: 2008. *Crit Care Med.* 2008;36:296-327.

Hospital-wide impact of a standardized order set for the management of bacteremic severe sepsis

Thiel SW, Asghar MF, Micek ST, et al (Washington Univ School of Medicine, St. Louis, MO; St. Luke's Hosp, St. Louis, MO; Barnes-Jewish Hosp, St. Louis, MO; Ctr for Healthcare Quality and Effectiveness, St. Louis, MO)

Crit Care Med 37:819-824, 2009

Objective.—To evaluate the hospital-wide impact of a standardized order set for the management of bacteremic severe sepsis on processes of medical care and patient outcomes.

Design.—Retrospective, before and after study design.

Setting.—Barnes-Jewish Hospital, a 1200-bed academic medical center.

Patients.—Bacteremic patients with severe sepsis (200 from the 18-month before period and 200 from the 18-month after period).

Interventions.—Hospital-wide implementation of a standardized order set for the management of bacteremic severe sepsis.

Measurements and Main Results.—A total of 400 patients with bacteremia and severe sepsis were selected at random within the specified time periods. Patients in the after group received more intravenous fluids in the first 12 hours after onset of hypotension (1627 ± 1862 mL vs. 2054 ± 2237 mL; $p = 0.04$) and were more likely to receive appropriate initial antibiotic therapy (53.0% vs. 65.5%, $p = 0.01$). In-hospital mortality was statistically decreased in the after group (55.0% vs.

39.5%, $p < 0.01$), as was the hospital length of stay (28.7 ± 30.1 days vs. 22.4 ± 20.9 days; $p = 0.02$). Compared with the before group, the after group had reduced occurrence of renal failure (49.0% vs. 36.0%, $p < 0.01$), cardiovascular failure (70.5% vs. 57.0%, $p < 0.01$), and were less likely to require vasopressors after initial fluid resuscitation (68.5% vs. 52.5%, $p < 0.01$).

Conclusions.—The implementation of a hospital-wide standardized order set for the management of bacteremic severe sepsis was associated with greater fluid administration, improved antibiotic therapy, decreased incidence of organ failure, and improved survival.

▶ Severe sepsis and septic shock are important causes of morbidity and mortality in critically ill patients. Standardization of evidence-based practices, such as those recommended by the Surviving Sepsis Campaign, have been an important step toward optimizing care and improving patient outcomes in sepsis.[1] In a previous study, Micek et al[2] showed that the implementation of a standardized order set for the management of severe sepsis in the emergency department was associated with improved process of care and patient outcomes. In the current study, the same group evaluated the impact of a hospital-wide standardized order set for the management of bacteremic severe sepsis. In a before-and-after study design, the investigators report greater fluid administration, shorter time to antibiotic administration, increased use of appropriate antibiotics, and increased compliance with hemodynamic endpoints of resuscitation in the intervention group. All this was associated with decreased hospital length of stay, decreased incidence of organ failure, and improved mortality. An interesting finding of this study was the fact that the impact on improved outcomes was greatest in ICU and emergency department patients and lowest in hospital ward patients. This suggests that caring for severe sepsis patients is more difficult on the hospital wards, and that there may be more barriers to the efficient implementation of evidence-based practices on the hospital wards. The results of this study continue to support the use of evidence-based guidelines applied in a systematic/protocolized way to all patients with severe sepsis. It also illustrates the importance of simple measures (timely antibiotics and fluids) in patient outcomes in severe sepsis.

S. L. Zanotti-Cavazzoni, MD

References

1. Dellinger RP, Levy MM, Carlet JM, et al. Surviving Sepsis Campaign: International guidelines for management of severe sepsis and septic shock. *Crit Care Med.* 2008;2008(36):296-327.
2. Micek ST, Roubinian N, Heuring T, et al. Before-after study of standardized hospital order set for the management of septic shock. *Crit Care Med.* 2006;34: 2707-2713.

Biomarkers of sepsis

Marshall JC, for the International Sepsis Forum (Li Ka Shing Knowledge Inst, Toronto, Ontario, Canada, St. Michael's Hosp, Toronto, Ontario, Canada, Univ of Toronto, Toronto, Ontario, Canada; Friedrich-Schiller Univ, Jena, Germany)
Crit Care Med 37:2290-2298, 2009

Background.—A complex network of biological mediators underlies the clinical syndrome of sepsis. The nonspecific physiologic criteria of sepsis syndrome or the systemic inflammatory response syndrome do not adequately identify patients who might benefit from either conventional anti-infective therapies or from novel therapies that target specific mediators of sepsis. Validated biomarkers of sepsis may improve diagnosis and therapeutic decision making for these high-risk patients.

Objectives.—To develop a methodologic framework for the identification and validation of biomarkers of sepsis.

Methods.—A small group meeting of experts in clinical epidemiology, biomarker development, and sepsis clinical trials; selective narrative review of the biomarker literature.

Results.—The utility of a biomarker is a function of the degree to which it adds value to the available clinical information in the domains of screening, diagnosis, risk stratification, and monitoring of the response to therapy. We identified needs for greater standardization of biomarker methodologies, greater methodologic rigor in biomarker studies, wider integration of biomarkers into clinical studies (in particular, early phase studies), and increased collaboration among investigators, pharmaceutical industry, biomarker industry, and regulatory agencies.

Conclusions.—Biomarkers promise to transform sepsis from a physiologic syndrome to a group of distinct biochemical disorders. This transformation could aid therapeutic decision making, and hence improve the prognosis for patients with sepsis, but will require an unprecedented degree of systematic investigation and collaboration.

▶ The sepsis syndrome remains a clinical challenge. The current definitions from systemic inflammatory response syndrome (SIRS) to septic shock lack specificity and mask the wide heterogeneity present among patients regarding disease process, clinical management, and outcome. Significant efforts have been made over the past decade to identify "biomarkers of sepsis" that could help establish early diagnosis and faster management. Despite positive laboratory and clinical trials, numerous potential barriers prevent translating these research advances and incorporating them in current clinical practice. In this interesting article, Marshall and Reinhart, based on expert colloquium, constructed a methodologic framework for identification and validation of biomarkers in sepsis.

If validated, biomarkers can transform our clinical approach to sepsis. Their use can extend from screening patients at increased risk to achieving more rapid and reliable diagnosis and implementing timely intervention, identifying subgroups through risk stratification, monitoring response to intervention, and establishing a surrogate endpoint.

However, biomarker validation faces obstacles at multiple levels. After 2 decades of studies on procalcitonin (PCT), a recent review concluded that the publications concerning its diagnostic and prognostic utility are contradictory. In addition, patient characteristic and clinical setting vary markedly, and data have been difficult to interpret and have often been extrapolated inappropriately to clinical usage. Further attempts at meta-analysis are greatly compromised by the divergence of circumstances of reported studies and the different timing of the PCT trials. This is one example among others that highlight the encountered obstacles:

1. The first level is the measurement variability and lack of standardization, including assay methodology, reagents, and site for sampling and other confounding effects (example: LUMItest for PCT vs the newer more sensitive assay Kryptor). Here the authors propose the use of likelihood ratios in the investigation and development of assays and understanding of results.

2. The second level is the absence of a gold standard with which the biomarker can be compared. A biomarker should discriminate patients with disease from those free of disease. This would allow risk stratification, timely intervention, and would assist in resource allocation. This highlights the need that controls and patients should be comparable in the clinical presentation and physiologic derangements when designing a study rather than using healthy volunteers as controls, which sets the ground for spectrum bias.

3. The third level occurs when demonstrating that the biomarker differentially identifies patients who experience benefit from a particular intervention. This requires the performance of adequately powered studies, a condition not easily available.

4. The fourth level is demonstrating that the measurement of the biomarker can inform a clinical decision that can lead to improved patient outcomes. That is, it must predict disease progression, be affected by therapy, and respond to the same biological process that is thought to mediate the clinical outcome.

The authors finally concluded that establishing the "biomarker of sepsis" will require an unprecedented degree of systemic investigation and collaboration among researchers and research institutions that address all the above-mentioned obstacles (Table 3 in the original article).

Following this detailed, well-organized framework, even though it requires extraordinary efforts, could set the ground for well-designed studies that can change our approach to sepsis from a physiologic syndrome to a group of distinct biochemical profiles that could provide patients with individualized therapy and better outcome, similar to oncology.

Z. A. Kobeissi, MD

S. L. Zanotti-Cavazzoni, MD

Granulocyte–Macrophage Colony-stimulating Factor to Reverse Sepsis-associated Immunosuppression: A Double-Blind, Randomized, Placebo-controlled Multicenter Trial

Meisel C, Schefold JC, Pschowski R, et al (Charité Campus Mitte, Berlin, Germany; Charité Campus Virchow, Berlin, Germany)
Am J Respir Crit Care Med 180:640-648, 2009

Rationale.—Sustained sepsis-associated immunosuppression is associated with uncontrolled infection, multiple organ dysfunction, and death.

Objectives.—In the first controlled biomarker-guided immunostimulatory trial in sepsis, we tested whether granulocyte–macrophage colony-stimulating factor (GM-CSF) reverses monocyte deactivation, a hallmark of sepsis-associated immunosuppression (primary endpoint), and improves the immunological and clinical course of patients with sepsis.

Methods.—In a prospective, randomized, double-blind, placebo-controlled, multicenter trial, 38 patients (19/group) with severe sepsis or septic shock and sepsis-associated immunosuppression (monocytic HLA-DR [mHLA-DR] < 8,000 monoclonal antibodies (mAb) per cell for 2 d) were treated with GM-CSF (4 μg/kg/d) or placebo for 8 days. The patients' clinical and immunological course was followed up for 28 days.

Measurements and Main Results.—Both groups showed comparable baseline mHLA-DR levels (5,609 ± 3,628 vs. 5,659 ± 3,332 mAb per cell), which significantly increased within 24 hours in the GM-CSF group. After GM-CSF treatment, mHLA-DR was normalized in 19/19 treated patients, whereas this occurred in 3/19 control subjects only ($P < 0.001$). GM-CSF also restored ex-vivo Toll-like receptor 2/4–induced proinflammatory monocytic cytokine production. In patients receiving GM-CSF, a shorter time of mechanical ventilation (148 ± 103 vs. 207 ± 58 h, $P = 0.04$), an improved Acute Physiology and Chronic Health Evaluation-II score ($P = 0.02$), and a shorter length of both intrahospital and intensive care unit stay was observed (59 ± 33 vs. 69 ± 46 and 41 ± 26 vs. 52 ± 39 d, respectively, both not significant). Side effects related to the intervention were not noted.

Conclusions.—Biomarker-guided GM-CSF therapy in sepsis is safe and effective for restoring monocytic immunocompetence. Use of GM-CSF may shorten the time of mechanical ventilation and hospital/intensive care unit stay. A multicenter trial powered for the improvement of clinical parameters and mortality as primary endpoints seems indicated.

Clinical trial registered with www.clinicaltrials.gov (NCT00252915).

▶ Sepsis remains an important cause of morbidity and mortality in the intensive care unit. Numerous trials have been conducted with novel agents aimed at modulating the proinflammatory host response. Unfortunately, the vast majority of these trials have failed. One possible explanation may lie in the fact that many patients with sepsis develop severe immunosuppression in the later course of their disease. This state, also known as "immunoparalysis," results from triggering of counter-regulatory, anti-inflammatory pathways, and is associated with impaired innate and adaptive immune responses. Survivors of sepsis spontaneously recover immune function. Several studies have shown an association between low levels of monocytic HLA-DR (mHLA-DR) surface expression and immune cell dysfunctions in patients with sepsis. Based on this finding, mHLA-DR expression has been proposed as a global biomarker of sepsis-induced immunoparalysis. In this randomized, double-blind, placebo-controlled trial, patients with sepsis-induced immunosuppression (as measured by mHLA-DR < 8000 monoclonal antibodies per cell for 2 consecutive days) were treated with granulocyte-macrophage colony-stimulating factor (GM-CSF) or placebo. The primary endpoint of the study was restoration of mHLA-DR expression. The study demonstrated that immunostimulation with GM-CSF in patients with immunosuppression effectively restores mHLA-DR expression. This restoration of immune function was associated with improved outcomes such as shorter mechanical ventilation time and decreased length of ICU and hospital stay. No side effects to treatment with GM-CSF were reported. A multicenter trial powered for patient-important outcomes (mortality) seems to be indicated based on these promising results. The most important contribution of this study is the use of a biomarker to identify a subpopulation of sepsis patients with a higher likelihood of responding to a specific treatment and using this biomarker in a longitudinal way to evaluate the response to treatment.

S. L. Zanotti-Cavazzoni, MD

8 Metabolism/ Gastrointestinal/ Nutrition/ Hematology-Oncology

Comparison of coagulation factor XIII content and concentration in cryoprecipitate and fresh-frozen plasma

Caudill JSC, Nichols WL, Plumhoff EA, et al (Mayo Clinic, Rochester, MN)

Transfusion 49:765-770, 2009

Background.—For patients with plasma coagulation factor XIII (pFXIII) deficiency, recommended means of replacement include infusions of fresh-frozen plasma (FFP), cryoprecipitate, or (where available) factor (F)XIII concentrates. Quantitative differences in pFXIII concentration in FFP and cryoprecipitate are not well defined and were, therefore, the subject of this study.

Study Design and Methods.—FFP and cryoprecipitate (10 bags each from blood group O donors) were analyzed to quantify pFXIII activity and antigen. Coagulation FVIII, fibrinogen, and von Willebrand factor (VWF) were also quantitated.

Results.—Mean ($\pm$ SD) pFXIII activity in cryoprecipitate and FFP bags was 60 ± 30 and 288 ± 77 U per bag, respectively, and pFXIII antigen and activity levels were concordant. Other comparisons (mean $\pm$ SD) between cryoprecipitate and FFP, respectively, were as follows: coagulation FVIII activity, 133 ± 37 and 265 ± 83 U per bag; fibrinogen content (Clauss kinetic assay), 183 ± 44 and 725 ± 199 mg per bag; VWF antigen content, 181 ± 53 and 218 ± 70 U per bag; VWF ristocetin cofactor activity, 168 ± 34 and 221 ± 65 U per bag; VWF collagen-binding activity, 164 ± 40 and 208 ± 71 U per bag; and fluid (plasma) volumes per bag, 21.3 ± 2.7 and 245 ± 29 mL.

Conclusion.—In contrast to other cryoprecipitable coagulation proteins, pFXIII is only mildly enriched in cryoprecipitate when compared with FFP (approx. two- to threefold). Although both products can provide effective pFXIII replacement, FFP may be preferred when infusion volume is not a major consideration and pFXIII concentrates are not available. VWF is substantially enriched in cryoprecipitate (approx. ninefold compared with its concentration in FFP), with VWF activity content exceeding that of FVIII by approximately 26 percent on average.

▶ The need to replace individual clotting factors or fibrinogen in patients with coagulopathy is a problem that intensivists face not infrequently. In this study, the investigators evaluated the overall content and concentration of factor XIII as well as a number of other clotting components (factor VIII, von Willebrand factor, fibrinogen) in cryoprecipitate and fresh-frozen plasma (FFP). The concentration of all these clotting components was found to be higher in cryoprecipitate. However, because of the greater volume of a typical bag of FFP, more, often substantially more, was present in the FFP. In patients requiring replacement of individual clotting factors or fibrinogen, the choice is not always straightforward. In patients in whom volume is an issue, a physiologically adequate dose can often be achieved using cryoprecipitate, but at the theoretical increased risk of exposure to a greater number of donors due to the pooled nature of this product. FFP often provides greater amounts of clotting factors with fewer donor exposures, but at lower concentrations and requiring larger volumes of administration, although in many critically ill patients this last issue may not necessarily be considered a negative. The decision as to which clotting factor preparation is appropriate must be individualized to the specific case and may benefit from the input of a hematologist before a final decision is made.

D. R. Gerber, DO

Intensive versus Conventional Glucose Control in Critically Ill Patients
The NICE-SUGAR Study Investigators (George Inst for International Health, New South Wales, Sydney; et al)
N Engl J Med 360:1283-1297, 2009

Background.—The optimal target range for blood glucose in critically ill patients remains unclear.

Methods.—Within 24 hours after admission to an intensive care unit (ICU), adults who were expected to require treatment in the ICU on 3 or more consecutive days were randomly assigned to undergo either intensive glucose control, with a target blood glucose range of 81 to 108 mg per deciliter (4.5 to 6.0 mmol per liter), or conventional glucose control, with a target of 180 mg or less per deciliter (10.0 mmol or less per liter). We defined the primary end point as death from any cause within 90 days after randomization.

Results.—Of the 6104 patients who underwent randomization, 3054 were assigned to undergo intensive control and 3050 to undergo conventional control; data with regard to the primary outcome at day 90 were available for 3010 and 3012 patients, respectively. The two groups had similar characteristics at baseline. A total of 829 patients (27.5%) in the intensive-control group and 751 (24.9%) in the conventional-control group died (odds ratio for intensive control, 1.14; 95% confidence interval, 1.02 to 1.28; P = 0.02). The treatment effect did not differ significantly between operative (surgical) patients and nonoperative (medical) patients (odds ratio for death in the intensive-control group, 1.31 and 1.07, respectively; P = 0.10). Severe hypoglycemia (blood glucose level, ≤40 mg per deciliter [2.2 mmol per liter]) was reported in 206 of 3016 patients (6.8%) in the intensive-control group and 15 of 3014 (0.5%) in the conventional-control group (P<0.001). There was no significant difference between the two treatment groups in the median number of days in the ICU (P = 0.84) or hospital (P = 0.86) or the median number of days of mechanical ventilation (P = 0.56) or renal-replacement therapy (P = 0.39).

Conclusions.—In this large, international, randomized trial, we found that intensive glucose control increased mortality among adults in the ICU: a blood glucose target of 180 mg or less per deciliter resulted in lower mortality than did a target of 81 to 108 mg per deciliter. (ClinicalTrials.gov number, NCT00220987.)

▶ This study of over 6000 critically ill patients calls into question the recent trend of tight glucose control. As can be seen in Fig 3, the overall mortality was significant (*P* = .02) for those patients treated with intensive glucose control as compared with more conventional control. The data also appear fairly homogenous for the point estimates across all subgroups, although there are some notable outliers like trauma patients and patients on steroids. As caution is required in instituting a tight glucose control regimen in ICU patients, caution is required in interpreting this study. As can be seen in Table 1 in the section on organ failure, the rate of respiratory, hepatic, cardiovascular, and renal failure is higher in the intensive control group, and the impact of subtle increases in these critical organ dysfunctions on outcomes is hard to assess. More important is the rate of hypoglycemia, which was 6.8% in the tight control groups compared with 0.5% in the conventional group. Clearly, it appears that hypoglycemia is associated with unfavorable outcomes, but does that mean tight control is also? This would only be true if the 2 are intimately linked when in fact they may not be. Of concern about the methods of this otherwise wonderful study is the fact that the frequency of glucose measurements could be extended to every 4 hours; thus, important episodes of less severe hypoglycemia were missed, and the duration and thus negative organ impact of significant hypoglycemia was extended. Some health systems are seeing very low rates of hypoglycemia, but these typically do glucose checks every hour routinely. Given these findings, however, it would seem prudent to be less strict with glucose control in most patient populations and that a range of 90 to 140 would seem reasonable. It is also worth noting that even in the conventional arm,

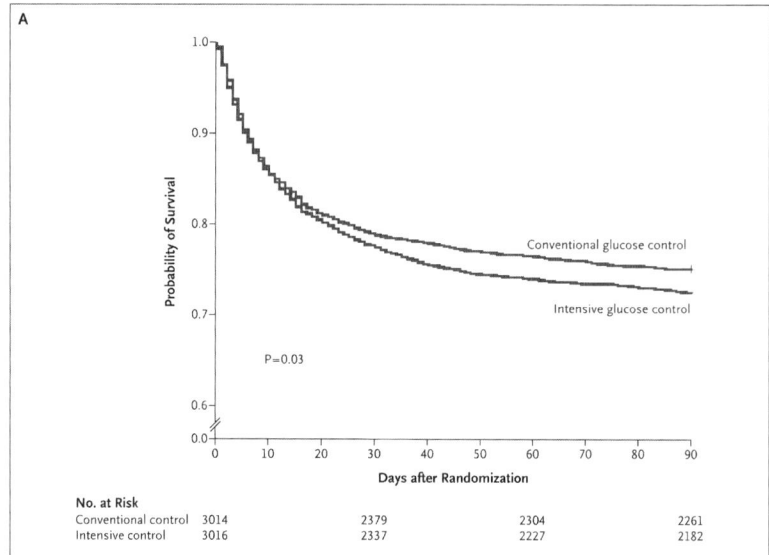

FIGURE 3.—Probability of survival and odds ratios for death, according to treatment group. Panel A shows Kaplan–Meier estimates for the probability of survival, which at 90 days was greater in the conventional-control group than in the intensive-control group (hazard ratio, 1.11; 95% confidence interval, 1.01 to 1.23; P = 0.03). Panel B shows the odds ratios (and 95% confidence intervals) for death from any cause in the intensive-control group as compared with the conventional-control group, among all patients and in six predefined pairs of subgroups. The size of the symbols indicates the relative numbers of deaths. The Acute Physiology and Chronic Health Evaluation II (APACHE II) score can range from 0 to 71, with higher scores indicating more severe organ dysfunction. (Reprinted from The NICE-SUGAR Study Investigators. Intensive versus conventional glucose control in critically Ill patients. *N Engl J Med.* 2009;360:1283-1297. Copyright 2009 Massachusetts Medical Society. All rights reserved.)

TABLE 1.—Baseline Characteristics of the Study Patients*

Variable	Intensive Glucose Control	Conventional Glucose Control
Age — yr	60.4±17.2	59.9±17.1
Female sex — no./total no. (%)	1128/3016 (37.4)	1079/3014 (35.8)
Weight — kg	80.7±21.4	80.9±21.2
Body-mass index†	27.9±7.7	28.0±7.2
Interval from ICU admission to randomization — hr	13.4±7.6	13.4±7.7
Reason for ICU admission — no./total no. (%)		
Operative	1112/3015 (36.9)	1121/3014 (37.2)
Nonoperative	1903/3015 (63.1)	1893/3014 (62.8)
Location before ICU admission — no./total no. (%)		
Emergency department	718/3015 (23.8)	749/3014 (24.9)
Hospital floor (or ward)		
Without previous ICU admission	640/3015 (21.2)	618/3014 (20.5)
With previous ICU admission	42/3015 (1.4)	30/3014 (1.0)
Another ICU	125/3015 (4.1)	102/3014 (3.4)
Another hospital	445/3015 (14.8)	453/3014 (15.0)
Operating room		
After emergency surgery	682/3015 (22.6)	671/3014 (22.3)
After elective surgery	363/3015 (12.0)	391/3014 (13.0)
APACHE II score	21.1±7.91	21.1±8.3
Blood glucose level — mg/dl	146±52.3	144±49.1
Organ failure or dysfunction — no./total no. (%)		
Respiratory		
Dysfunction (SOFA score, 1–2)	1207/2993 (40.3)	1222/2990 (40.9)
Failure (SOFA score, 3–4)	1526/2993 (51.0)	1521/2990 (50.9)
Coagulatory		
Dysfunction (SOFA score, 1–2)	947/2987 (31.7)	874/2989 (29.2)
Failure (SOFA score, 3–4)	128/2987 (4.3)	137/2989 (4.6)
Hepatic		
Dysfunction (SOFA score, 1–2)	831/2807 (29.6)	834/2802 (29.8)
Failure (SOFA score, 3–4)	70/2807 (2.5)	50/2802 (1.8)
Cardiovascular		
Dysfunction (SOFA score, 1–2)	583/3011 (19.4)	614/3012 (20.4)
Failure (SOFA score, 3–4)	1726/3011 (57.3)	1695/3012 (56.3)
Renal		
Dysfunction (SOFA score, 1–2)	1042/2981 (35.0)	1071/2974 (36.0)
Failure (SOFA score, 3–4)	249/2981 (8.4)	228/2974 (7.7)
Mechanical ventilation — no./total no. (%)	2825/3014 (93.7)	2793/3014 (92.7)
Renal-replacement therapy — no./total no. (%)	179/3014 (5.9)	165/3014 (5.5)
History of diabetes mellitus — no./total no. (%)	615/3015 (20.4)	596/3014 (19.8)
Type I diabetes	50/615 (8.1)	42/596 (7.0)
Type II diabetes	565/615 (91.9)	554/596 (93.0)
Previous treatment with insulin	183/615 (29.8)	163/596 (27.3)
Previous treatment with systemic corticosteroids — no./total no. (%)	393/3014 (13.0)	378/3014 (12.5)
Subgroup classification — no./total no. (%)		
Severe sepsis at randomization	676/3014 (22.4)	626/3014 (20.8)
Trauma	422/3014 (14.0)	466/3014 (15.5)
APACHE II score ≥25	929/3013 (30.8)	945/3012 (31.4)

*Plus–minus values are means ±SD. Acute Physiology and Chronic Health Evaluation II (APACHE II) scores can range from 0 to 71, with higher scores indicating more severe illness, and Sequential Organ Failure Assessment (SOFA) scores can range from 0 to 4 for each organ system, with higher scores indicating more severe organ dysfunction. Severe sepsis was defined according to the consensus-conference criteria of the American College of Chest Physicians–Society of Critical Care Medicine.[28] To convert the values for blood glucose to millimoles per liter, multiply by 0.05551. ICU denotes intensive care unit. Editor's Note: Please refer to original journal article for full reference.
†The body-mass index is the weight in kilograms divided by the square of the height in meters.

glucoses were much better controlled than only a few years ago when many patients were allowed to stay in the 180 to 250 range for prolonged periods of time.

T. Dorman, MD

Accuracy of AccuChek glucose measurement in intensive care patients
Meynaar IA, van Spreuwel M, Tangkau PL, et al (Reinier de Graaf Hosp, Delft, Netherlands; et al)
Crit Care Med 37:2691-2696, 2009

Objective.—To evaluate the accuracy of the AccuChek Inform point-of-care glucose measurement device as compared with central laboratory glucose measurement.

Design.—Prospective, observational study.

Setting.—A ten-bed mixed closed format intensive care unit in a 500-bed general hospital. The unit has a computerized insulin protocol aiming for 81 to 135 mg/dL.

Patients.—All intensive care unit patients were eligible.

Interventions.—None.

Measurements and Main Results.—Paired samples (AccuChek glucose in whole blood calibrated to give whole blood results and central laboratory glucose in serum) were taken simultaneously. In 32 critically ill patients, we obtained the following information: mean ± standard deviation age 71.6 ± 11.9 yrs; mean Acute Physiology and Chronic Health Evaluation II score at admission 17.8 ± 6.7; 239 paired samples were taken from arterial catheters. Mean AccuChek whole blood glucose was 126 ± 36 mg/dL (7.0 ± 2.0 mmol/L); mean central laboratory serum glucose was 137 ± 38 mg/dL (7.6 ± 2.1 mmol/L). Mean difference was 11 mg/dL (0.61 mmol/L) (8%) (95% Confidence Interval = 9–13 mg/dL, $p < .001$). ISO 15197 guideline requires 95% of point-of-care measurements to be within 15 mg/dL margins with reference <75 mg/dL or within 20% if reference is higher. In total, 216 (90.4%) of AccuChek measurements were within ISO 15197 margins. Because AccuChek was calibrated to give whole blood results, we calculated a correction factor of 1.086 from the two mean values to correct whole blood AccuChek into serum-like results. This is almost the same as the correction factor of 1.080 given by Roche Diagnostics. By multiplying AccuChek whole blood results with 1.086, 225 (94.1%) of results were within the ISO 15197 margins. Hematocrit did not influence AccuChek results in the 0.20 to 0.44 range. Beyond this range, there were not enough data to draw conclusions.

Conclusions.—In critically ill patients, the accuracy of AccuChek glucose measurement calibrated to give serum-like results with blood samples derived from arterial catheters is acceptable but falls short by about 1% of complying with the ISO 15197 guideline.

▶ Since the publication of a landmark trial by van den Berghe and collaboratively,[1] tight glycemic control in the intensive care unit has become an increasingly common practice. The initial enthusiasm for tight glycemic control has decreased in light of more recent publications that have raised questions regarding the risks of tight glycemic control. How tight glucose control should be in critically ill patients is still a matter of debate. This debate centers around concerns for increased risks of hypoglycemia. Furthermore, concerns have been raised in the literature regarding the accuracy and reliability of point-of-care glucose measurement. Critchell et al[2] compared AccuChek catheter glucose measurements with serum glucose measurements in critically ill patients. In this study, the authors found significant discrepancies between fingerstick AccuChecks and central laboratory glucose levels and recommended against the use of AccuChecks in critically ill patients undergoing tight glycemic control. Other studies have reported different results, and part of this might be related to difference in methodologies and location of blood sampling for point-of-care testing. If one considers that glycemic control remains a common practice in the intensive care unit, it becomes very important for clinicians to understand the potential limitations of bedside point-of-care glucose measuring. In this prospective study, the investigators evaluated the accuracy of glucose measurements by AccuChek from whole blood compared with central laboratory measurements from serum glucose. The authors found that AccuChek glucose measurements in whole blood with a correction factor to give serum-like values shortly fails to comply with ISO 15197 guidelines. However, they concluded that it had acceptable accuracy for use in intensive care units with protocols that aim for glucose values between 81 and 135 mg/dL and with blood samples derived from arterial catheters. They also found that hematocrit levels within a range of 0.20 to 0.44 did not have any influence on the AccuCheck results. The results of this study do not resolve questions remaining on the appropriate use of tight glycemic control or on the best place to monitor patient's glucose at the bedside. However, clinicians can take home the message that if glucose is monitored by AccuChek and blood obtained from arterial lines, there seems to be an acceptable accuracy when compared with serum glucose measured in the central laboratory. Clinicians should also recognize that to achieve that accuracy, there is a conversion factor that needs to be calculated.

S. L. Zanotti-Cavazzoni, MD

References

1. van de Berghe G, Wouters P, Weekers F, et al. Intensive insulin therapy in the critically ill patients. *N Engl J Med.* 2001;345:1359-1367.
2. Critchell CD, Savarese V, Callahan A, Aboud C, Jabbour S, Marik P. Accuracy of bedside capillary blood glucose measurements in critically ill patients. *Intensive Care Med.* 2007;33:2079-2084.

The Effects of Platelet Transfusions Evaluated Using Rotational Thromboelastometry

Flisberg P, Rundgren M, Engström M (Lund Univ Hosp, Sweden; Halmstad Central Hosp, Sweden)
Anesth Analg 108:1430-1432, 2009

Background.—In this study, we assessed the immediate effects of platelet transfusion on whole blood coagulation.

Methods.—Ten thrombocytopenic patients given a single unit platelet transfusion of $200-300 \times 10^9$ platelets had their coagulation status assessed before and immediately after transfusion using rotational thromboelastometry.

Results.—Transfusion increased the median platelet count from 31.5 to 43.5×10^9/L. Clot formation time decreased by 32% ($P = 0.005$), whereas maximum clot strength increased by 47% ($P = 0.005$).

Conclusion.—Statistically significant improvements in rotational thromboelastometry-measured parameters were observed in association with a mean increase of 12×109/L in platelet count after platelet transfusion in these patients.

▶ Thrombocytopenia is a commonly encountered problem in the critical care setting, and clinicians are often faced with the question of how aggressively to replace platelets in anticipation of an invasive procedure, and how best to time such replacement. In this investigation the authors evaluated the impact of infusion of one unit of platelets on the platelet count, clotting time, and mechanical clot characteristics in thrombocytopenic patients requiring central venous catheter placement. Not only was the anticipated increase in platelet count and decrease in time to clot formation noted, but there was also a significant and rapid increase in clot strength demonstrated as well following the administration of a single unit of platelets. While no clinical evaluation for bleeding or other complications was performed as part of this investigation, this study suggests that platelet transfusion, even at small volumes, provides significant hemostatic benefit in thrombocytopenic patients, and that these effects occur very soon after transfusion. As the authors point out, clinical evaluation of these effects are needed.

D. R. Gerber, DO

Leucocyte depletion of perioperative blood transfusion does not affect long-term survival and recurrence in patients with gastrointestinal cancer

Lange MM, cooperative clinical investigators of the Cancer Recurrence And Blood Transfusion (CRAB) study and the Transfusion Associated Complications = Transfusion Induced Complications? (TACTIC) study (Leiden Univ Med Centre, The Netherlands; et al)
Br J Surg 96:734-740, 2009

Background.—Perioperative red blood cell (RBC) transfusion may be associated with a poor prognosis in cancer surgery. Allogeneic leucocytes are assumed to play a causal role. This study evaluated the long-term effect of transfusion with leucocyte-depleted (LD) blood in patients with gastrointestinal cancer.

Methods.—The Transfusion Associated Complications = Transfusion Induced Complications? (TACTIC) study is a multicentre randomized controlled trial evaluating the short-term benefits of LD *versus* non-LD RBC transfusions. The present study evaluated 5-year survival and cancer recurrence among 512 patients with gastrointestinal cancer included in the TACTIC study.

Results.—Some 89·2 per cent of patients had a primary tumour and 79·7 per cent underwent surgery with curative intent; 243 patients received perioperative RBC transfusion (median 3 units). The 5-year overall survival rate of patients with any type of gastrointestinal cancer was 50·8 per cent in the LD group and 45·8 per cent in the non-LD group ($P = 0·191$). Corresponding 5-year disease-free survival rates were 60·0 and 56·6 per cent ($P = 0·482$), and recurrence rates 32·9 and 34·3 per cent ($P = 0·864$).

Conclusion.—Leucocyte depletion is not associated with better long-term survival and lower recurrence rates in patients with gastrointestinal cancer.

▶ The potential for transfused packed red blood cells (PRBC) to exert an immunomodulatory effect on the recipient has been an area of concern and research for several decades now. Data have suggested that this intervention may increase the risk of solid tumor recurrence and decrease the incidence of rejection of renal allografts, as well as increase the risk of infection. While the presence of white blood cells (WBC) in transfused blood has often been postulated as a significant factor in mediating any alterations in host immune responses, in recent years the vast majority of transfused blood has been depleted of these cells. To date, the data are unclear as to the contribution WBC make to any immunomodulation that occurs as a result of PRBC transfusion. In this study patients undergoing surgery for a variety of gastrointestinal malignancies were transfused with either leukocyte-depleted or nondepleted red cells and observed over a 5-year period for a variety of outcome parameters, including recurrence of their cancer, disease-free survival, and overall survival. The presence or absence of leukocytes from PRBC did not appear to be a factor in any of these outcome parameters. While leukocytes are clearly a factor in such processes as acute transfusion reactions, it remains uncertain whether vigorous leukocyte depletion offers significant benefit, despite the hypothetical advantages of such a process. Tartter et al demonstrated a significant decrease in the postoperative infection rate among patients receiving WBC-depleted PRBC compared with those receiveving standard red cells, while Titlestad et al could not replicate these findings.[1,2] Hébert et al reported a small but significant reduction in mortality following the introduction of a universal leukoreduction program.[3] While these investigators noted a decrease in febrile episodes, they could not identify a decrease in the incidence of serious nosocomial infections. The use of leukocyte reduction in a critically ill population, while hypothetically appealing, thus remains unconfirmed, and would likely benefit from prospective evaluation.

D. R. Gerber, DO

References

1. Tartter PI, Mohandas K, Azar P, Endres J, Kaplan J, Spivack M. Randomized trial comparing packed red cell blood transfusion with and without leukocyte depletion for gastrointestinal surgery. *Am J Surg.* 1998;176:462-466.
2. Titlestad IL, Ebbesen LS, Ainsworth AP, Lillevang ST, Qvist N, Georgsen J. Leukocyte-depletion of blood components does not significantly reduce the risk of infectious complications. results of a double-blinded, randomized study. *Int J Colorectal Dis.* 2001;16:147-153.
3. Hébert PC, Fergusson D, Blajchman MA, et al. Clinical outcomes following institution of the Canadian universal leukoreduction program for red blood cell transfusions. *JAMA.* 2003;289:1950-1956.

The Influence of the Preoperative Immune Response on Blood Transfusion Requirements in Patients Undergoing Cardiac Surgery

Leal-Noval SR, Arellano V, Vallejo A, et al (Univ of Seville, Spain; et al)
J Cardiothorac Vasc Anesth 23:330-335, 2009

Objective.—The purpose of this study was to evaluate the influence of preoperative type I and II immune responses on blood transfusion requirements.

Design.—A prospective and observational trial.

Setting.—A postcardiac surgery unit of a university hospital.

Participants.—Seventy-one consecutive patients undergoing elective cardiac surgery.

Interventions.—Blood samples drawn for laboratory analysis and immunologic study.

Measurements and Main Results.—Patients were divided into 2 groups according to blood transfusion requirements: ≤ 2 units (n = 35) and >2 units of red blood cells (n = 36). The preoperative immune response was assessed by flow cytometry, measuring the proportion of CD4 + T helper cells producing cytokines, including Th1 response (interferon-γ and tumor necrosis factor-α [TNF-α]) and Th2 response (interleukin 4 and 10). Two logistic regression analyses (including and not including immunologic variables) were used to select and weight perioperative variables associated with an increased risk of transfusion. Three variables were found to be independent predictors of transfusion requirements when immunologic variables were not included: preoperative platelet count, preoperative hemoglobin, and hypertension. When all the variables were included, preoperative hemoglobin, cardiopulmonary bypass time, and the preoperative proportion of CD4+ T cells producing TNF-α were associated with an increased risk of transfusion (Hosmer-Lemeshow, 0.33; c-index, 0.93), but preoperative platelet count and hypertension were not.

Conclusions.—A low preoperative Th1 immune response, as assessed by the proportion of CD4+ T-helper–producing TNF-α, was associated with a higher blood transfusion rate.

▶ Although an extensive body of literature has accumulated indicating that perioperative transfusion is often detrimental in patients undergoing cardiac surgery, and recent guidelines have been published supporting restrictive transfusion practices in cardiothoracic surgical patients, packed red blood cell (PRBC) transfusion remains common in such patients. The ability to identify patients at increased risk of perioperative bleeding and potentially preventing such bleeding, with the ultimate goal of avoiding PRBC transfusion, is therefore a worthwhile endeavor. In this study, the authors attempted to evaluate the possible influence of preoperative immunological factors on the risk of perioperative bleed requiring transfusion in cardiac surgical patients undergoing cardiopulmonary bypass. In addition to such traditionally recognized risk factors as preoperative hemoglobin and duration of bypass time, the proportion of lipopolysaccharide-stimulated tumor necrosis factor-α (TNF-α) producing CD4+ cells was found to be a significant risk factor for bleeding. Although a small, preliminary study, these findings are potentially of great clinical consequence. If patients at increased risk of perioperative risk bleeding can be identified preoperatively, it may be possible to intervene, depending on the pathophysiology involved, to decrease the risk of such bleeding, thereby decreasing the need for perioperative transfusion with its associated risks and complications.

D. R. Gerber, DO

Transfusion insurgency: practice change through education and evidence-based recommendations
Brandt M-M, Rubinfeld I, Jordan J, et al (Henry Ford Hosp, Detroit, MI)
Am J Surg 197:279-283, 2009

Background.—In 2000, we implemented an evidence-based guideline in the surgical intensive care unit (SICU) using a transfusion threshold of hemoglobin <8 g/dL. We hypothesized that continual education on the transfusion protocol would decrease transfusions.

Methods.—We analyzed 2-month samples of admissions in even-numbered years from 1998 to 2006. Any infusion of packed red blood cells (PRBCs) was included.

Results.—We analyzed data from 2,138 patients resulting in 5,130 transfusions. Thirty-six patients received >20 U of blood. The only difference between groups occurred in 2006 when renal failure increased. Transfusions decreased from 3.2 ± 0.34 (SE) to 1.7 ± 0.2. The number of patients who received blood also decreased. Mortality and length of stay (LOS) were not different among the groups. Every unit of blood transfused increased the mortality risk by 14%.

Conclusions.—Implementation of an evidence-based transfusion guideline reduced the number of infused units and patients transfused without an increase in mortality.

▶ Despite the ever-increasing body of literature indicating that a restrictive approach to packed red blood cell (PRBC) transfusion in the critically ill is well tolerated and possibly even beneficial, the adoption of such strategies through formal protocols has been limited. In this article, the authors report on their experience in a high-acuity tertiary care surgical ICU, after establishing a series of transfusion guidelines and establishing an ongoing educational program for the house staff detailing the evolving evidence regarding the safety and benefits of a restrictive approach to PRBC transfusion. The guidelines established a routine threshold hemoglobin of 8 gm/dL for PRBC transfusion in their unit. Data were collected on transfusion practices, demographics, and numerous outcome parameters at several intervals over an 8-year period, beginning before the institution of the protocol and educational program. The authors found a significant reduction in the average number of units of blood transfused per patient. Compared with the year before the introduction of the program, the final year of the study also showed significant reductions in the percentage of patients transfused, the percentage of patients receiving over 10 units of blood, and the percentage receiving over 20 units of blood. Although there also appeared to be a decline in mortality, this did not achieve significance. This interesting and important study lends further support to the basic concept that at the very least a restrictive transfusion strategy is not harmful in a high-acuity critically ill patient population. At least as importantly, it also demonstrates that it is feasible to alter practice over extended periods of time through the establishment of defined, evidence-based guidelines, especially if supported by ongoing educational reinforcement. These results can serve as a foundation for other institutions to evaluate their transfusion practices and to consider methods to best address this issue according to their specific needs and circumstances.

D. R. Gerber, DO

Noninfectious Serious Hazards of Transfusion

Hendrickson JE, Hillyer CD (Emory Univ School of Medicine, Atlanta, GA)
Anesth Analg 108:759-769, 2009

As infectious complications from blood transfusion have decreased because of improved donor questionnaires and sophisticated infectious disease blood screening, noninfectious serious hazards of transfusion (NISHOTs) have emerged as the most common complications of transfusion. The category of NISHOTs is very broad, including everything from well-described and categorized transfusion reactions (hemolytic, febrile, septic, and allergic/urticarial/anaphylactic) to lesser known complications. These include mistransfusion, transfusion-related acute lung injury, transfusion-associated circulatory overload, posttransfusion purpura, transfusion-associated graft versus host disease, microchimerism, transfusion-related immunomodulation, alloimmunization, metabolic derangements, coagulopathic complications of massive transfusion, complications from red cell storage lesions, complications from over or undertransfusion, and iron overload.

In recent years, NISHOTs have attracted more attention than ever before, both in the lay press and in the scientific community. As the list of potential complications from blood transfusion grows, investigators have focused on the morbidity and mortality of liberal versus restrictive red blood cell transfusion, as well as the potential dangers of transfusing "older" versus "younger" blood. In this article, we review NISHOTs, focusing on the most recent concerns and literature.

▶ The potential for transfusion to expose recipients to the risk of infectious complications is well, perhaps over recognized, given the vanishingly low incidence of transmission of viral pathogens in the blood supply of developed countries. While some serious noninfectious complications are well known, if not always well recognized (eg, tranfusion-associated lung injury, hemolytic, and febrile nonhemolytic transfusions reactions), many others are underappreciated or essentially unknown. A key example of these would be septic transfusion reactions, reportedly the cause of 14% of transfusion-related deaths from 2001-2003. Numerous other serious transfusion reactions occur as well, including but not limited to transfusion-associated circulatory overload, transfusion-associated graft-versus-host disease, transfusion-related immunomodulation, and a host of metabolic derangements associated with transfusion, to name a few. In this article, the authors comprehesively review the array of noninfectious hazards of transfusion and their implications for clinical practice. In light of the increasing body of literature suggesting limited use of and potential adverse effects of liberal transfusion in the critical care population, the information contained in this review may provide yet further grounds for even more cautious use of red blood cell transfusion, with a better understanding of the potential hazards associated with such intervention.

D. R. Gerber, DO

Time course and etiology of death in patients with severe anemia

Tobian AAR, Ness PM, Noveck H, et al (The Johns Hopkins Hosp, Baltimore, MD; Univ of Medicine and Dentistry of New Jersey, New Brunswick)
Transfusion 49:1395-1399, 2009

Background.—Mortality increases as hemoglobin (Hb) levels fall. Among severely anemic patients, the clinical course, cause of death, and whether there are any warning signs before death are unknown.

Study Design and Methods.—A retrospective cohort study was performed of surgical patients who refused red blood cell transfusions for religious reasons and died with a Hb concentration 6 g/dL or less. Mortality was defined as death that occurred during hospitalization.

Results.—Among the 1958 Jehovah's Witness patients that had surgery, 117 (5.6%) had a postoperative Hb level of 6 g/dL or less and 39 (33.3%) of these individuals died in the hospital. The median number of days from surgery to the lowest Hb level was 3 days (range, 0-22 days; interquartile range, 1-8 days) and from the lowest postoperative Hb level to death was 2 days (range, 0-40 days; interquartile range, 1-12 days). Individuals with a Hb level of 2.0 g/dL or less had on median 1.0 (interquartile range, 0.5-1.5) day from their lowest Hb to death while individuals with their lowest Hb ranging between 4.1 and 5.0 g/dL had on median 11 (interquartile range, 1-23) days from their lowest Hb to death. Except for anemia, no single etiology of death was predominant.

Conclusions.—While there does not appear to be any single etiology that can be predictive or preventative of mortality for anemic patients, individuals with very low Hb concentrations often do not die quickly. Thus, there appears to be a potential time window where transfusion medicine physicians may intervene.

▶ Anemia is well recognized as a risk factor for poor outcomes for patients undergoing a variety of interventions, including major surgical procedures. In this study, the investigators retrospectively reviewed data on nearly 2000 Jehovah's Witness patients who had major surgical procedures from 1981 through 1994, with the goal of identifying any clinical indicators (other than anemia) to predict an increased likelihood of death, and to identify a possible time period before death wherein intervention may have been helpful. One hundred and seventeen of the 1958 patients identified in the study had hemoglobins less than 6 g/dL, and 39 of those died in-hospital (with hemoglobins ranging from 1.5-5.7 g/dL). Overall, the authors could not identify a clear association between lowest hemoglobin level and time of death, although most patients with levels over 3 g/dL had at least 4.5 days from the date of their lowest hemoglobin until their date of death. The authors reviewed the records to identify the cause of death in each case and to classify these as hypoxic or not, presumably on the principle that severe anemia is an etiology of cellular hypoxia. Causes of hypoxic death were listed as respiratory failure, bleeding, arrhythmia, myocardial infarction, anoxic encephalopathy, do not resuscitate (DNR) order on a ventilator with decreasing blood pressure, and metabolic acidosis. While many of these deaths may have been related to tissue hypoxia directly or indirectly due to anemia, it is impossible to specifically implicate cellular hypoxia as a result of anemia in individual cases, making such conclusions speculative. While intuitively it seems reasonable to expect that such a window allows time to intervene and prevent a significant proportion of these deaths, such a conclusion also remains hypothetical. Without knowing when the reported complications and terminal events occurred, we don't know if interventions would be aimed at prevention or reversal of effects. Even in severely anemic patients, not everyone requires intervention, as evidenced by the fact that 67% of those with hemoglobins less than 6 g/dL survived. With the well-documented shortcomings of packed red blood cells, the use of transfusion in this population, while likely to be greater than in most, would still need to weighed against the risk of unnecessary transfusion in those who seem to do well with no intervention. As far as nontransfusion interventions (eg, erythropoietin), such therapies take too long to take effect to be useful in these situations. Finally, as the authors point out, these data are not only retrospective, but also at their most recent, 15 years old, and much has changed in techniques and management in the intervening years. Nevertheless, these findings are extremely interesting and provide an incentive for prospective evaluation of the impact of severe anemia on outcome in critically ill patients and the potential role for aggressive intervention through various mechanisms.

D. R. Gerber, DO

Acid–base disorders evaluation in critically ill patients: we can improve our diagnostic ability
Boniatti MM, Cardoso PRC, Castilho RK, et al (Hosp de Clínicas de Porto Alegre, Brazil)
Intensive Care Med 35:1377-1382, 2009

Purpose.—To determine whether Stewart's approach can improve our ability to diagnose acid–base disorders compared to the traditional model.

Methods.—This prospective cohort study took place in a university-affiliated hospital during the period of February–May 2007. We recorded clinical data and acid–base variables from one hundred seventy-five patients at intensive care unit admission.

Results.—Of the 68 patients with normal standard base excess (SBE) (SBE between −4.9 and +4.9), most ($n = 59$; 86.8%) had a lower effective strong ion difference (SIDe), and of these, 15 (25.4%) had SIDe < 30 mEq/L. Thus, the evaluation according to Stewart's method would allow an additional diagnosis of metabolic disorder in 33.7% patients.

Conclusions.—The Stewart approach, compared to the traditional evaluation, results in identification of more patients with major acid–base disturbances.

▶ Acid-base disorders frequently exist in ICU patients. Correct interpretation of electrolytes and blood gases is critical to the diagnosis and management of

TABLE 3.—Examples of acid–base disorders

	Patient 1	Patient 2
Measured variables		
Sodium (mmol/L)	151	146
Potassium (mmol/L)	3.4	3.8
Calcium (mg/dl)	7.0	7.2
Magnesium (mmol/L)	2.0	1.8
Phosphate (mmol/L)	1.0	2.0
Albumin (g/L)	27.0	27.0
Chloride (mmol/L)	121	124
pH	7.48	7.43
$PaCO_2$ (mmHg)	29.0	30.2
Lactate (mmol/L)	2.0	1.3
Derived variables		
HCO_3 (mmol/L)	21.5	20.0
SBE (mmol/L)	−0.7	−3.8
AG (mmol/L)	12.4	6.3
SIDa (mmol/L)	34.4	27.4
SIDe (mmol/L)	29.9	28.8
SIG (mmol/L)	4.5	−1.4

HCO_3 serum bicarbonate, *SBE* standard base excess, *AG* anion gap, SID_a apparent strong ion difference, SID_e effective strong ion difference, *SIG* strong ion gap.

critically ill patients. This authors stated in the Methods section that they intended to compare 3 methods; base excess (BE), anion gap (AG), and strong ion difference (SID), also known as the Stewart method. Table 3 shows an example of 2 patients with slightly alkalotic pHs, bicarbonates that are the lower limits of normal, BEs that are essentially normal, yet identifiable extra anions using SID. The fact that the BE is not very useful in critically ill patients has been long appreciated and is not a new finding. The fact that many continue to use this in their daily practice is of concern, however. Use of SID has been previously shown to improve diagnostic ability. The reason it has not been widely adopted is secondary to major reasons. First, it is quite cumbersome to calculate and thus has frequent calculation errors associated. When it identifies an extra anion that would have been missed, it commonly identifies an anion that does not lead to alterations in management. In both cases in Table 3 the extra anion is chloride, which was known simply by looking at the chloride concentrations on the electrolyte panel. It would have been nice to see a table that listed every patient with a direct comparison, case by case of all the variables mentioned in the methods, including corrected AG, but these data were not available for review in the article. Thus, until prospectively obtained data show meaningful benefit from the use of SID in all cases that outweigh its limitations, it seems prudent that one uses the corrected AG approach for its simplicity and user friendliness.

T. Dorman, MD

Effect of early nutrition on deaths due to severe traumatic brain injury

Härtl R, Gerber LM, Ni Q, et al (Weill Cornell Med College, NY; et al)
J Neurosurg 109:50-56, 2008

Object.—Traumatic brain injury (TBI) remains a serious public health crisis requiring continuous improvement in prehospital and inhospital care. This condition results in a hypermetabolic state that increases systemic and cerebral energy requirements, but achieving adequate nutrition to meet this demand has not been a priority in reducing death due to TBI. The effect of timing and quantity of nutrition on death within the first 2 weeks of injury was analyzed in a large prospective database of adult patients with severe TBI in New York State.

Methods.—The study is based on 797 patients with severe TBI (Glasgow Coma Scale [GCS] score < 9) treated at 22 trauma centers enrolled in a New York State quality improvement program between 2000 and 2006. The inhospital section of the prospectively collected database includes information on age, initial GCS score, weight and height, results of CT scanning, and daily parameters such as pupillary status, arterial hypotension, GCS score, and number of calories fed per day.

Results.—Patients who were not fed within 5 and 7 days after TBI had a 2- and 4-fold increased likelihood of death, respectively. The amount of nutrition in the first 5 days was related to death; every 10-kcal/kg decrease in caloric intake was associated with a 30–40% increase in mortality rates. This held up even after controlling for factors known to affect mortality, including arterial hypotension, age, pupillary status, initial GCS score, and CT scan findings.

Conclusions.—Nutrition is a significant predictor of death due to TBI. Together with prevention of arterial hypotension, hypoxia, and intracranial hypertension it is one of the few therapeutic interventions that can directly affect TBI outcome.

▶ This study evaluated the effects of early nutrition on mortality in patients who suffered a traumatic brain injury. As stated in the article, approximately 85% of the 52 000 patients die within 2 weeks of sustaining their injury. Studies to date focus on maintaining cerebral perfusion, hemodynamic support, and tissue oxygenation as critical interventions that reduce mortality in this period. Traumatic brain injury results in a hypermetabolic state that increases systemic and cerebral energy requirements. Smaller studies suggest a benefit to early nutritional support. This study examined the effect of timing and quantity of nutrition on mortality within 2 weeks of sustaining the brain injury.

Dr Härtl et al conducted a review of prospectively collected information in the Brain Trauma Foundation database involving several centers in New York State. Ultimately, 797 patients were included in the study. Sixty-one percent of patients were fed within 3 to 5 days. The results were quite impressive. The mortality at 2 weeks was significantly higher in patients where nutrition was delayed or withheld. Patients who were not fed the recommended target amount also had a higher risk of death at 2 weeks. The mortality was decreased in patients with elevated intracranial pressure who were fed early.

This study, which gleaned information from a large database of patients, strongly suggests that early feeding is beneficial. As the author states, a prospectively designed study would be ethically difficult to conduct. Early nutritional support is beneficial in critically ill patients. Traumatic injuries, sepsis, and patients admitted to the intensive care unit often have hypermetabolic states with increased energy requirements. Patient nutritional reserves may be used quickly, and detrimental effects may ensue if calories are not supplied. This study has intriguing implications not only for patients with brain injury, but also for critically ill patients with different disease states. Nutrition is initially often overlooked in a critically ill, unstable patient. Dr Härtl et al have suggested that early nutritional support, as demonstrated in traumatic brain injury patients, may be just as important as other initial interventions.

C. W. Deitch, MD

Decontamination of the Digestive Tract and Oropharynx in ICU Patients
de Smet AMGA, Kluytmans JAJW, Cooper BS, et al (Univ Med Ctr, Utrecht, the Netherlands; Amphia Hosp, Breda, the Netherlands; Centre for Infections Health Protection Agency Statistics, London; et al)
N Engl J Med 360:20-31, 2009

Background.—Selective digestive tract decontamination (SDD) and selective oropharyngeal decontamination (SOD) are infection-prevention measures used in the treatment of some patients in intensive care, but reported effects on patient outcome are conflicting.

Methods.—We evaluated the effectiveness of SDD and SOD in a crossover study using cluster randomization in 13 intensive care units (ICUs), all in the Netherlands. Patients with an expected duration of intubation of more than 48 hours or an expected ICU stay of more than 72 hours were eligible. In each ICU, three regimens (SDD, SOD, and standard care) were applied in random order over the course of 6 months. Mortality at day 28 was the primary end point. SDD consisted of 4 days of intravenous cefotaxime and topical application of tobramycin, colistin, and amphotericin B in the oropharynx and stomach. SOD consisted of oropharyngeal application only of the same antibiotics. Monthly point-prevalence studies were performed to analyze antibiotic resistance.

Results.—A total of 5939 patients were enrolled in the study, with 1990 assigned to standard care, 1904 to SOD, and 2045 to SDD; crude mortality in the groups at day 28 was 27.5%, 26.6%, and 26.9%, respectively. In a random-effects logistic-regression model with age, sex, Acute Physiology and Chronic Health Evaluation (APACHE II) score, intubation status, and medical specialty used as covariates, odds ratios for death at day 28 in the SOD and SDD groups, as compared with the standard-care group, were 0.86 (95% confidence interval [CI], 0.74 to 0.99) and 0.83 (95% CI, 0.72 to 0.97), respectively.

Conclusions.—In an ICU population in which the mortality rate associated with standard care was 27.5% at day 28, the rate was reduced by an estimated 3.5 percentage points with SDD and by 2.9 percentage points with SOD. (Controlled Clinical Trials number, ISRCTN35176830.)

▶ Infection control is of the utmost importance in an intensive care unit where significant mortality is due to septic complications. Simple hygiene measures among health care professionals, as well as the adherence to sterile procedures where applicable, are common practices in ICU settings. Novel therapies such as decontamination of the oropharynx and the gastrointestinal tract are appealing additions to offset septic complications in the ICU. However, outcomes in studies to date have yielded conflicting results, and as such, no standard exists regarding this aspect of infection control. These studies have lacked the statistical power to show a survival benefit.

This article is a prospectively controlled crossover study that enrolled 5939 patients in several intensive care settings across the Netherlands. The primary endpoint was mortality at 28 days. Secondary endpoints included in-hospital mortality, prevalence of resistance, duration of mechanical ventilation, length of ICU stay, and overall hospital stay. The patients were assigned to control, selective digestive tract decontamination (SDD), and selective oropharyngeal decontamination (SOD). The crude mortality rates at day 28 were 27.5%, 26.9%, and 26.6% respectively. There was a tendency for lower rates of ICU bacteremia and candidiasis, but not reaching statistical significance. Resistance was not seen in the duration of this relatively short study.

This study highlights an important issue in critical care medicine, namely the plausibility of conferring a survival benefit with a relatively simple intervention. By selective statistical methods the authors were able to define a reduction in mortality of 3.5% with SDD and 2.9% with SOD. The crude mortality differences were not as impressive. It is intriguing, however, to contemplate relatively low cost interventions and their impact on a very difficult population to study and to demonstrate a mortality benefit. Bacterial resistance is a potential drawback to widespread use of decontamination, although it was not seen in this study. The authors do suggest that resistance may be more of an issue in regions with high prevalence of resistance among bacterial isolates. Given the large population included in this study, selection bias may potentially hinder the results, and a study that addresses such a topic would need validation before it is accepted as a widespread standard of intensive care.

C. W. Deitch, MD

Impact of Radiologic Intervention on Mortality in Necrotizing Pancreatitis: The Role of Organ Failure

Rocha FG, Benoit E, Zinner MJ, et al (Brigham and Women's Hosp, Boston, MA)
Arch Surg 144:261-265, 2009

Background.—Our group previously reported that organ failure and mortality in necrotizing pancreatitis (NP) are not different between patients with infected and sterile necrosis. Since that report, management of this disease has evolved to include image-guided percutaneous catheter drainage (PCD) to improve morbidity and mortality. We evaluated the effect of PCD on mortality in NP.

Design.—Retrospective analysis.

Setting.—Tertiary care referral center.

Patients.—A total of 689 consecutive patients treated for acute pancreatitis between 2001 and 2005, of whom 64 (9.3%) had pancreatic necrosis documented on contrast-enhanced computed tomography.

Main Outcome Measures.—Mortality and organ failure.

Results.—In the 64 patients with documented NP, overall mortality was 16%. Thirty-six patients (56%) had organ failure according to the Atlanta classification. Compared with patients with sterile necrosis, those with infected necrosis did not have an increased prevalence of organ failure or increased need for intubation, pressors, or dialysis but had an increased mortality. Mortality in patients treated conservatively was 1 of 29 (3%); in those with PCD alone, 6 of 11 (55%); in those with PCD and surgery, 2 of 17 (12%); and in those with surgery alone, 1 of 7 (14%). All patients treated with PCD alone had organ failure, whereas 10 (59%) of those with PCD and surgery had organ failure.

Conclusion.—The use of PCD did not improve the mortality of NP among patients with organ failure.

▶ The role of invasive intervention in severe pancreatitis is complicated. Radiographic and clinical findings may identify a subset of patients with higher morbidity and mortality. Complications of severe pancreatitis include necrosis, pseudocyst formation, fistulae, bleeding, and multisystem organ dysfunction. Contrast imaging can delineate viable pancreas from necrotic tissue. Patients with necrotizing pancreatitis are at risk for infection, which can be determined with fine needle aspiration of the necrotic tissue. Treatment of infected necrosis is either surgical debridement or percutaneous drainage with the aid of an interventional radiologist. This study is a retrospective analysis at a tertiary care hospital evaluating the impact of percutaneous catheter drainage (PCD) and surgical debridement on mortality and organ failure.

A total of 689 patients were identified, 64 of which had evidence of necrosis. Forty-nine had sterile necrosis whereas 15 had infected necrosis. The mortality was higher in the patients with infected necrosis, and was higher in patients with multisystem organ failure. The authors note an overall increase in the use of PCD at their institution. However, they failed to notice any improvement in overall mortality. The authors compared these results with their previous study and noted no difference in the prevalence of necrotizing pancreatitis, organ failure, or mortality.

There is an increased use of interventional radiologists in the approach to severe pancreatitis. The percutaneous placement of catheters that aid in the drainage of an infected necrotic pancreas serves to treat patients who may be too unstable to tolerate the stress of surgical debridement, and in some cases may act as a bridge to surgery when a patient's clinical condition stabilizes. This study reflected on a small number of patients. A prospective randomized trial that enrolls patients with necrotizing pancreatitis may further clarify the role and clinical impact of percutaneous drainage compared with surgery. Furthermore, it would be interesting to evaluate if early percutaneous drainage of sterile necrosis has a role in preventing the development of the systemic inflammatory response syndrome and possibly impacting on the organ dysfunction associated with both sterile and infected necrosis of the pancreas.

C. W. Deitch, MD

A simple prognostic score for risk assessment in patients with acute pancreatitis

Gonzálvez-Gasch A, de Casasola GG, Martín RB, et al (USP Hosp San Jaime, Alicante, Spain; Hosp Infanta Cristina, Madrid, Spain; et al)
Eur J Intern Med 20:e43-e48, 2009

Background.—Acute pancreatitis (AP) is a common disease that poses potential serious problems. Its clinical course is often unpredictable. Identification of high risk patients enables early appropriate treatment.

Methods.—We conducted a prospective study to develop a new prognostic method that can objectively and easily grade the severity of AP within the first 72 h of admission. The prediction rule was based on clinical and analytical parameters in 308 patients admitted in a community-based hospital. We validated the score in 193 additional patients in the same hospital.

Results.—Independent prognostic factors related to poor prognosis were age >65 years, leucocytes >13,000/mm^3, albumin <2.5 mg/dL, calcium <8.5 mg/dL and reactive C protein > 150 mg/dL. We assigned points to each of the independent factors for complicated AP in proportion to the regression coefficients. We defined three different risk groups according to the points obtained in the prediction rule. Low risk, 0 points (18% patients, 0% risk), moderate, 1–3 points (56% patients, 19% risk) and high, 4–6 points (26% patients, 73% risk). The sensitivity of this formula was 90% with specificity of 63%. The positive and negative predictive values were 50% and 94% respectively.

Conclusions.—Our simple prediction rule is an additional tool that may help physicians stratifying the severity of AP. Patients with high risk for complicated AP should be kept under close surveillance whereas low risk patients would not need special monitoring.

▶ Multiple scoring systems are available in clinical practice that attempt to stratify and define the risk of severity in patients who present with acute pancreatitis. The common parameters used include the well-known Ranson's criteria, the acute physiology and chronic health evaluation (APACHE) II score, and the Atlanta criteria. These systems all have limitations that preclude their acceptance as the standard approach to patients with pancreatitis. Some criticisms suggest these systems are outdated or too cumbersome to use in everyday clinical practice, or that the advances in intensive care medicine prevent these systems from making accurate predictions of morbidity and mortality.

The study by Dr Gonzálvez-Gasch et al is a prospectively designed trial that enrolled 308 patients in a community-based hospital with acute pancreatitis. Twenty-four clinical variables were initially collected, and an arbitrary definition of severe pancreatitis was employed using common clinical parameters normally associated with severe disease. A univariate statistical analysis was used, followed by a multivariate logistic regression analysis that identified 5 factors associated with a complicated hospital course. These included age > 65, leukocyte > 13 000, albumin < 2.5 mg/dL, calcium < 8.5 mg/dL, and an elevated C reactive protein > 150 mg/dL. These variables were entered into a statistical formula to determine the probability of suffering a complicated course of acute pancreatitis. The results suggested a score of 1 to 3 predicted moderate risk, and a score of 4 to 6 predicted a high risk of severity. The scoring system was subsequently validated in a second cohort of patients prospectively enrolled and included in the final discussion of this study.

The high negative predictive value of the collected data is beneficial in identifying patients who are at low risk of suffering complicated disease. The low positive predictive value, however, prevents this scoring system from accurately predicting patients who are at high risk for severity. The low mortality and low percentage of patients suffering from pancreatic necrosis may also account for the lack of inclusion of commonly used variables of severity such as hypoxemia, renal insufficiency, and persistent organ dysfunction. The authors used a CT severity index to help define severe pancreatitis. However, the question that beckons is: should an imaging index of severity be used to stratify patients' risk upon initial presentation to the hospital? Tissue necrosis noted on imaging studies obtained early during the hospital course commonly predicts organ damage, infection, and prolonged hospital stays.

The authors of this study accurately assess the need for a simple risk-stratifying system that can be used across a range of clinical settings as well as for the different etiologies of acute pancreatitis. This scoring evaluation is simple to obtain and calculate. It will be interesting to follow up confirmatory studies that validate this system in the future. Ultimately, the objective is to identify a set of scoring parameters that accurately identify and predict early disease severity in patients with acute pancreatitis. This will allow proper triage of patients and efficient allocation of health care resources.

C. W. Deitch, MD

A Prospective Evaluation of the Bedside Index for Severity in Acute Pancreatitis Score in Assessing Mortality and Intermediate Markers of Severity in Acute Pancreatitis

Singh VK, Wu BU, Bollen TL, et al (Brigham and Women's Hosp, Boston, MA; et al)
Am J Gastroenterol 104:966-971, 2009

Objectives.—Our aim was to prospectively evaluate the ability of the bedside index for severity in acute pancreatitis (BISAP) score to predict mortality as well as intermediate markers of severity in a tertiary center.

Methods.—The BISAP score was evaluated among 397 consecutive cases of acute pancreatitis admitted to our institution between June 2005 and December 2007. BISAP scores were calculated on all cases using data within 24 h of presentation. The ability of the BISAP score to predict mortality was evaluated using trend and discrimination analysis. The optimal cutoff score for mortality from the receiver operating curve was used to evaluate the development of organ failure, persistent organ failure, and pancreatic necrosis.

Results.—Among 397 cases, there were 14 (3.5%) deaths. There was a statistically significant trend for increasing mortality ($P < 0.0001$) with increasing BISAP score. The area under the receiver operating curve for mortality by BISAP score in the prospective cohort was 0.82 (95% confidence interval: 0.70, 0.95), which was similar to that of the previously published validation cohort. A BISAP score ≥3 was associated with an increased risk of developing organ failure (odds ratio = 7.4, 95% confidence interval: 2.8, 19.5), persistent organ failure (odds ratio = 12.7, 95% confidence interval: 4.7, 33.9), and pancreatic necrosis (odds ratio = 3.8, 95% confidence interval: 1.8, 8.5).

Conclusions.—The BISAP score represents a simple way to identify patients at risk of increased mortality and the development of intermediate markers of severity within 24 h of presentation. This risk stratification capability can be utilized to improve clinical care and facilitate enrollment in clinical trials.

▶ Multiple scoring systems exist to predict the severity of acute pancreatitis in hospitalized patients. The well-known systems include Ranson's criteria, the Acute Physiology and Chronic Health Evaluation (APACHE) II score, and the Atlanta criteria. The problems with these systems include the time needed to calculate a score, the population included in the initial studies describing these scoring systems not correlating to the acute population in the hospital, and the improvement in critical care making some of the variables outdated. Simplified accurate scoring systems are needed to predict which patients are at risk for morbidity and mortality from acute pancreatitis. A validated, widely applicable system may allow for proper triage and care of patients suffering from acute pancreatitis, as well as a judicious allocation of health care resources. The Bedside Index for Severity in Acute Pancreatitis score (BISAP) is a previously described score that suggests data can be collected within 24 hours of admission that has reliable prognostic information regarding necrosis and death.

The study by Dr Singh et al is a prospectively designed assessment of 397 cases of pancreatitis admitted to an academic tertiary care center with known excellence in biliary tract disease. The data were collected up to 7 days on each patient. The BISAP score consists of 5 variables: blood urea nitrogen (BUN), alteration in the mental status, pleural effusion, evidence of the systemic inflammatory response syndrome, and age. The scores were calculated within 24 hours of admission. The results suggested that a significant percentage of patients had a higher risk of necrosis, persistent organ failure, and death if the BISAP score was greater than or equal to 3.

The validated features of the BISAP are comparable with the APACHE II score. The BISAP system is easier to calculate both in the intensive care setting and on the general hospital wards. Simple scoring systems are necessary to identify and stratify patients at risk for mortality from acute pancreatitis. Those patients at risk for persistent organ dysfunction and pancreatic necrosis who are identified upon admission, or early in the hospital course, should be triaged to a more intense level of initial care. Early intervention may offer a survival advantage, or may diminish the associated morbidity associated with severe acute pancreatitis. These important endpoints await future trials in patients identified as high risk for severe pancreatitis.

C. W. Deitch, MD

Prophylactic endotracheal intubation in critically ill patients undergoing endoscopy for upper GI hemorrhage

Rehman A, Iscimen R, Yilmaz M, et al (Mayo Clinic, Rochester, MN; Uludag Univ, Bursa, Turkey; Akdeniz Univ, Antalya, Turkey)
Gastrointest Endosc 69:e55-e59, 2009

Background.—Cardiopulmonary complications are common after endoscopy for upper GI (UGI) hemorrhage in the intensive care unit (ICU).

Objective.—To evaluate the practice and outcome of elective prophylactic endotracheal intubation before endoscopy for UGI hemorrhage in the ICU.

Design.—Retrospective, propensity-matched case-control study.

Setting.—A 24-bed medical ICU in a tertiary center.

Patients.—ICU patients who underwent endoscopy for UGI hemorrhage.

Main Outcome Measurements.—Cardiopulmonary complications, ICU and hospital length of stay, and mortality. In a propensity analysis, patients who were intubated for airway protection before UGI endoscopy were matched by probability of intubation to controls who were not intubated before UGI endoscopy.

Results.—Of 307 patients, 53 underwent elective prophylactic intubation before UGI endoscopy. The probability of intubation depended on the Acute Physiology and Chronic Health Evaluation III (APACHE III) score (OR 1.4; 95% CI, 1.2-1.6), age (OR 0.97; 95% CI, 0.95-0.09), the presence of hemetemesis (OR 1.9; 95% CI, 0.8-5.1), previous lung disease (OR 2.1; 95% CI, 0.8-4.9), and the number of transfusions (OR 1.1; 95% CI, 1.0-1.1 per unit). Nonintubated matched controls were identified for all but 4 patients with active massive hemetemesis, who were excluded from matched analysis. Cumulative incidence of cardiopulmonary complications (53% vs 45%, $P = .414$), ICU length of stay (median 2.2 vs 1.8 days, $P = .138$), hospital length of stay (6.9 vs 5.9 days, $P = .785$), and hospital mortality (14% vs 20%, $P = .366$) were similar.

Conclusions.—Cardiopulmonary complications are frequent after endoscopy for acute UGI bleeding in ICU patients and are largely unaffected by the practice of prophylactic intubation.

▶ The complication rates of diagnostic upper endoscopy are very low-ranging from under 1%. However, the incidence of complications rises when performing these examinations in the acute setting for upper gastrointestinal hemorrhage. The primary risk is cardiac and pulmonary complications. Twenty percent of patients undergoing endoscopy for acute interventions develop pulmonary infiltrates with associated leukocytosis and fever. Airway protection is often deemed prudent in such cases where gastric contents may be aspirated into the lungs.

This study by Dr Rehman et al is a retrospective review of 307 patients in 1 tertiary care ICU, who were admitted for upper gastrointestinal hemorrhage. Fifty-seven patients were intubated prophylactically for airway protection. The patients included in the study suffered from a severe bleeding episode. The primary outcome was the cumulative incidence of cardiopulmonary complications such as myocardial infarction, cardiac arrest, aspiration, pneumonia, ARDS, and pulmonary edema. The results suggested that the likelihood of patients being intubated was influenced by the severity of the illness, age, the presence of hematemesis, history of chronic lung disease, and the number of transfusions. Compared with the control population, there was no difference in cardiopulmonary complications, ICU, and hospital stay nor in ICU and hospital mortality.

This study shows a large variation in physicians' perception as to when to intubate patients admitted with upper gastrointestinal bleed. The retrospective design of the study suggests that the decision to intubate patients was subjective and likely influenced by the physicians called to make that decision upon the patients' presentation. A trial that randomizes patients prospectively and measures similar outcomes may offer more reliable results. Until such data exist there will be no accepted standard of care and the decision to protect the patient's airway during an endoscopy for gastrointestinal bleeding will rest upon the decision of the physician.

C. W. Deitch, MD

Fulminant *Clostridium difficile* Colitis: Patterns of Care and Predictors of Mortality

Sailhamer EA, Carson K, Chang Y, et al (Massachusetts General Hosp, Boston)
Arch Surg 144:433-439, 2009

Hypothesis.—There exist predictors of mortality and the need for colectomy among patients with fulminant *Clostridium difficile* colitis.

Design.—Retrospective study.

Setting.—Academic tertiary referral center.

Patients.—We reviewed the records of 4796 inpatients diagnosed as having *C difficile* colitis from January 1, 1996, to December 31, 2007, and identified 199 (4.1%) with fulminant *C difficile* colitis, as defined by the need for colectomy or admission to the intensive care unit for *C difficile* colitis.

Main Outcome Measures.—Risk of inpatient mortality was determined by multivariate analysis according to clinical predictors, colectomy, and medical team.

Results.—The inhospital mortality rate for fulminant *C difficile* colitis was 34.7%. Independent predictors of mortality included the following: (1) age of 70 years or older, (2) severe leukocytosis or leukopenia (white blood cell count, $\geq 35\,000/\mu L$ or $<4000/\mu L$) or bandemia (neutrophil bands, $\geq 10\%$), and (3) cardiorespiratory failure (intubation or vasopressors). When all 3 factors were present, the mortality rate was 57.1%; when all 3 were absent, the mortality rate was 0%. Patients who underwent colectomy had a trend toward decreased mortality rates (odds ratio, 0.49; 95% confidence interval, 0.21-1.1; $P=.08$). Among patients admitted primarily for fulminant *C difficile* colitis, care in the surgical department compared with the nonsurgical department resulted in a higher rate of operation (85.1% vs 11.2%; $P<.001$) and lower mortality rates (12.8% vs 39.3%; $P=.001$). Patients admitted directly to the surgical department had a shorter mean (SD) interval from admission to operation (0 vs 1.7 [2.8] days; $P=.001$).

Conclusions.—Despite awareness and treatment, fulminant *C difficile* colitis remains a highly lethal disease. Reliable predictors of mortality exist and should be used to prompt aggressive surgical intervention. Survival rates are higher in patients who were cared for by surgical vs nonsurgical departments, possibly because of more frequent and earlier operations.

▶ *Clostridium difficile* colitis is the most common nosocomial infection of the gastrointestinal tract. Hospitals have seen increasing incidence, and increased severity of the disease, with emergence of more virulent strains of *Clostridium* species. This increases the burden on health care resources and expenditures. Medical therapy is sufficient in most cases. Surgery is reserved for fulminant disease, defined as toxic megacolon, shock, colectomy, and intensive care use.

This study is a retrospective analysis of fulminant *C difficile* colitis at an academic tertiary care center. The authors included 199 patients in the study out of 4796 total cases. These patients were cared for by surgical and non-surgical teams. Seventy-five underwent surgery and 124 were treated medically with metronidazole, vancomycin, or a combination of antibiotics. The primary outcome was inpatient mortality. The secondary outcome was the need for a colectomy. The patients in this study were more likely to undergo a colectomy if they had a physical exam consistent with peritonitis or impending catastrophic abdominal consequences of their disease, elevated leukocyte count, an abnormal CT scan, or required intubation.

The inpatient mortality was 34.7%. A univariate analysis followed by multiple logistic regression models identified 3 predictors of mortality: age > 70, elevated or depressed WBC, and requirement for intubation or pressor support. If all 3 factors were present, the mortality was 57.1%. If the patient lacked all 3 criteria, the mortality was 0%. Those who underwent a colectomy had 32% mortality. However, those who underwent surgery were 2 times more likely to survive than those who were treated conservatively. Mortality tended to be higher in patients cared for by nonsurgical teams, but the surgery tends to select out patients who are sicker, older, and with marginal nutritional status. The use of vancomycin increased the odds of survival by 4 fold and statistically trended toward decreasing mortality.

Although the retrospective design of this study may limit the conclusions, one cannot argue with the overall salient findings presented. The incidence and virulence of *C difficile* colitis are increasing, and objective criteria to stratify patients at risk for fulminant disease are lacking. The parameters presented in this study are easy to identify and can be obtained in virtually all patients with this disease. Patients presenting with these characteristics should be considered for early surgical intervention and early use of vancomycin.

A prospective study may be better suited to assess the need for aggressive medical therapy compared with colectomy in high-risk individuals. Advanced serologic and microbiologic testing for strains with high virulence may also add to our ability to stratify risk and offer more aggressive therapy where appropriate. Any potential identification of increased risk to patients with *C difficile* colitis would potentially offer decreased mortality and a survival benefit.

C. W. Deitch, MD

Duodenal versus gastric feeding in medical intensive care unit patients: A prospective, randomized, clinical study

Hsu C-W, Sun S-F, Lin S-L, et al (Kaohsiung Veterans General Hosp, Taiwan; et al)
Crit Care Med 37:1866-1872, 2009

Objective.—To determine whether medical intensive care unit (ICU) patients receiving nasoduodenal (ND) feedings achieve optimal nutritional support and better clinical outcomes compared with patients receiving nasogastric (NG) feedings.

Design.—A prospective, randomized, clinical study.

Setting.—Medical ICU of a university-affiliated tertiary medical center.

Patients.—One hundred twenty-one medical ICU patients required enteral feeding.

Interventions.—Patients were randomized to receive enteral feeding. One group received ND feedings and the other group received NG feedings. All patients followed the same protocol.

Measurements and Main Results.—The primary outcome of optimal nutritional support was assessed by measurement of time to goal tube feed rate and daily calorie and protein intake. Secondary clinical outcomes included number of ICU, hospital and ventilator days, number of the days in the study, blood–glucose levels, incidence of vomiting, diarrhea, gastrointestinal bleeding, tube replaced, tube clogged, fever, bacteremia, and ventilator-associated pneumonia (VAP), and mortality rate. Results showed that the ND group had a higher average daily calorie and protein intake compared with NG group and achieved nutritional goals earlier. In terms of clinical outcomes, patients in the ND group had a lower rate of vomiting and VAP. The other clinical outcomes such as number of ICU days, hospital days, ventilator days, blood–glucose level, tube replaced or clogged, diarrhea, gastrointestinal bleeding, fever, bacteremia, and mortality rate were not significantly different between two groups.

Conclusions.—Patients who received ND feedings achieved nutritional goals earlier than those who received NG feeding. ND feeding group also has a lower rate of vomiting and VAP in the medical ICU setting.

▶ Enteral feeding has shown consistent benefits when compared with parenteral nutritional support. As the authors point out, early enteral feeding is associated with enhancing the gut mucosal barrier. This has the potential benefit of preventing translocation of bacteria and endotoxemia. Overall the medical literature suggests an advantage of enteral feeding in ICU patients with respect to infection rates, length of hospital stay, and total use of health care resources.

This article by Dr Hsu et al is a prospective, randomized clinical trial comparing the benefits in 2 methods of enteral feeding. A total of 121 patients were randomized to receive enteral feeding with a tube placed into the stomach (nasogastric [NG]) versus a tube advanced into the duodenum (nasoduodenal [ND]). The baseline demographics were similar, but the results revealed some intriguing differences. The ND group had higher calorie intakes and higher protein intakes compared with the NG cohort. The ND group also had a significantly lower incidence of vomiting, as well as a lower rate of ventilator-associated pneumonia (VAP). There was a trend toward decreased diarrhea, gastrointestinal bleeding, and residual volumes in the ND group that did not reach clinical significance. There was no difference in mortality.

Enteral feeding should be the primary objective in patients who are unable to meet their caloric goals by oral feeding. Total parenteral nutrition should be reserved for patients who are unable to tolerate nutrition by enteral means. This study underlines important aspects of enteral feeding in critically ill patients. One must keep in mind the risks associated with enteral feeding, namely aspiration and pneumonia, both of which contribute to morbidity and mortality in the ICU. This study elucidates that feeding beyond the pylorus decreases gastric residual volume and may allow for tighter glycemic control. Labile blood sugar is associated with decreased gastrointestinal motility, which can increase aspiration risks. The ND group also received significantly more calories and protein than the NG group. This has importance in critically ill patients who are often catabolic and do not receive adequate nutrition to meet their increased energy requirements.

Overall, enteral feeding, when possible, should be adopted as the primary means for nutritional replacement in the hospitalized patient. Larger, multi-centered trials must be conducted to validate the findings in Dr Hsu's study.

C. W. Deitch, MD

A 6-year review of total parenteral nutrition use and association with late-onset acute respiratory distress syndrome among ventilated trauma victims

Plurad D, Green D, Inaba K, et al (Univ of Southern California and Los Angeles County Hosp Div of Trauma/Surgical Critical Care)
Injury 40:511-515, 2009

Aim.—To establish whether total parenteral nutrition (TPN) for ventilated trauma victims is associated with late-onset acute respiratory distress syndrome (ARDS) independent of ventilation and transfusion parameters.

Method.—Intensive care unit data over 6 years from a level I centre regarding all trauma victims ≥16 years old who underwent mechanical ventilation within the first 48 h of admission were examined. Patients were prospectively followed for late ARDS. Variables were examined for significant changes over time and independent associations with late ARDS were determined.

Results.—Of 2346 eligible patients among whom 404 (17.2%) were exposed to TPN, 192 (8.2%) met criteria for late ARDS. The incidence of late ARDS among those exposed to TPN was 28.7% (116/404) compared with 3.9% (76/1942) among those not so exposed. Adjustments for potential confounding associated risk factors were made.

Conclusions.—TPN administration is independently associated with late ARDS, and its use among critically ill trauma victims should be carefully scrutinized.

▶ The acute respiratory distress syndrome (ARDS) is a complication seen in ICU settings. It results from a variety of conditions including trauma, sepsis, and pneumonia. The authors differentiate early onset versus late-onset ARDS. Late-onset ARDS has a higher associated morbidity. The incidence of this complication seems to be decreasing over the last several years. There may be multiple considerations to account for this favorable trend. Total parenteral nutrition (TPN) has been associated with increased length of ICU stay, prolonged mechanical ventilation, and worsening pulmonary dysfunction. Lipid infusions seem to be especially harmful in patients with existing ARDS, and may increase morbidity and mortality in such patients.

This study included trauma victims who were intubated and exposed to TPN before the development of ARDS. Of 2346 patients included in the analysis, 404 of them were exposed to TPN, and 192 developed late onset ARDS. The overall incidence of ARDS associated with TPN exposure was 28.7% compared with 3.9% of patients who developed ARDS in the absence of TPN. The patients who were in the late ARDS and TPN group generally had a higher injury severity score (ISS), received more blood products, and higher peak inspiratory pressures and higher fluid balance. They also had a higher incidence of penetrating trauma, elevated body mass index, were more likely to be hypotensive on admission, and had a lower Glasgow coma score than the group that developed ARDS without TPN exposure. Data were not collected regarding lung injury, pneumonia, sepsis, and organ failure.

This study highlights a potential future shift in the approach to nutritional replacement in ICU patients. Although this was a retrospective analysis, the data are compelling. There are multiple variables that are associated with the development of ARDS. Apart from the possible role of TPN, transfusions, excess fluids, hypotension, and sepsis may all pose cumulative risks in critically ill patients. The reasons for prolonged parenteral feeding were not included in this retrospective review. The authors note a decrease in the incidence of ARDS from 2000 to 2005. Again there is no clear reason for this favorable trend. Intensive care has improved, patients are generally admitted with lower peak inspiratory pressures, are decreasing blood transfusions and ventilation protocols are changing. The authors also note a decreased use of TPN in their institution.

Overall, this intriguing report suggests the need for prospective analyses of the risks of TPN in critically ill patients, regardless of the etiology. Enteral nutrition is associated with more beneficial outcomes in hospitalized patients, and this study may stimulate further research into this important aspect of critical care.

C. W. Deitch, MD

9 Renal

Acquired hypernatraemia is an independent predictor of mortality in critically ill patients
O'Donoghue SD, Dulhunty JM, Bandeshe HK, et al (Royal Brisbane and Women's Hosp, Queensland, Australia)
Anaesthesia 64:514-520, 2009

This study reports the incidence and associated mortality of acquired hypernatraemia (Na > 150 mmol. l^{-1}) in a general medical/surgical intensive care unit. Patients admitted over a 5-year period with normal sodium values were eligible for inclusion; exclusions were made for burn/neurosurgical diagnoses and for hypertonic saline therapy. From 3475 admissions (3317 patients), 266 (7.7%) episodes of hypernatraemia were observed. Hospital mortality was 33.5% in the hypernatraemic group and 7.7% in the normonatraemic group (p < 0.001). Acquired hypernatraemia was

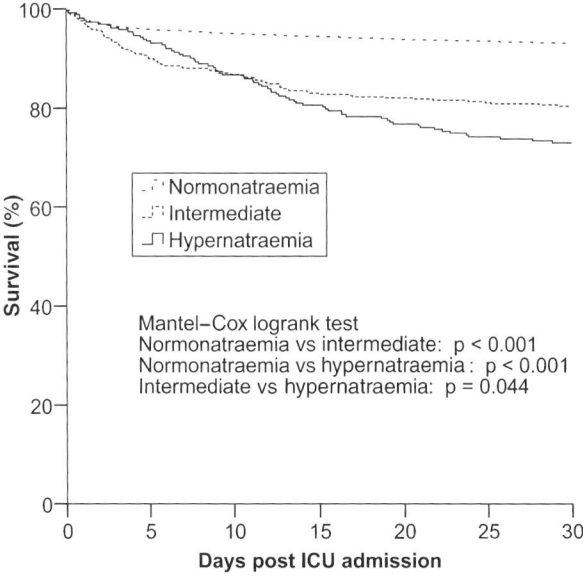

FIGURE 1.—Kaplan–Meier curve of ICU survival to 30 days by sodium group. (Reprinted from O'Donoghue SD, Dulhunty JM, Bandeshe HK, et al. Acquired hypernatraemia is an independent predictor of mortality in critically ill patients. *Anaesthesia*. 2009;64:514-520, with permission of John Wiley & Sons, Inc.)

TABLE 1.—Demographic and Outcome Characteristics by Sodium Group

Characteristic	Hypernatraemia (n = 263 with 266 admissions)	Intermediate (n = 419 with 427 admissions)	Normonatraemia (n = 2239 with 2293 admissions)	Hn vs Nn p value
Age; mean (SD)	60.0 (16.6)	59.7 (18.5)	57.8 (19.0)	0.075
Sex (males); n (%)	157 (59.7)	255 (60.9)	1306 (58.3)	0.67
APACHE II score*; mean (SD)	24.7 (8.1)	22.2 (8.0)†	16.1 (7.3)	< 0.001
Median (IQR [range])	24 (19–30 [8–54])	21 (16–27 [5–49])	15 (11–19 [0–59])	–
Admission category*; n (%)				
Cardiovascular	43 (16.5)	99 (23.5)†	627 (27.6)	< 0.001
Pneumonia	33 (12.6)	37 (8.8)	70 (3.1)	< 0.001
Other respiratory	43 (16.5)	48 (11.4)	340 (14.9)	0.51
Sepsis	42 (16.1)	57 (13.5)	102 (4.5)	< 0.001
Gastrointestinal	64 (24.5)	80 (19.0)	410 (18.0)	0.011
Trauma	12 (4.6)	34 (8.1)	167 (7.3)	0.10
Miscellaneous‡	24 (9.2)	67 (15.9)†	559 (24.6)	< 0.001
Chronic respiratory disease; n (%)	33 (12.5)	26 (6.2)†	125 (5.6)	< 0.001
Heart failure; n (%)	25 (9.5)	24 (7.5)†	143 (6.4)	0.056
Liver failure; n (%)	13 (4.9)	16 (3.8)	30 (1.3)	< 0.001
Chronic renal failure; n (%)	11 (4.2)	15 (3.6)	80 (3.6)	0.62
Immuno-compromise; n (%)	43 (16.3)	35 (8.4)†	137 (6.1)	< 0.001
Lymphoma; n (%)	8 (3.0)	8 (1.9)	25 (1.1)	0.018
Metastatic cancer; n (%)	15 (5.7)	15 (3.6)	168 (7.5)	0.29
Leukaemia / myeloma; n (%)	13 (4.9)	12 (2.9)	26 (1.2)	< 0.001
Postoperative admission*; n (%)	65 (24.4)	154 (36.1)†	1339 (58.4)	< 0.001
Emergency surgery*; n (%)	48 (18.0)	99 (23.2)	352 (15.4)	0.25
Dialysis*; n (%)	42 (15.8)	51 (11.9)	55 (2.4)	< 0.001
Parenteral nutrition*; n (%)	57 (21.4)	49 (11.5)†	49 (2.1)	< 0.001
Frusemide*; n (%)	225 (84.6)	275 (64.4)†	568 (24.8)	< 0.001
ICU LOS (days)*; mean (SD)	13.3 (13.7)	6.6 (7.7)†	1.6 (2.7)	< 0.001
Median (IQR [range])	9.1 (5.1–15 [0.05–99])	4.1 (1.8–8.0 [0.08–54])	1.0 (0.8–1.8 [0.03–104])	–
Hospital LOS (days); mean (SD)	45.1 (61.8)	39.5 (57.3)	18.8 (29.2)	< 0.001
Median (IQR; range)	29 (15–52 [0.6–515])	21 (11–44 [0.2–512])	9.9 (5.1–21 [0.1–491])	–
ICU mortality*; n (%)	57 (21.9)	57 (14.5)	77 (3.4)	< 0.001

(*Continued*)

TABLE 1. *(continued)*

Characteristic	Hypernatraemia (*n* = 263 with 266 admissions)	Intermediate (*n* = 419 with 427 admissions)	Normonatraemia (*n* = 2239 with 2293 admissions)	Hn vs Nn p value
In-hospital mortality; *n* (%)	88 (33.5)	88 (21.0)†	173 (7.7)	< 0.001

Hn, hypernatraemic group; Nn, normonatraemic group; APACHE, acute physiology and chronic health evaluation; ICU, intensive care unit; LOS, length of stay.
*Number of admissions used in the denominator.
†Significant difference (p < 0.05) between hypernatraemic group and intermediate group.
‡Miscellaneous: includes drug overdose (5 in hypernatraemic group vs 26 vs 175 in other groups) and hysterectomy (1 in hypernatraemic group vs 1 vs 90 in other groups).

an independent risk factor for in-hospital mortality (OR 1.97, 95% CI 1.37–2.82, p < 0.001). Intermediate sodium levels (145–150 mmol l⁻¹) were associated with increased mortality (OR 1.42, 95% CI 1.02–1.98). Uncorrected sodium at discharge (p = 0.001) and peak sodium (p = 0.001) were better predictors of mortality than time to onset (p = 0.71) and duration of hypernatraemia (p = 1.0). Hypernatraemia avoidance is justified, but determinants of hypernatraemia and benefits of targeted treatment strategies require further elucidation.

▶ This is an important observational study of over 7000 ICU admissions at a single center. Like all good observational studies this does not attempt to answer a question, but it indeed raises many. As can be seen in Fig 1, the mortality rate of patients that developed hypernatremia while in the ICU is significantly higher as compared with those that did not and in addition, those with intermediate sodium concentrations had intermediate mortality similar to the appearance of a dose-response effect. This apparent dose-response effect adds some degree of validity to the base observation. It is important to note that certain patient types were excluded, and these included those with burns, neurosurgical diagnoses, and patients in whom hypertonic saline was administered. One should not interpret these results as causative until a well-done prospective trial is conducted, and in fact some of the data from this observational study should cause one to wonder if this association is indeed clinically relevant. In Table 1 it should be noted that there is a higher rate of pneumonia, chronic respiratory disease, sepsis, liver failure, dialytic therapy, immunocompromised state, and the use of total parenteral nutrition (TPN) in the hypernatremic group, and these in combination may have contributed to the higher mortality. In addition, a protective factor of being admitted postoperatively was more than 2-fold more common in the normonatraemic group. Finally, the exact causative pathway by which elevated sodium levels may worsen mortality is unclear.

T. Dorman, MD

Acquired hypernatraemia is an independent predictor of mortality in critically ill patients
O'Donoghue SD, Dulhunty JM, Bandeshe HK, et al (Royal Brisbane and Women's Hosp, Queensland, Australia)
Anaesthesia 64:514-520, 2009

This study reports the incidence and associated mortality of acquired hypernatraemia (Na > 150 mmol.l^{-1}) in a general medical/surgical intensive care unit. Patients admitted over a 5-year period with normal sodium values were eligible for inclusion; exclusions were made for burn/neurosurgical diagnoses and for hypertonic saline therapy. From 3475 admissions (3317 patients), 266 (7.7%) episodes of hypernatraemia were observed. Hospital mortality was 33.5% in the hypernatraemic group and 7.7% in the normonatraemic group (p < 0.001). Acquired hypernatraemia was an independent risk factor for in-hospital mortality (OR 1.97, 95% CI 1.37–2.82, p < 0.001). Intermediate sodium levels (145–150 mmol.l^{-1}) were associated with increased mortality (OR 1.42, 95% CI 1.02–1.98). Uncorrected sodium at discharge (p = 0.001) and peak sodium (p = 0.001) were better predictors of mortality than time to onset (p = 0.71) and duration of hypernatraemia (p = 1.0). Hypernatraemia avoidance is justified, but determinants of hypernatraemia and benefits of targeted treatment strategies require further elucidation.

▶ The development of hypernatremia (Na > 150 mmol/L) in hospitalized patients has been reported to be low (around 2%), but mortality in this group seems to be exceedingly high (40%-60%). In critically ill patients admitted to the intensive care unit, the incidence and impact on outcomes of hypernatremia are not well defined. In this retrospective study, a large database (over 3000 critically ill patients) was evaluated to determine the incidence of ICU-acquired hypernatremia and its impact on patient outcomes. This is the largest study to date to investigate the incidence and patient outcomes of hypernatremia acquired in the ICU. In this study, the incidence of hypernatremia was 7.7%. The associated mortality in patients with hypernatremia was high (33.5%). Furthermore, in a multivariate analysis, hypernatremia was shown to be an independent predictor of mortality. There was a graded increase in mortality associated with the degree of hypernatremia. The major limitation of this study lies in its retrospective nature, which precludes us from determining hypernatremia as a cause of increased mortality. However, despite this limitation, these results should encourage clinicians to proactively prevent and treat hypernatremia in critically ill patients.

S. L. Zanotti-Cavazzoni, MD

Acute kidney injury in septic shock: clinical outcomes and impact of duration of hypotension prior to initiation of antimicrobial therapy

Bagshaw SM, The Cooperative Antimicrobial Therapy of Septic Shock (CATSS) Database Research Group (Univ of Alberta, Edmonton, Canada; et al)

Intensive Care Med 35:871-881, 2009

Objective.—To describe the incidence and outcomes associated with early acute kidney injury (AKI) in septic shock and explore the association between duration from hypotension onset to effective antimicrobial therapy and AKI.

Design.—Retrospective cohort study.

Subjects.—A total of 4,532 adult patients with septic shock from 1989 to 2005.

Setting.—Intensive care units of 22 academic and community hospitals in Canada, the United States and Saudi Arabia.

Measurements and Main Results.—In total, 64.4% of patients with septic shock developed early AKI (i.e., within 24 h after onset of hypotension). By RIFLE criteria, 16.3% had risk, 29.4% had injury and 18.7% had failure. AKI patients were older, more likely female, with more comorbid disease and greater severity of illness. Of 3,373 patients (74.4%) with hypotension prior to receiving effective antimicrobial therapy, the median (IQR) time from hypotension onset to antimicrobial therapy was 5.5 h (2.0–13.3). Patients with AKI were more likely to have longer delays to receiving antimicrobial therapy compared to those with no AKI [6.0 (2.3–15.3) h for AKI vs. 4.3 (1.5–10.8) h for no AKI, $P < 0.0001$]. A longer duration to antimicrobial therapy was also associated an increase in odds of AKI [odds ratio (OR) 1.14, 95% CI 1.10–1.20, $P < 0.001$, per hour (log-transformed) delay]. AKI was associated with significantly higher odds of death in both ICU (OR 1.73, 95% CI 1.60–1.9, $P < 0.0001$) and hospital (OR 1.62, 95% CI, 1.5–1.7, $P < 0.0001$). By Cox proportional hazards analysis, including propensity score-adjustment, each RIFLE category was independently associated with a greater hazard ratio for death (risk 1.31; injury 1.45; failure 1.56).

Conclusion.—Early AKI is common in septic shock. Delays to appropriate antimicrobial therapy may contribute to significant increases in the incidence of AKI. Survival was considerably lower for septic shock associated with early AKI, with increasing severity of AKI, and with increasing delays to appropriate antimicrobial therapy.

▶ Sepsis is the most common cause of death[1] and the predominant cause of acute renal failure[2] in critically ill patients. Progressive delay in the administration of antibiotics to patients with septic shock is associated with a graded increase in the risk of death.[3] Numerous studies over the past few years have shown that acute kidney injury (AKI) is associated with an increase in mortality.[2,4-6] It is logical, then, to ask whether a delay in antibiotic administration to patients with septic shock might be associated with the development of AKI.

Bagshaw et al analyzed the Cooperative Antimicrobial Therapy of Septic Shock (CATSS) database to answer that question.[7] In their observational study of patients admitted to 22 institutions over the years 1989-2005, they found that patients who developed AKI (by RIFLE criteria) were more likely to have had a delay in initiation of antibiotics (defined as the duration of hypotension) compared with the group without AKI. Moreover, the hazard ratio for AKI increased progressively with increasing delay. The group with AKI was older and sicker than the group without, and they had a higher mortality, even when adjusted for comorbidities and propensity for death.

The study is observational, which is clearly an appropriate design for the question at hand, but one that opens the door to various types of bias— a point the authors concede. Furthermore, the criterion for AKI uses a 24-hour time point, allowing inclusion of patients whose AKI might be only brief. This, along with the imputation of a normal baseline creatinine concentration in the cases of missing data, would only tend to dilute the AKI population. These latter limitations, therefore, render the observed associations all the more credible. In that light, the study further emphasizes the importance of early antimicrobial therapy in patients with septic shock, in this case to prevent AKI.

J. S. Rachoin, MD

L. S. Weisberg, MD

References

1. Hotchkiss RS, Karl IE. The pathophysiology and treatment of sepsis. *N Engl J Med.* 2003;348:138-150.
2. Bagshaw SW, Uchino D, Bellomo R, et al. Beginning and Ending Supportive Therapy for the Kidney (BEST Kidney) Investigators. Septic acute kidney injury in critically ill patients: clinical characteristics and outcomes. *Clin J Am Soc Nephrol.* 2007;2:431-439.
3. Kumar A, Roberts D, Wood KE, et al. Duration of hypotension before initiation of effective antimicrobial therapy is the critical determinant of survival in human septic shock. *Crit Care Med.* 2006;34:1589-1596.
4. Uchino S, Kellum JA, Bellomo R, et al. Beginning and Ending Supportive Therapy for the Kidney (BEST Kidney) Investigators. Acute renal failure in critically ill patients: a multinational, multicenter study. *JAMA.* 2005;294:813-818.
5. Hoste EA, Clermont G, Kersten A, et al. RIFLE criteria for acute kidney injury are associated with hospital mortality in critically ill patients: a cohort analysis. *Crit Care.* 2006;10:R73.
6. Lassnigg A, Schmid ER, Hiesmayr M, et al. Impact of minimal increases in serum creatinine on outcome in patients after cardiothoracic surgery: do we have to revise current definitions of acute renal failure? *Crit Care Med.* 2008;36: 1129-1137.
7. Bagshaw SM, Lapinsky S, Dial S, et al. Cooperative Antimicrobial Therapy of Septic Shock (CATSS) Database Research Group. Acute kidney injury in septic shock: clinical outcomes and impact of duration of hypotension prior to initiation of antimicrobial therapy. *Intensive Care Med.* 2009;35:871-881.

Early Use of Polymyxin B Hemoperfusion in Abdominal Septic Shock: The EUPHAS Randomized Controlled Trial

Cruz DN, Antonelli M, Fumagalli R, et al (St Bortolo Hosp and International Renal Res Inst Vicenza; Catholic Univ of Sacred Heart, Rome; Milano Bicocca Univ, Monza; et al)
JAMA 301:2445-2452, 2009

Context.—Polymyxin B fiber column is a medical device designed to reduce blood endotoxin levels in sepsis. Gram-negative–induced abdominal sepsis is likely associated with high circulating endotoxin. Reducing circulating endotoxin levels with polymyxin B hemoperfusion could potentially improve patient clinical outcomes.

Objective.—To determine whether polymyxin B hemoperfusion added to conventional medical therapy improves clinical outcomes (mean arterial pressure [MAP], vasopressor requirement, oxygenation, organ dysfunction) and mortality compared with conventional therapy alone.

Design, Setting, and Patients.—A prospective, multicenter, randomized controlled trial (Early Use of Polymyxin B Hemoperfusion in Abdominal Sepsis [EUPHAS]) conducted at 10 Italian tertiary care intensive care units between December 2004 and December 2007. Sixty-four patients were enrolled with severe sepsis or septic shock who underwent emergency surgery for intra-abdominal infection.

Intervention.—Patients were randomized to either conventional therapy (n=30) or conventional therapy plus 2 sessions of polymyxin B hemoperfusion (n=34).

Main Outcome Measures.—Primary outcome was change in MAP and vasopressor requirement, and secondary outcomes were PaO_2/FIO_2 (fraction of inspired oxygen) ratio, change in organ dysfunction measured using Sequential Organ Failure Assessment (SOFA) scores, and 28-day mortality.

Results.—MAP increased (76 to 84 mm Hg; $P = .001$) and vasopressor requirement decreased (inotropic score, 29.9 to 6.8; $P < .001$) at 72 hours in the polymyxin B group but not in the conventional therapy group (MAP, 74 to 77 mm Hg; $P = .37$; inotropic score, 28.6 to 22.4; $P = .14$). The PaO_2/FIO_2 ratio increased slightly (235 to 264; $P = .049$) in the polymyxin B group but not in the conventional therapy group (217 to 228; $P = .79$). SOFA scores improved in the polymyxin B group but not in the conventional therapy group (change in SOFA, -3.4 vs -0.1; $P < .001$), and 28-day mortality was 32% (11/34 patients) in the polymyxin B group and 53% (16/30 patients) in the conventional therapy group (unadjusted hazard ratio [HR], 0.43; 95% confidence interval [CI], 0.20-0.94; adjusted HR, 0.36; 95% CI, 0.16-0.80).

Conclusion.—In this preliminary study, polymyxin B hemoperfusion added to conventional therapy significantly improved hemodynamics and organ dysfunction and reduced 28-day mortality in a targeted population with severe sepsis and/or septic shock from intra-abdominal gram-negative infections.

Trial Registration.—clinicaltrials.gov Identifier: NCT00629382.

▶ The single most common cause of acute kidney injury (AKI) and failure in critically ill patients is sepsis.[1] Moreover, sepsis-associated AKI carries a higher mortality than AKI in other settings.[2] For these, and other obvious reasons, the treatment of sepsis has been the target of intensive investigation in the past decade.

Severe sepsis (infection-induced organ dysfunction), in the setting of gram-negative bacterial infection, is the consequence of endotoxin (or lipopolysaccharide [LPS]) binding to toll-like receptors and the ensuing inflammatory and coagulation cascade.[3] High levels of endotoxin have been associated with increased mortality and are found not only in gram-negative infections but also culture-negative or gram-positive infections.[4] Given the central role of LPS in the pathogenesis of sepsis, it is not surprising that it has featured prominently in the history of clinical research in sepsis.

Several methods have been evaluated for the effectiveness of removing or inactivating endotoxin, such as lipid A analog, phospholipid emulsion, ethyl pyruvate, a variety of LPS-binding proteins, and polymyxin B.[4] This last compound is an antimicrobial that binds to the lipid A moiety of LPS. A systematic review of small, heterogeneous clinical trials in patients with sepsis suggested a beneficial effect of hemoperfusion using a membrane to which polymyxin B was bound.[5] With that encouragement, a large, multicenter, randomized trial of polymyxin B hemoperfusion in sepsis was undertaken and reviewed here.[6]

In this trial, Cruz et al randomized 64 patients with abdominal sepsis to polymyxin B hemoperfusion or conventional therapy.[6] Patients assigned to the polymyxin B hemoperfusion arm had a significant increase in mean arterial pressure, a reduction in vasopressor use, and an improvement in sequential organ failure assessment (SOFA) scores, compared with the control group. Mortality at 28 days was significantly lower in the polymyxin B group (adjusted hazard ratio [HR] 0.36). This reduction in mortality was detected at a scheduled interim analysis and prompted early termination of the study. There was no difference between groups in any renal endpoints.

These impressive results must be viewed with some caution for 2 reasons. First, because the trial was stopped early and included a smaller number of patients than originally intended, there is a greater chance of a type I error. Second, for logistical reasons, the study was not blinded, creating the opportunity for bias. Nevertheless, these preliminary results are encouraging and open the way for larger trials, perhaps including patients with more diverse causes of sepsis.

J. S. Rachoin, MD
L. S. Weisberg, MD

References

1. Uchino S, Bellomo R, Morimatsu H, et al. External validation of severity scoring systems for acute renal failure using a multinational database. *Crit Care Med.* 2005;33:1961-1967.

2. Bagshaw SM, Uchino S, Bellomo R, et al. Septic acute kidney injury in critically ill patients: clinical characteristics and outcomes. *Clin J Am Soc Nephrol.* 2007;2: 431-439.
3. Cinel I, Dellinger RP. Advances in pathogenesis and management of sepsis. *Curr Opin Infect Dis.* 2007;20:345-352.
4. Nahra R, Dellinger RP. Targeting the lipopolysaccharides: still a matter of debate? *Curr Opin Anaesthesiol.* 2008;21:98-104.
5. Cruz DN, Perazella MA, Bellomo R, et al. Effectiveness of polymyxin B-immobilized fiber column in sepsis: a systematic review. *Crit Care.* 2007;11:R47.
6. Cruz DN, Antonelli M, Fumagalli R, et al. Early use of polymyxin B hemoperfusion in abdominal septic shock: the EUPHAS randomized controlled trial. *JAMA.* 2009;301:2445-2452.

Angiotensin converting enzyme insertion/deletion genetic polymorphism: Its impact on renal function in critically ill patients

du Cheyron D, Fradin S, Ramakers M, et al (Service de Réanimation Médicale, Caen, France; Laboratoire de Biochimie, Caen, France)
Crit Care Med 36:3178-3183, 2008

Objective.—Previous clinical studies have suggested an association between the insertion/deletion (I/D) genetic polymorphism of angiotensin converting enzyme and acute or chronic diseases. We aimed to test the prognostic value of the I-allele, which is associated with lower angiotensin converting enzyme activity, on acute kidney injury.

Design.—Prospective 6-month noninterventional study.

Setting.—Intensive care unit of a University Hospital.

Patients and Methods.—One hundred eighty consecutive admitted white patients for an expected intensive care unit stay >48 hr. Angiotensin converting enzyme genetic polymorphism was screened for genotype (I/D polymorphism analysis by polymerase chain reaction amplification) and phenotype (measurement of the circulating rate of angiotensin converting enzyme by spectrophotometry). Acute kidney injury was assessed according to Risk, Injury, Failure, Loss, and End-stage Kidney classification.

Intervention.—None.

Results.—II, ID, and DD genotype frequencies were 25%, 48%, and 27%, respectively. II and ID genotypes were associated with lower baseline circulating rates of angiotensin converting enzyme (20 ± 14 and 22 ± 18 U/L, respectively, vs. 30 ± 23 U/L for DD genotype; $p = 0.04$). Repartition of angiotensin converting enzyme genotypes were different in patients with and without acute kidney injury ($p < 0.0001$), with greater II genotype proportion in acute kidney injury patients (42% vs. 13% for those without acute kidney injury). After adjustment on the identified prognostic factors, II genotype was independently associated with increased risk of acute kidney injury (adjusted odds ratio, 6.5; 95% confidence interval, 2.4–17.7; $p = 0.0002$), then death among patients with acute kidney injury (adjusted odds ratio, 1.7; 95% confidence ratio, 1.1–2.6; $p = 0.02$).

Conclusion.—These data confirm the key role of the renin-angiotensin system to maintain glomerular filtration rate, and highlight an association between a genetic factor and susceptibility to and prognosis of acute kidney disease.

▶ Acute renal failure (ARF) in critically ill patients is associated with a substantially increased risk of death.[1] One popular notion, although far from confirmed, holds that prevention of ARF will reduce mortality.[2,3] There is a consensus, however, that the key to successful prevention of ARF is the application of prophylactic interventions as early as possible in the course of illness. This strategy, in turn, depends on identification of patients at risk of ARF. Although advances have been made in this regard, particularly in well-defined circumstances,[4,5] it is clear that the risk factors for ARF in most critically ill patients are incompletely understood.

One missing piece of the risk puzzle might reside in the genotypic background of the patient. This notion is not new: Genotype has been linked to chronic illnesses such as hypertension, cardiovascular disease, and more recently, end-stage renal disease. One of the genes that has been extensively studied is the gene coding for angiotensin-converting enzyme (ACE).[6]

The ACE gene, located on chromosome 17, exhibits polymorphism reflecting the insertion (I) or deletion (D) of a 287 base-pair sequence, resulting in the genotypic variations II, ID, and DD.[7] Circulating ACE levels are higher in patients with the DD genotype than with the II.[8] The II genotype has been found to be protective against diabetic nephropathy[6] and associated with better survival in patient with idiopathic cardiomyopathy.[9]

In this prospective, noninterventional study,[10] du Cheyron et al characterized the ACE genotype of 180 critically ill patients and monitored them for the development of acute kidney injury. They found that, after adjusting for known risk factors, the II genotype was independently associated with increased risk of ARF. Furthermore, among patients who developed acute kidney injury, the II genotype was independently associated with death. Circulating ACE levels were lower in patients with the II and ID genotypes than with the DD genotype.

These results are consistent with the observation that inhibition of ACE in patients with hypovolemia or decompensated congestive heart failure predisposes to ARF by impairing the kidney's capacity to autoregulate its blood flow and glomerular filtration.[11,12] Why ACE polymorphism in this study was associated with increased mortality among patients with acute kidney injury remains to be elucidated.

Given the study population's modest size and ethnic homogeneity, the results of the study can only be considered preliminary. It may, nonetheless, portend a new era in clinical medicine in which the genotype may comprise an important part of the patient's risk profile, opening the way to tailored preventive strategies.

J. S. Rachoin, MD
L. S. Weisberg, MD

References

1. Hoste EA, Clermont G, Kersten A, et al. RIFLE criteria for acute kidney injury are associated with hospital mortality in critically ill patients: a cohort analysis. *Crit Care.* 2006;10:R73.
2. Kellum JA, Angus DC. Patients are dying of acute renal failure. *Crit Care Med.* 2002;30:2156-2157.
3. Rudnick M, Feldman H. Contrast-induced nephropathy: what are the true clinical consequences? *Clin J Am Soc Nephrol.* 2008;3:263-272.
4. Conlon P, Stafford-Smith M, White W, et al. Acute renal failure following cardiac surgery. *Nephrol Dial Transplant.* 1999;14:1158-1162.
5. Pannu N, Wiebe N, Tonelli M. Prophylaxis strategies for contrast-induced nephropathy. *JAMA.* 2006;295:2765-2779.
6. Ruggenenti P, Bettinaglio P, Pinares F, Remuzzi G. Angiotensin converting enzyme insertion/deletion polymorphism and renoprotection in diabetic and nondiabetic nephropathies. *Clin J Am Soc Nephrol.* 2008;3:1511-1525.
7. Rigat B, Hubert C, Corvol P, Soubrier F. PCR detection of the insertion/deletion polymorphism of the human angiotensin converting enzyme gene (DCP1) (dipeptidyl carboxypeptidase 1). *Nucleic Acids Res.* 1992;20:1433.
8. Rigat B, Hubert C, Alhenc-Gelas F, Cambien F, Corvol P, Soubrier F. An insertion/deletion polymorphism in the angiotensin I-converting enzyme gene accounting for half the variance of serum enzyme levels. *J Clin Invest.* 1990; 86:1343-1346.
9. Andersson B, Sylven C. The DD genotype of the angiotensin-converting enzyme gene is associated with increased mortality in idiopathic heart failure. *J Am Coll Cardiol.* 1996;28:162-167.
10. du Cheyron D, Fradin S, Ramakers M, et al. Angiotensin converting enzyme insertion/deletion genetic polymorphism: its impact on renal function in critically ill patients. *Crit Care Med.* 2008;36:3178-3183.
11. Abuelo JG. Normotensive ischemic acute renal failure. *N Engl J Med.* 2007;357: 797-805.
12. Hricik DE, Dunn MJ. Angiotensin-converting enzyme inhibitor-induced renal failure: causes, consequences, and diagnostic uses. *J Am Soc Nephrol.* 1990;1: 845-858.

Acid–base disorders evaluation in critically ill patients: we can improve our diagnostic ability

Boniatti MM, Cardoso PRC, Castilho RK, et al (Hosp de Clínicas de Porto Alegre, Brazil)
Intensive Care Med 35:1377-1382, 2009

Purpose.—To determine whether Stewart's approach can improve our ability to diagnose acid–base disorders compared to the traditional model.

Methods.—This prospective cohort study took place in a university-affiliated hospital during the period of February–May 2007. We recorded clinical data and acid–base variables from one hundred seventy-five patients at intensive care unit admission.

Results.—Of the 68 patients with normal standard base excess (SBE) (SBE between -4.9 and $+4.9$), most ($n = 59$; 86.8%) had a lower effective strong ion difference (SIDe), and of these, 15 (25.4%) had SIDe < 30 mEq/L.

Thus, the evaluation according to Stewart's method would allow an additional diagnosis of metabolic disorder in 33.7% patients.

Conclusions.—The Stewart approach, compared to the traditional evaluation, results in identification of more patients with major acid–base disturbances.

▶ Acid-base disorders are common in critically ill patients. Traditionally, intensivists have diagnosed and identified primary acid-base disorders by using formulas and concepts proposed by Henderson and Hasselbach. This traditional method identifies the prescience of a metabolic acidosis based on the determination of the anion gap (AG), standard base excess (SBE), and bicarbonate (HCO_3). Although this method is widely used, some have pointed out that it may oversimplify complex acid-base derangements and hence may not perform well in critically ill patients with extreme abnormalities. More recently, various critical care physicians have proposed an alternative method for the evaluation of acid-base disorders – the Stewart method. The Stewart method is a mathematical model based on psychochemical principles. This model proposes 3 variables that independently determine the concentration of hydrogen ($H+$) and, consequently, define the pH. These variables are the strong ion difference (difference between fully dissociated anions and cations, SID), the total weak acid concentration (especially albumin and phosphate), and $PaCO_2$. In this model only these 3 variables are important, because if they don't change, there cannot be a change in $H+$ or HCO_3. In this article, the authors conducted a prospective cohort study in critically ill patients to determine whether the application of the Stewart method could improve diagnosis of acid-base disorders in critically ill patients. They report increased sensitivity with the Stewart method in identifying metabolic acidosis, particularly in patients with significant abnormalities in albumin and phosphate. Although it would seem that, based on these results, the Stewart method outperforms the traditional Henderson and Hasselbach method, most of the missed metabolic acidosis can be identified if one corrects the AG for albumin and phosphate. It is likely that both methods will still have their proponents and detractors as this study and the current literature don't show a significant clinical benefit on patient care with one particular method. For the clinician, understanding one method and applying it well at the bedside is perhaps the most important take-home message.

S. L. Zanotti-Cavazzoni, MD

Fluid accumulation, survival and recovery of kidney function in critically ill patients with acute kidney injury

Bouchard J, Program to Improve Care in Acute Renal Disease (PICARD) Study Group (Univ of California San Diego; et al)
Kidney Int 76:422-427, 2009

Fluid accumulation is associated with adverse outcomes in critically ill patients. Here, we sought to determine if fluid accumulation is associated with mortality and non-recovery of kidney function in critically ill adults with acute kidney injury. Fluid overload was defined as more than a 10% increase in body weight relative to baseline, measured in 618 patients enrolled in a prospective multicenter observational study. Patients with fluid overload experienced significantly higher mortality within 60 days of enrollment. Among dialyzed patients, survivors had significantly lower fluid accumulation when dialysis was initiated compared to non-survivors after adjustments for dialysis modality and severity score. The adjusted odds ratio for death associated with fluid overload at dialysis initiation was 2.07. In non-dialyzed patients, survivors had significantly less fluid accumulation at the peak of their serum creatinine. Fluid over-load at the time of diagnosis of acute kidney injury was not associated with recovery of kidney function. However, patients with fluid overload when their serum creatinine reached its peak were significantly less likely to recover kidney function. Our study shows that in patients with acute kidney injury, fluid overload was independently associated with mortality. Whether the fluid overload was the result of a more severe renal failure or it contributed to its cause will require clinical trials in which the role of fluid administration to such patients is directly tested.

▶ Early goal-directed therapy, with aggressive fluid resuscitation, reduces mortality in patients with severe sepsis.[1] Generalizing this fluid management approach to patients with diagnoses other than severe sepsis may be inadvisable, however. Indeed, patients with acute lung injury[2] or recent surgery[3] randomized to a liberal fluid administration regimen fared worse than patients randomized to a conservative fluid strategy, with respect to several important outcomes. Given the difficulties in the fluid management of patients with acute kidney injury (AKI), it would be important to know whether fluid balance has an impact on clinical outcomes in this population.

Program to Improve Care in Acute Renal Disease (PICARD) is a multicenter research consortium established to conduct observational studies of factors associated with clinical outcomes in a cohort of 618 critically ill patients with AKI. The most recent study by these respected investigators tries to address the role of fluid balance in this population.[4] They found that, among patients who required renal replacement therapy, fluid accumulation was lower in patients who survived for 30 days than those who died. Fluid overload (defined as accumulation of at least 10% of body weight in fluid) was associated with a doubling of the odds of death. Even among patients who did not require dialysis, the odds of death were higher in those who accumulated more fluid. These relationships held after adjustment for Acute Physiology and Chronic Health Evaluation III (APACHE III) score.

It is tempting to infer from these results that positive fluid balance in patients with AKI prejudices against survival. Such an inference must be made with great caution from this observational study, however. One must ask, for example, whether the fluids were administered for reasons which might, in themselves, have increased mortality. In that regard, the evidence shows that the group with fluid overload much more commonly had sepsis or septic shock. Thus, clinicians would do well to wait for the sort of randomized controlled trials that have guided fluid management in other populations[2,3] before altering their care of patients with AKI in the ICU based on the results of this study.

J. S. Rachoin, MD
L. S. Weisberg, MD

References

1. Rivers E, Nguyen B, Havstad S, et al. Early Goal-Directed Therapy Collaborative Group. Early goal-directed therapy in the treatment of severe sepsis and septic shock. *N Engl J Med*. 2001;345:1368-1377.
2. Wiedemann HP, Wheeler AP, Bernard GR, et al. Comparison of two fluid-management strategies in acute lung injury. *N Engl J Med*. 2006;354:2564-2575.
3. Stewart RM, Park PK, Hunt JP, et al. Less is more: improved outcomes in surgical patients with conservative fluid administration and central venous catheter monitoring. *J Am Coll Surg*. 2009;208:725-735.
4. Bouchard J, Soroko SB, Chertow GM, et al. Program to Improve Care in Acute Renal Disease (PICARD) Study Group. Fluid accumulation, survival and recovery of kidney function in critically ill patients with acute kidney injury. *Kidney Int*. 2009;76:422-427.

Novel and conventional serum biomarkers predicting acute kidney injury in adult cardiac surgery—A prospective cohort study
Haase-Fielitz A, Bellomo R, Devarajan P, et al (Austin Health, Melbourne, Australia; Cincinnati Children's Hosp Med Ctr, OH; et al)
Crit Care Med 37:553-560, 2009

Objective.—To compare the value of novel with conventional serum biomarkers in the prediction of acute kidney injury (AKI) in adult cardiac surgical patients according to preoperative renal function.

Design.—Single-center, prospective observational study.

Setting.—Tertiary hospital.

Patients.—One hundred adult cardiac surgical patients.

Measurements and Main Results.—We measured concentrations of plasma neutrophil gelatinase-associated lipocalin (NGAL), and serum cystatin C, and creatinine and urea at baseline, on arrival in the intensive care unit (ICU) and at 24 hours postoperatively. We assessed such biomarkers in relation to the development of AKI (>50% increase in creatinine from baseline) and to a composite end point (need for renal replacement therapy and in-hospital mortality). We defined an area under the receiver operating characteristic curve of 0.60–0.69 as poor, 0.70–0.79 as fair, 0.80–0.89 as good, and 0.90–1.00 as excellent in terms of predictive value. On arrival in ICU, plasma NGAL and serum cystatin C were of good predictive value, but creatinine and urea were of poor predictive value. After exclusion of patients with preoperative renal impairment (estimated glomerular filtration rate <60 mL/min), the predictive performance for AKI of all renal biomarkers on arrival in ICU remained unchanged except for cystatin C, which was of fair value in such patients. At 24 hours postoperatively, all renal biomarkers were of good predictive value. On arrival in ICU, novel biomarkers were superior to conventional biomarkers ($p < 0.05$). Plasma NGAL ($p = 0.015$) and serum cystatin C ($p = 0.007$) were independent predictors of AKI and of excellent value in the prediction of the composite end point.

Conclusions.—Early postoperative measurement of plasma NGAL was of good value in identifying patients who developed AKI after adult cardiac surgery. Plasma NGAL and serum cystatin C were superior to conventional biomarkers in the prediction of AKI and were also of prognostic value in this setting.

▶ Acute kidney injury (AKI) is common in critically ill patients.[1] The first consensus definition of AKI, based on a change in serum creatinine concentration over 7 days (the RIFLE criteria[2]), revealed a proportional relationship between severity of AKI and mortality.[3,4] With the recognition that a very small change in serum creatinine concentration over a short time was associated with adverse outcomes,[5,6] a new definition of AKI was proposed: the AKIN criteria.[7] This shortened the time interval of definition to 48 hours. Both these definitions rely on changes in serum creatinine concentration and are subject to the inherent limitations of this marker, not the least of which is the time required for creatinine's detectable accumulation in the circulation.[8] There is a belief, as yet unsubstantiated, that the earlier one can diagnose AKI, the better one's chance to intervene and improve the patient's outcome. This has spurred the effort to detect AKI as early as possible using new biomarkers.[8]

Ideally, a biomarker should not only be disease-specific (such as troponin for myocardial infarction), but also highly sensitive (to avoid underdiagnosis).[9] Among the most promising candidate biomarkers are neutrophil gelatinase-associated lipocalin (NGAL)[10] and cystatin C.[11] Cystatin C is produced by all nucleated cells, is freely filtered by the glomerulus, and is reabsorbed and degraded by the proximal tubules cells.[11] The serum concentration, unlike that of creatinine, is not affected by age, sex, or race. NGAL is synthesized in a number of organs, and circulating levels are increased in AKI, especially with renal tubular injury.[10] The simultaneous use of those biomarkers could provide better information than each alone: NGAL might indicate tubular injury, whereas cystatin C could reflect the impairment of glomerular filtration.

In this study, Haase-Fielitz et al showed that, in patients who developed AKI (using a liberal definition) after open-heart surgery, serum NGAL and cystatin C levels increased earlier than traditional makers of AKI, serum urea, and creatinine (see Fig 1 in the original article).[12] It is important to note, however, that when applied to their whole population, the positive predictive value of these novel biomarkers was poor, and no better than that of the conventional markers. This seems to be due to their low specificity, seen mainly in the patients with underlying chronic kidney disease. It is exactly that subgroup, however, that is at greatest risk of postoperative AKI. Nonetheless, this article provides a glimmer of hope that a panel of novel biomarkers, including NGAL and cystatin C, might lead to earlier diagnosis of AKI, and set the stage for fruitful intervention.

J. S. Rachoin, MD
L. S. Weisberg, MD

References

1. Uchino S, Kellum JA, Bellomo R, et al. Ending Supportive Therapy for the Kidney (BEST Kidney) Investigators. Acute renal failure in critically ill patients: a multinational, multicenter study. *JAMA.* 2005;294:813-818.
2. Bellomo R, Ronco C, Kellum JA, Mehta RL, Palevsky P. Acute Dialysis Quality Initiative workgroup. Acute renal failure—definition, outcome measures, animal models, fluid therapy and information technology needs: the second international consensus conference of the Acute Dialysis Quality Initiative (ADQI) Group. *Crit Care.* 2004;8:R204-R212.
3. Hoste EA, Clermont G, Kersten A, et al. RIFLE criteria for acute kidney injury are associated with hospital mortality in critically ill patients: a cohort analysis. *Crit Care.* 2006;10:R73.
4. Uchino S, Bellomo R, Goldsmith D, Bates S, Ronco C. An assessment of the RIFLE criteria for acute renal failure in hospitalized patients. *Crit Care Med.* 2006;34:1913-1917.
5. Kuitunen A, Vento A, Suojaranta-Ylinen R, Pettilä V. Acute renal failure after cardiac surgery: evaluation of the RIFLE classification. *Ann Thorac Surg.* 2006;81:542-546.
6. Lassnigg A, Schmidlin D, Mouhieddine M, et al. Minimal changes of serum creatinine predict prognosis in patients after cardiothoracic surgery: a prospective cohort study. *J Am Soc Nephrol.* 2004;15:1597-1605.
7. Mehta RL, Kellum JA, Shah SV, et al. Acute Kidney Injury Network: report of an initiative to improve outcomes in acute kidney injury. *Crit Care.* 2007;11:R31.
8. Parikh CR, Devarajan P. New biomarkers of acute kidney injury. *Crit Care Med.* 2008;36:S159-S165.
9. Hewitt SM, Dear J, Star RA. Discovery of protein biomarkers for renal diseases. *J Am Soc Nephrol.* 2004;15:1677-1689.
10. Wheeler DS, Devarajan P, Ma Q, et al. Serum neutrophil gelatinase-associated lipocalin (NGAL) as a marker of acute kidney injury in critically ill children with septic shock. *Crit Care Med.* 2008;36:1297-1303.
11. Herget-Rosenthal S, Marggraf G, Hüsing J, et al. Early detection of acute renal failure by serum cystatin C. *Kidney Int.* 2004;66:1115-1122.
12. Haase-Fielitz A, Bellomo R, Devarajan P, et al. The predictive performance of plasma neutrophil gelatinase-associated lipocalin (NGAL) increases with grade of acute kidney injury. *Nephrol Dial Transplant.* 2009;24:3349-3354.

Timing of renal replacement therapy and clinical outcomes in critically ill patients with severe acute kidney injury

Bagshaw SM, for the Beginning and Ending Supportive Therapy for the Kidney (BEST Kidney) Investigators (Austin and Repatriation Med Centre, Melbourne, Australia; et al)

J Crit Care 24:129-140, 2009

Purpose.—The aim of this study is to evaluate the relationship between timing of renal replacement therapy (RRT) in severe acute kidney injury and clinical outcomes.

Methods.—This was a prospective multicenter observational study conducted at 54 intensive care units (ICUs) in 23 countries enrolling 1238 patients.

Results.—Timing of RRT was stratified into "early" and "late" by median urea and creatinine at the time RRT was started. Timing was also categorized temporally from ICU admission into early (<2 days), delayed (2-5 days), and late (>5 days). Renal replacement therapy timing by serum urea showed no significant difference in crude (63.4% for urea ≤24.2 mmol/L vs 61.4% for urea >24.2 mmol/L; odds ratio [OR], 0.92; 95% confidence interval [CI], 0.73-1.15; $P = .48$) or covariate-adjusted mortality (OR, 1.25; 95% CI, 0.91-1.70; $P = .16$). When stratified by creatinine, late RRT was associated with lower crude (53.4% for creatinine >309 μmol/L vs 71.4% for creatinine ≤309 μmol/L; OR, 0.46; 95% CI, 0.36-0.58; $P < .0001$) and covariate-adjusted mortality (OR, 0.51; 95% CI, 0.37-0.69; $P < .001$). However, for timing relative to ICU admission, late RRT was associated with greater crude (72.8% vs 62.3% vs 59%, $P < .001$) and covariate-adjusted mortality (OR, 1.95; 95% CI, 1.30-2.92; $P = .001$). Overall, late RRT was associated with a longer duration of RRT and stay in hospital and greater dialysis dependence.

Conclusion.—Timing of RRT, a potentially modifiable factor, might exert an important influence on patient survival. However, this largely depended on its definition. Late RRT (days from admission) was associated with a longer duration of RRT, longer hospital stay, and higher dialysis dependence.

▶ Many critically ill patients with acute renal failure (ARF) require renal replacement therapy (RRT). The proportion of patients with ARF who eventually undergo RRT varies considerably from one study to another.[1] There are many reasons for this variability, including the characteristics of the study population and local practice patterns. The latter factor is influenced by availability of resources and by an understanding of the indications for RRT. Most clinicians agree that RRT is indicated for intractable volume overload, refractory acidemia, life-threatening hyperkalemia, or overt uremia. Most clinicians also agree, however, that waiting for those "absolute" indications places the patient at unnecessary risk. What, then, is the optimal timing for initiation of RRT in ARF?

TABLE 6.—Summary of Mortality by Timing of RRT

Timing of RRT	Crude Mortality (%)	OR for Death (95% CI) Crude	Multivariate Adjusted
Timing by median serum urea			
Early (≤24 mmol/L)	63.4	1.0[a]	1.0[a]
Late (>24 mmol/L)	61.4	0.92 (0.73-1.15)	1.25 (0.91-1.70)
Timing by median SCr			
Early (≤309 μmol/L)	71.4	1.0[a]	1.0[a]
Late (>309 μmol/L)	53.4	0.46 (0.36-0.58)	0.51 (0.38-0.69)
Timing by median Δurea			
Early (≤3.1 mmol/L)	62.7	1.0[a]	1.0[a]
Late (>3.1 mmol/L)	62.1	0.97 (0.77-1.23)	0.87 (0.63-1.19)
Timing by median ΔSCr			
Early (≤163 μmol/L)	70.3	1.0[a]	1.0[a]
Late (>163 μmol/L)	55.6	0.53 (0.41-0.69)	0.56 (0.40-0.80)
Timing relative to ICU admission			
Early (<2 d)	58.9	1.0[a]	1.0[a]
Delayed (2-5 d)	62.1	1.14 (0.82-1.60)	1.19 (0.78-1.82)
Late (>5 d)	72.8	1.87 (1.38-2.53)	2.20 (1.44-3.37)

[a]Reference indicator variable.

More than 20 studies have examined "early versus late" initiation of RRT. Unfortunately, very few studies that examined this issue were randomized. Randomized trials account for fewer than 10% of all patients studied. Clouding the issue further are the many different definitions of "early" initiation, some using temporal criteria (days to initiation) and others using biochemical criteria (absolute magnitude or change in concentration of urea and creatinine). A recent meta-analysis suggested a trend toward a survival benefit with earlier initiation of RRT, but the analysis was limited by the poor quality of most of the included studies.[2]

To shed more light on this murky topic, Bagshaw et al performed a large prospective observational trial and compared patient outcomes with "early" versus "late" RRT.[3] They defined "timing" temporally and biochemically. They found that starting RRT at higher serum creatinine was associated with better outcomes, but if RRT was initiated more than 5 days into the ICU stay, there was higher mortality (Table 6).

These results might seem contradictory, but have at least 2 possible explanations: First, the patients whose RRT was initiated after 5 days might have developed ARF late in their stay, a condition previously observed to be associated with poor outcome.[4] Second, the patients with higher serum creatinine at initiation of RRT were more likely to have underlying chronic kidney disease, and thus have a lower threshold for development of ARF and initiation of RRT. As with all observational studies, the results are likely to be confounded by assignment to the various treatment strategies in ways that are not amenable to post hoc adjustment.

This study reemphasizes the problems inherent in studying this crucial topic in critical care nephrology. The issue of "early" versus "late" initiation of RRT will be resolved only by a large randomized, prospective trial. Even in such a trial, care will have to be taken to avoid enrolling patients into the "early" RRT group who would uneventfully recover renal function without RRT. To that end, the development of biomarkers of ARF with strong positive predictive value will be essential.

J. S. Rachoin, MD

L. S. Weisberg, MD

References

1. Hoste EA, Schurgers M. Epidemiology of acute kidney injury: how big is the problem? *Crit Care Med.* 2008;36:S146-S151.
2. Seabra VF, Balk EM, Liangos O, Sosa MA, Cendoroglo M, Jaber BL. Timing of renal replacement therapy initiation in acute renal failure: a meta-analysis. *Am J Kidney Dis.* 2008;52:272-284.
3. Bagshaw SM, Uchino S, Bellomo R, et al. Beginning and Ending Supportive Therapy for the Kidney (BEST Kidney) Investigators. Timing of renal replacement therapy and clinical outcomes in critically ill patients with severe acute kidney injury. *J Crit Care.* 2009;24:129-140.
4. Guerin C, Girard R, Selli JM, Perdrix JP, Ayzac L. Initial versus delayed acute renal failure in the intensive care unit. A multicenter prospective epidemiological study. Rhône-Alpes Area Study Group on Acute Renal Failure. *Am J Respir Crit Care Med.* 2000;161:872-879.

10 Trauma and Overdose

Western Trauma Association (WTA) Critical Decisions in Trauma: Management of Adult Blunt Splenic Trauma
Moore FA, Davis JW, Moore EE Jr, et al (The Weill Cornell Med College, NY; Univ of California, San Francisco; Univ of Colorado Health Science Ctr, Denver; et al)
J Trauma 65:1007-1011, 2008

This is a position article from members of the Western Trauma Association (WTA). Because there are no prospective randomized trials, the algorithm is based on the expert opinion of WTA members and published observational studies. We recognize that variability in decision making will continue. We hope this management algorithm will encourage institutions to develop local protocols based on the resources that are available and local expert consensus opinion to apply the safest, most reliable management strategies for their patients. What works at one institution may not work at another. The algorithm contains letters A through K, which corresponds to lettered text. This text is intentionally concise and its purpose is to navigate the reader through the algorithm and to identify and discuss the gray zones in the logic of this decision making. This annotated algorithm is intended to (a) serve as a quick reference for bedside clinicians, (b) foster more detailed patient care protocols that will allow for prospective collection of data to identify best practices, and (c) generate research projects to answer specific questions concerning decision making in the management of adult blunt splenic trauma.

▶ Most splenic injuries today are managed using nonoperative means. This approach began in pediatric surgical practice and was gradually adapted to the care of adult patients with splenic injury. Nonoperative management is now used in as many as 85% of patients with blunt splenic injury. Failure rates are consistently under 10% and mortality under 5%. The figure provided is a consensus report from the Western Trauma Association. In literature reviewed by these authors, the rate of angiography for splenic injury ranged from 0% to 81% with a failure rate after 2000 of 2% to 9%. Mortality for reported series having this data was 1% to 5%.

Several observations are appropriate for the algorithm presented (Fig 1). Perhaps, the critical observation of these authors is that management of splenic injury should be determined not by anatomic grade of injury but rather on associated hemodynamic instability (Table 2). Patients are moved through the algorithm based on hemodynamic response to injury rather than specific anatomy of

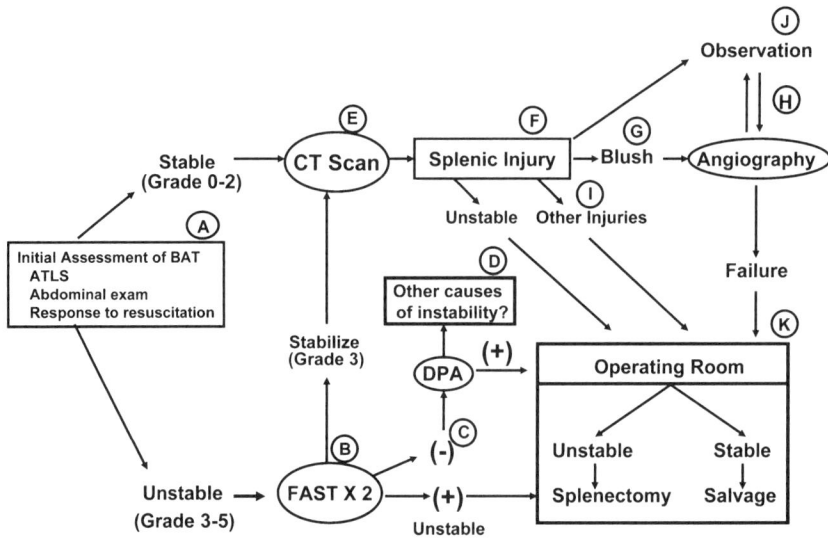

FIGURE 1.—Adult blunt splenic trauma. Editor's Note: Essential steps follow in alphabetical order. The essential observation in this algorithm rests on patient response to crystalloid and colloid resuscitation. The stable patient receives anatomic imaging complemented by angiography and operation, if necessary, while the unstable patient (grades 3-5) is quickly evaluated for intra-abdominal hemorrhage and taken to the operating room. Splenic salvage is inappropriate in the unstable patient. (Courtesy of Moore FA, Davis JW, Moore EE Jr, et al. Western Trauma Association (WTA) critical decisions in trauma: management of adult blunt splenic trauma. *J Trauma.* 2008;65:1007-1011.)

TABLE 2.—Hemodynamic Instability Score[38]

Grade 0: No significant hypotension (systolic blood pressure [SBP] <90 mm Hg) or serious tachycardia (heart rate [HR] >130)
Grade 1: Hypotension or tachycardia by report but none recorded in emergency department (ED)
Grade 2: Hypotension or tachycardia responsive to initial volume loading with no ongoing fluid or PRBC requirement
Grade 3: Hypotension or tachycardia responsive to initial volume loading with modest ongoing fluid (<250 mL/h) or PRBC requirement
Grade 4: Hypotension or tachycardia only responsive to >2 L of volume loading and the need for vigorous ongoing fluid infusion (>250 mL/h) and PRBC transfusion
Grade 5: Hypotension unresponsive to fluid and PRBC transfusion

Editor's Note: Please refer to original journal article for full references.

splenic trauma. I was surprised to see the authors using diagnostic peritoneal aspiration (DPA) or diagnostic peritoneal lavage (DPL). This technique is infrequently used in most trauma centers and many trainees and staff surgeons are sufficiently unfamiliar with DPA or DPL. Another controversy is the response to the "blush" seen on computed tomography. Vascular "blush" is felt consistent with vascular injury but does not necessarily warrant angiographic intervention. The Western Trauma Association recommends angiography for patients with hemodynamic instability and vascular blush on CT imaging. The authors make no comment on the percentage of patients who are candidates for angiography. Noting the varied use of angiography reviewed by these authors, an optimal rate of angiography is not addressed. Despite the variable use of angiography, mortality rate is little affected in centers reporting these data.[1,2]

Finally, blunt splenic injury is associated with a low rate of late hemorrhage, probably due to delayed rupture of splenic artery pseudoaneurysms.[3,4] Management of this problem remains controversial. A high rate of follow-up splenectomy is typically seen. Some authors have recommended delayed CT imaging to identify patients at risk for late hemorrhage. While identifying this controversy, the Western Trauma Association authors do not make a final recommendation.

D. J. Dries, MSE, MD

References

1. Wei B, Hemmila MR, Arbabi S, Taheri PA, Wahl WL. Angioembolization reduces operative intervention for blunt splenic injury. *J Trauma*. 2008;64:1472-1477.
2. Smith HE, Biffl WL, Majercik SD, Jednacz J, Lambiase R, Cioffi WG. Splenic artery embolization: have we gone too far? *J Trauma*. 2006;61:541-546.
3. Gamblin TC, Wall CE Jr, Royer GM, Dalton ML, Ashley DW. Delayed splenic rupture: case reprots and review of the literature. *J Trauma*. 2005;59:1231-1234.
4. Weinberg JA, Magnotti LJ, Croce MA, Edwards NM, Fabian TC. The utility of serial computed tomography imaging of blunt splenic injury: still worth a second look? *J Trauma*. 2007;62:1143-1148.

The presence of the adult respiratory distress syndrome does not worsen mortality or discharge disability in blunt trauma patients with severe traumatic brain injury

Salim A, Martin M, Brown C, et al (Univ of Southern California Keck School of Medicine and the Los Angeles County + Univ of Southern California Med Ctr, Los Angeles)
Injury 39:30-35, 2008

Purpose.—To evaluate the prevalence of the acute respiratory distress syndrome (ARDS) among blunt trauma patients with severe traumatic brain injury (TBI) and to determine if ARDS is associated with higher mortality, morbidity and worse discharge outcome.

Methods.—Blunt trauma patients with TBI (head abbreviated injury score {AIS} $\geq$ 4) who developed predefined ARDS criteria between January 2000 and December 2004 were prospectively collected as part of an ongoing ARDS database. Each patient in the TBI + ARDS group was matched with two control TBI patients based on age, injury severity score (ISS) and head AIS. Outcomes including complications, mortality and discharge disability were compared between the two groups.

Results.—Among 362 TBI patients, 28 (7.7%) developed ARDS. There were no differences between the two groups with respect to age, sex, ISS, Glasgow coma score (GCS), head, abdomen and extremity AIS. The

TBI + ARDS group had significantly more patients with chest AIS ≥ 3 (57.1% versus 32.1%, $p = 0.03$). There was no difference with respect to overall mortality between the TBI + ARDS group (50.0%) and the TBI group (51.8%) (OR 0.79: 95% CI 0.31–2.03, $p = 0.63$). There was no significant difference with respect to discharge functional capacity between the two groups. There were significantly more overall complications in the TBI + ARDS group (42.9%) compared to the TBI group (16.1%) (OR 3.66: 95% CI 1.19–11.24, $p = 0.02$). The TBI + ARDS group had an overall mean intensive care unit (ICU) length of stay of 15.6 days, versus 8.4 days in the TBI group ($p < 0.01$). The TBI + ARDS group had significantly higher hospital charges than the TBI group ($210,097 versus $115,342, $p < 0.01$).

Conclusion.—The presence of ARDS was not associated with higher mortality or worse discharge disability. It was, however, associated with higher hospital morbidity, longer ICU and hospital length of stay.

▶ In a prospective study published in 2003, Holland and coworkers noted worse outcome in patients with isolated head trauma who developed acute lung injury based on international criteria.[1] Remarkably, they found no association between Injury Severity Score, arterial hypotension at admission or the amount of blood transfused, and mortality. The authors explain this contradictory set of results by invoking development of neurogenic pulmonary edema with catecholamine release after injury to the brain and brain stem. They also suggest that acute lung injury may be a secondary response to aggressive maintenance of brain perfusion with fluid administration and vasoactive drugs. The present article argues that mortality is not affected, but acute respiratory distress syndrome (ARDS) in the setting of severe traumatic brain injury does require increased hospital stay and resource consumption. This observation is consistent with other reports in the trauma literature.[2,3]

Several additional observations can be made. ARDS is a classic example of hypoxemic lung injury. While hypotension and hypoxia have historically been proposed as markers of poorer outcome in the setting of brain injury, the evidence implicating hypoxemia as a particular negative factor is relatively weak in recent studies.[4] In fact, hypoxia may not be a powerful determinant of adverse outcome. Hypoxemic respiratory failure is typically managed with small tidal volumes and elevated PEEP. Because ARDS is associated with poor respiratory system compliance, therapy with PEEP should have little effect on cerebral or systemic hemodynamics.[5] Even hypercarbia may be tolerated in selected patients, but intracranial pressure must be monitored. Patients in the present study are matched for age. Advancing age has been identified as a marker for adverse outcome related to ARDS in the setting of injury.[6] Finally, while patients experiencing ARDS in this trial required longer hospital stay and greater resource consumption, the trauma patient population as a whole may have better outcome with prolonged ICU stay than other patient groups.[7]

Perhaps the most important conclusion is that we lack sensitive markers of cerebral resuscitation and oxygen delivery in the setting of injury.[8,9] Until we are better able to assess tissue oxygen transport in the setting of acute organ insults, we will be left with contradictory messages regarding the effect of respiratory failure. Outcome of injury to the head remains the vital consideration in multisystem trauma.[10]

D. J. Dries, MSE, MD

References

1. Holland MC, Mackersie RC, Morabito D, et al. The development of acute lung injury is associated with worse neurologic outcome in patients with severe traumatic brain injury. *J Trauma*. 2003;55:106-111.
2. Salim A, Martin M, Constantinou C, et al. Acute respiratory distress syndrome in the trauma intensive care unit: morbid but not mortal. *Arch Surg*. 2006;141: 655-658.
3. Manley G, Knudson MM, Morabito D, Damson S, Ericson V, Pitts L. Hypotension, hypoxia, and head injury: frequency, duration, and consequences. *Arch Surg*. 2001;136:1118-1123.
4. Jeremitsky E, Omert L, Dunham CM, Protech J, Rodriguez A. Harbingers of poor outcome the day after severe brain injury: hypothermia, hypoxia, and hypoperfusion. *J Trauma*. 2003;54:312-319.
5. Caricato A, Conti G, Della Corte F, et al. Effects of PEEP on the intracranial system of patients with head injury and subarachnoid hemorrhage: the role of respiratory system compliance. *J Trauma*. 2005;58:571-576.
6. Johnston CJ, Rubenfeld GD, Hudson LD. Effect of age on the development of ARDS in trauma patients. *Chest*. 2003;124:653-659.
7. Trottier V, McKenney MG, Beninati M, Manning R, Schulman CI. Survival after prolonged length of stay in a trauma intensive care unit. *J Trauma*. 2007;62: 147-150.
8. Gracias VH, Guillamondegui OD, Stiefel MF, et al. Cerebral cortical oxygenation: a pilot study. *J Trauma*. 2004;56:469-474.
9. Nicholls TP, Shoemaker WC, Wo CC, Gruen JP, Amar A, Dany AB. Survival, hemodynamics, and tissue oxygenation after head trauma. *J Am Col Surg*. 2006;202:120-130.
10. Lefering R, Paffrath T, Linker R, et al. Head injury and outcome – what influence do concomitant injuries have? *J Trauma*. 2008;65:1036-1044.

A high ratio of plasma and platelets to packed red blood cells in the first 6 hours of massive transfusion improves outcomes in a large multicenter study
Zink KA, Sambasivan CN, Holcomb JB, et al (Oregon Health & Science Univ, Portland)
Am J Surg 197:565-570, 2009

Background.—In trauma, most hemorrhagic deaths occur within the first 6 hours. This study examined the effect on survival of high ratios of fresh frozen plasma (FFP) and platelets (PLTs) to packed red blood cells (PRBCs) in the first 6 hours.

Methods.—Records of 466 massive transfusion trauma patients (≥10 U of PRBCs in 24 hours) at 16 level 1 trauma centers were reviewed. Transfusion ratios in the first 6 hours were correlated with outcome.

Results.—All groups had similar baseline characteristics. Higher 6-hour ratios of FFP:PRBCs and PLTs:PRBCs lead to improved 6-hour mortality

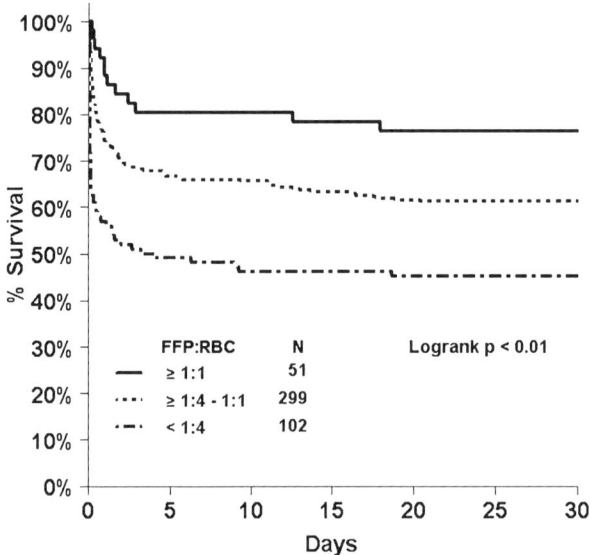

FIGURE 1.—Survival by FFP:red blood cell ratio. (Reprinted from Zink KA, Sambasivan CN, Holcomb JB, et al. A high ratio of plasma and platelets to packed red blood cells in the first 6 hours of massive transfusion improves outcomes in a large multicenter study. *Am J Surg.* 2009;197:565-570, with permission from Elsevier.)

(from 37.3 [in the lowest ratio group] to 15.7 [in the middle ratio group] to 2.0% [in the highest ratio group] and 22.8% to 19.0% to 3.2%, respectively) and in-hospital mortality (from 54.9 to 41.1 to 25.5% and 43.7% to 46.8% to 27.4%, respectively). Initial higher ratios of FFP:PRBCs and PLTs:PRBCs decreased overall PRBC transfusion.

Conclusions.—The early administration of high ratios of FFP and platelets improves survival and decreases overall PRBC need in massively transfused patients. The largest difference in mortality occurs during the first 6 hours after admission, suggesting that the early administration of FFP and platelets is critical.

▶ The authors add civilian data to a growing military experience suggesting that aggressive provision of platelets and fresh frozen plasma (FFP) (in ratios comparable with packed red blood cells) is associated with rapid resolution of life-threatening coagulopathy occurring after trauma and improved outcome (Figs 1 and 2). Coagulopathy has been associated with a combination of soft-tissue injury and ischemia. The combined effect of these insults is a hematologic disorder, which cannot be addressed by simple transfusion of packed red blood cells.

As nicely reviewed by Hess and coworkers, there may be 6 or more mechanisms involved in development of traumatic coagulopathy: tissue trauma, shock, hemodilution, hypothermia, acidemia, and inflammation.[1] Shock may be the main driver of early coagulopathy, but tissue injury with associated

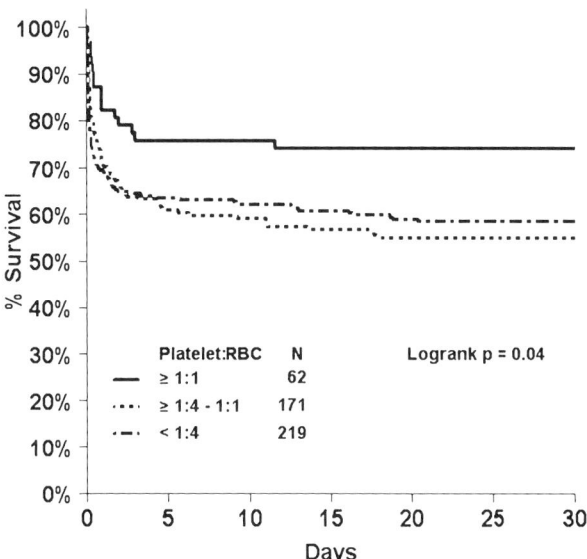

FIGURE 2.—Survival by PLT:red blood cell ratio. (Reprinted from Zink KA, Sambasivan CN, Holcomb JB, et al. A high ratio of plasma and platelets to packed red blood cells in the first 6 hours of massive transfusion improves outcomes in a large multicenter study. *Am J Surg.* 2009;197:565-570, with permission from Elsevier.)

insults to the vascular bed is a trigger. With inadequate blood replacement, hemodilution may exacerbate hemostatic derangement. Hypothermia and acidemia may aggravate an established coagulopathy. Inflammation is also associated with soft-tissue injury and is present in proportion to tissue lost. The mechanisms linking inflammation to coagulopathy after injury are under further investigation.

The authors respond to the obvious limitations in this retrospective work. First is variation in practice between 16 participating trauma centers. Second is a lack of exact timing of component delivery data. There is the potential for clinical practice differences across centers in addition to differing transfusion strategies.

This work brings into clearer focus the means to resolve the apparent contradiction in the surgical literature between transfusion risk and the need for massive transfusion in active hemorrhage.[2,3] It begins to appear that the patient with active bleeding needs early aggressive comprehensive blood product administration. These products must be given rapidly to achieve clotting factor and cell levels sufficient for organ preservation and hemostasis. Blood transfusion in the resuscitated patient or transfusion delayed or spread out over hours and days after injury defeats the goal of factor concentration and increases the risk of transfusion-related complications as described by many authors.[2]

D. J. Dries, MSE, MD

References

1. Hess JR, Brohi K, Dutton RP, et al. The coagulopathy of trauma: a review of mechanisms. *J Trauma*. 2008;65:748-754.
2. Napolitano L. Cumulative risks of early red blood cell transfusion. *J Trauma*. 2006;60:S26-S34.
3. Kauvar DS, Lefering R, Wade CE. Impact of hemorrhage on trauma outcome: an overview of epidemiology, clinical presentations, and therapeutic considerations. *J Trauma*. 2006;60:S3-S11.

A high ratio of plasma and platelets to packed red blood cells in the first 6 hours of massive transfusion improves outcomes in a large multicenter study

Zink KA, Sambasivan CN, Holcomb JB, et al (Oregon Health and Science Univ, Portland)

Am J Surg 197:565-570, 2009

Background.—In trauma, most hemorrhagic deaths occur within the first 6 hours. This study examined the effect on survival of high ratios of fresh frozen plasma (FFP) and platelets (PLTs) to packed red blood cells (PRBCs) in the first 6 hours.

Methods.—Records of 466 massive transfusion trauma patients ($\geq$10 U of PRBCs in 24 hours) at 16 level 1 trauma centers were reviewed. Transfusion ratios in the first 6 hours were correlated with outcome.

Results.—All groups had similar baseline characteristics. Higher 6-hour ratios of FFP:PRBCs and PLTs:PRBCs lead to improved 6-hour mortality (from 37.3 [in the lowest ratio group] to 15.7 [in the middle ratio group] to 2.0% [in the highest ratio group] and 22.8% to 19.0% to 3.2%, respectively) and in-hospital mortality (from 54.9 to 41.1 to 25.5% and 43.7% to 46.8% to 27.4%, respectively). Initial higher ratios of FFP:PRBCs and PLTs:PRBCs decreased overall PRBC transfusion.

Conclusions.—The early administration of high ratios of FFP and platelets improves survival and decreases overall PRBC need in massively transfused patients. The largest difference in mortality occurs during the first 6 hours after admission, suggesting that the early administration of FFP and platelets is critical.

▶ Efforts to limit the use of packed red blood cells have become more widespread in recent years, as the limitations and potential complications of such interventions have become more widely recognized and accepted. Application of such an approach to the trauma patient is particularly problematic due to the obvious issues of acute hemorrhage, which must be confronted on a routine basis in this population. As a result, the development of massive transfusion protocols, emphasizing the early, aggressive administration of platelets, fresh-frozen plasma, and sometimes other clotting factors has become an important area of interest in this population. This large, multicenter retrospective evaluation of data from the trauma registries of 16 level 1 centers demonstrated that early administration of blood components aimed at correcting coagulopathy (platelets and fresh-frozen plasma) was associated with a significant decrease in the need for packed red blood cell transfusion. Such interventions were also associated with improved outcomes as measured by mortality, and, among those in the high platelet, red cell group, ventilator-free days. While it is likely that a significant proportion of the improvement in outcome, particularly the improvement noted in early mortality, can be attributed to decreased bleeding by better hemostasis brought about by more aggressive repletion of platelets and clotting factors, what remains uncertain is how much of the effect on outcome is attributable to decreased exposure to red blood cells or to other potential beneficial effects of platelets or fresh-frozen plasma. As reported by Banbury et al in a study of cardiac surgical patients, platelets and fresh-frozen plasma appeared to have a modest but identifiable impact on reducing the incidence of postoperative infection, which was seen in transfused patients in that study.[1] Whether such a phenomenon is at work in trauma patients remains to be seen. In any event, these data strongly suggest that massive transfusion protocols incorporating early aggressive use of platelets and fresh-frozen plasma in actively bleeding trauma patients result in a decreased need for packed red blood cell transfusion and better overall outcomes.

D. R. Gerber, DO

Reference

1. Banbury MK, Brizzio ME, Rajeswaran J, Lytle BW, Blackstone EH. Transfusion increases the risk of postoperative infection after cardiovascular surgery. *J Am Coll Surg.* 2006;202:131-138.

Effect of whole-body CT during trauma resuscitation on survival: a retrospective, multicentre study
Huber-Wagner S, on behalf of the Working Group on Polytrauma of the German Trauma Society (Ludwig-Maximilians-Univ, Munich, Germany; et al)
Lancet 373:1455-1461, 2009

Background.—The number of trauma centres using whole-body CT for early assessment of primary trauma is increasing. There is no evidence to suggest that use of whole-body CT has any effect on the outcome of patients with major trauma. We therefore compared the probability of survival in patients with blunt trauma who had whole-body CT during resuscitation with those who had not.

Methods.—In a retrospective, multicentre study, we used the data recorded in the trauma registry of the German Trauma Society to calculate the probability of survival according to the trauma and injury severity score (TRISS), revised injury severity classification (RISC) score, and standardised mortality ratio (SMR, ratio of recorded to expected mortality) for 4621 patients with blunt trauma given whole-body or non-whole-body CT.

Findings.—1494 (32%) of 4621 patients were given whole-body CT. Mean age was 42·6 years (SD 20·7), 3364 (73%) were men, and mean injury-severity score was 29·7 (13·0). SMR based on TRISS was 0·745 (95% CI 0·633–0·859) for patients given whole-body CT versus 1·023 (0·909–1·137) for those given non-whole-body CT (p<0·001). SMR based on the RISC score was 0·865 (0·774–0·956) for patients given whole-body CT versus 1·034 (0·959–1·109) for those given non-whole-body CT (p=0·017). The relative reduction in mortality based on TRISS was 25% (14–37) versus 13% (4–23) based on RISC score. Multivariate adjustment for hospital level, year of trauma, and potential centre effects confirmed that whole-body CT is an independent predictor for survival (p≤0·002). The number needed to scan was 17 based on TRISS and 32 based on RISC calculation.

Interpretation.—Integration of whole-body CT into early trauma care significantly increased the probability of survival in patients with polytrauma. Whole-body CT is recommended as a standard diagnostic method during the early resuscitation phase for patients with polytrauma.

▶ This retrospective review uses the massive trauma registry of the German Trauma Society to examine outcomes related to whole-body CT. Because of the massive database and (possibly) gaps in the data system used, whole-body CT is associated with improved outcomes.

The most important immediate observation is that no one was ever cured by a CT scan. CT scan technique use is as effective as the clinical decisions and treatments evolving from the information produced. I suspect that centers with a whole-body CT imaging protocol in the German trauma system also have the most efficient clinical practice. This is suggested by the rapidity with which whole-body CT imaging can be completed. We also can infer that whole-body CT is performed in more sophisticated centers because the severity of injury in referred patients is higher in the whole-body CT population. Trauma systems are designed to refer patients with greatest injury severity to centers providing optimal resources.

The United States is examining the role for aggressive CT imaging in patients sustaining blunt and penetrating trauma. There are many attractive opportunities for this technology even in complex problems, including blunt and penetrating torso injury.[1,2] However, growing concern is being voiced for cancer risk associated with CT imaging. Cancer risk is disproportionately high in the first 3 decades of life.[3,4]

Finally, I believe that whole-body CT is a marker for high-effectiveness centers in the German trauma system. These data suggest that whole-body CT must be considered as a part of the treatment protocol in such centers. Unfortunately, limited demographic data or data on trauma centers are supplied to make clearer statements on the use of CT in light of its associated radiation risks.

D. J. Dries, MSE, MD

References

1. Salim A, Sangthong B, Martin M, Brown C, Plurad D, Demetriades D. Whole body imaging in blunt multisystem trauma patients without obvious signs of injury: results of a prospective study. *Arch Surg.* 2006;141:468-475.
2. Deunk J, Dekker HM, Brink M, van Vugt R, Edwards MJ, van Vugt AB. The value of indicated computed tomography scan of the chest and abdomen in addition to the conventional radiologic work-up for blunt trauma patients. *J Trauma.* 2007; 63:757-763.
3. Tien HC, Tremblay LN, Rizoli SB, et al. Radiation exposure from diagnostic imaging in severely injured trauma patients. *J Trauma.* 2007;62:151-156.
4. Brenner DJ, Hall EJ. Computed tomography-an increasing source of radiation exposure. *N Engl J Med.* 2007;357:2277-2284.

Transfusion, Not Just Injury Severity, Leads to Posttrauma Infection: A Matched Cohort Study

Sadjadi J, Cureton EL, Twomey P, et al (Univ of California San Francisco-East Bay)
Am Surg 75:307-312, 2009

Blood transfusion has been associated with infection; however, the collinearity of injury severity has not been clearly addressed to show a direct relationship. Using more rigorous analysis, we aimed to untangle the effect of injury severity from transfusion leading to sepsis. We hypothesized that blood transfusion independently increases infection in massively transfused *versus* nontransfused patients with matched Injury Severity Scores (ISSs). We performed a matched cohort study measuring infection rates in trauma patients receiving massive transfusion. Control subjects were contemporaneous patients with matched ISS receiving no blood. Infection was defined as intraperitoneal or intrathoracic abscesses, pneumonia, urinary tract infection, or bacteremia. Multivariate logistic and univariate analysis was completed. Infection rate was 61 per cent in 44 transfused patients *versus* 20 per cent in 44 control subjects ($P = 0.001$). Odds of infection were eightfold greater in transfused patients (OR, 7.97; 95% CI, 2.3 to 27.5; $P < 0.001$) independent of ISS, Glasgow Coma Scale, mechanism, and age. Infection was most associated with transfusion of packed red blood cells (PRBCs), although transfusion of other blood products had strong collinearity with PRBCs. Transfused patients had eight times the risk of infection independent of ISS; this appears to be the result of PRBC transfusion. Modifying the ratio of components in transfusion protocols favoring plasma may cause less infection after injury.

▶ This article adds statistical data to support the assertion that transfusion provides incremental risk in the setting of injury. The risk of infection appears to increase in proportion to blood product use and red blood cell use. It is very important to note, however, that the authors have selected a cohort of massively transfused (at least 10 units of packed red blood cells in the first 24 hours) patients to compare with patients who do not receive any

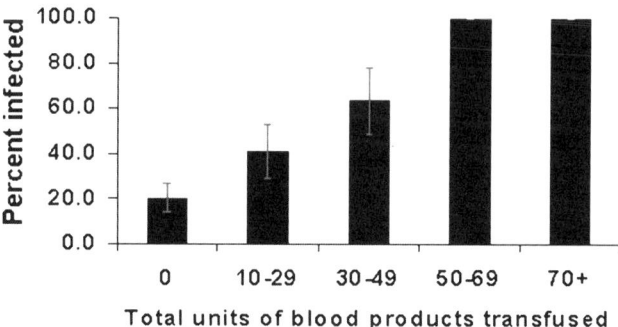

FIGURE 2.—Infection rate *vs* total units transfused. Univariate analysis shows a dose-dependent increase in infection rate with increasing units of total units of blood products transfused ($P < 0.01$, Cochrane-Armitage trend test). Error bars represent se. (Reprinted from Sadjadi J, Cureton EL, Twomey P, et al. Transfusion, not just injury severity, leads to posttrauma infection: a matched cohort study. *Am Surg.* 2009;75:307-312.)

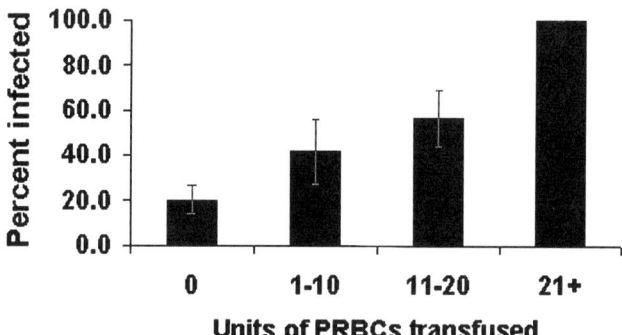

FIGURE 3.—Infection rate *versus* units packed red blood cells transfused. Univariate analysis shows a dose-dependent increase in infection rate with increasing units of packed red blood cells (PRBCs) transfused ($P < 0.01$, Cochrane-Armitage trend test). The multivariate analysis shows that when controlling for other blood products, PRBCs are independent risk factors for infection (see Table 3). Error bars represent SE. (Reprinted from Sadjadi J, Cureton EL, Twomey P, et al. Transfusion, not just injury severity, leads to posttrauma infection: a matched cohort study. *Am Surg.* 2009;75:307-312.)

transfusion. Thus, the outcome differences between the experimental groups should be dramatic.[1]

The figures demonstrate the incremental effect of transfusion of any blood product and aggregate transfusion on the incidence of infection using standard definitions. We are not given significant detail regarding these definitions. The potential lack of detail is always troubling in a retrospective registry trial. I should also note that mortality risk varies with Injury Severity Scores (ISSs) of comparable magnitude. For example, a high ISS that involves the head is associated with poorer outcome than a similar ISS where components of the ISS come from different body regions. Thus, simply stratifying by Glasgow Coma Score, which can be affected by substance use, and ISS may not lead to comparable patient groups.

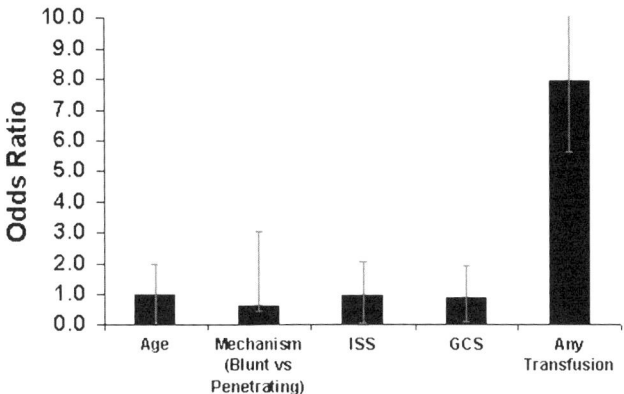

FIGURE 4.—Clinical covariates and infection odds ratios. Multivariate analysis showed that transfusion is an independent risk factor for infection (OR, 7.97; 95% CI, 2.3 to 27.5; $P < 0.001$). Age, mechanism (blunt/penetrating), Injury Severity Score (ISS), and Glasgow Coma Scale (GCS) were not independent risk factors for infection. Error bars represent CIs. (Reprinted from Sadjadi J, Cureton EL, Twomey P, et al. Transfusion, not just injury severity, leads to posttrauma infection: a matched cohort study. *Am Surg.* 2009;75:307-312.)

If one recognizes the clear bias in this study design and the limitations of retrospective data as used here, the message regarding adverse outcomes related to blood product use appears strong. Finally, I should note that we are told little about the blood products. For example, is the blood old or new?[2-4] Newer blood products are less likely to have the storage lesions (cytokine accumulation associated with prolonged storage) seen in fresh units. The strongest association of blood product use to outcome comes with the administration of packed red blood cells. However, details regarding administration of different blood components are not included (Figs 2-4).

D. J. Dries, MSE, MD

References

1. Bernard AC, Davenport DL, Chang PK, Vaughan TB, Zwischenberger JB. Intraoperative transfusion of 1 U to 2 U packed red blood cells is associated with increased 30-day mortality, surgical-site infection, pneumonia, and sepsis in general surgery patients. *J Am Coll Surg.* 2009;208:931-939.
2. Rael LT, Bar-Or R, Ambruso DR, et al. The effect of storage on the accumulation of oxidative biomarkers in donated packed red blood cells. *J Trauma.* 2009;66: 76-81.
3. Kiraly LN, Underwood S, Differding JA, Schreiber MA. Transfusion of aged packed red blood cells results in decreased tissue oxygenation in critically injured trauma patients. *J Trauma.* 2009;67:29-32.
4. Marik PE, Corwin HL. Acute lung injury following blood transfusion: expanding the definition. *Crit Care Med.* 2008;36:3080-3084.

Transfusion, Not Just Injury Severity, Leads to Posttrauma Infection: A Matched Cohort Study

Sadjadi J, Cureton EL, Twomey P, et al (Univ of California San Francisco–East Bay, Oakland)
Am Surg 75:307-312, 2009

Blood transfusion has been associated with infection; however, the collinearity of injury severity has not been clearly addressed to show a direct relationship. Using more rigorous analysis, we aimed to untangle the effect of injury severity from transfusion leading to sepsis. We hypothesized that blood transfusion independently increases infection in massively transfused *versus* nontransfused patients with matched Injury Severity Scores (ISSs). We performed a matched cohort study measuring infection rates in trauma patients receiving massive transfusion. Control subjects were contemporaneous patients with matched ISS receiving no blood. Infection was defined as intraperitoneal or intrathoracic abscesses, pneumonia, urinary tract infection, or bacteremia. Multivariate logistic and univariate analysis was completed. Infection rate was 61 per cent in 44 transfused patients *versus* 20 per cent in 44 control subjects ($P = 0.001$). Odds of infection were eightfold greater in transfused patients (OR, 7.97; 95% CI, 2.3 to 27.5; $P < 0.001$) independent of ISS, Glasgow Coma Scale, mechanism, and age. Infection was most associated with transfusion of packed red blood cells (PRBCs), although transfusion of other blood products had strong collinearity with PRBCs. Transfused patients had eight times the risk of infection independent of ISS; this appears to be the result of PRBC transfusion. Modifying the ratio of components in transfusion protocols favoring plasma may cause less infection after injury.

▶ This is yet another study indicating a strong relationship betwen packed red blood cell (PRBC) transfusion and the subsequent development of infection. In this study, the investigators compared the rates of infection in massively transfused (>10 units) versus nontransfused trauma patients, and found significantly greater rates of pneumonias, abscesses, and line infections in the transfused group. Infection seemed to be more or less linearly related to the number of units of blood transfused, and seemed to be associated only with PRBC, but not with other blood products. Because of this fact the authors suggest that in trauma (perhaps in other bleeding situations as well?) higher fresh-frozen plasma (FFP) to PRBC ratios may be appropriate. This may result in diminished bleeding and in a need for a smaller volume of PRBC transfusion with fewer attendant complication, including infection and potentially transfusion reactions. As the authors point out, the precise ratio of blood products, particularly for massive transfusion protocols, remains to be determined. However, given the shortcomings associated with transfused PRBCs, any strategies that could safely reduce their use in bleeding patients would be welcome.

D. R. Gerber, DO

Western Trauma Association Critical Decisions in Trauma: Management of Pelvic Fracture With Hemodynamic Instability

Davis JW, Moore FA, McIntyre RC Jr, et al (UCSF/Fresno, CA; Methodist Hosp, Houston, TX; Univ of Colorado, Health Sciences Ctr, Denver; et al)
J Trauma 65:1012-1015, 2008

The management of patients with hemodynamic instability from pelvic fracture is challenging and controversial. Mortality rates have ranged from 18% to 40% in reported series and death within the first 24 hours of injury was most often a result of acute blood loss. Significant decreases in mortality rates have been shown with adoption of algorithms for management of these injuries.

The key issues in management are identifying the site(s) of hemorrhage and then controlling the bleeding. Bleeding from pelvic fractures occurs from three major sources; arterial, venous, and cancellous bone. A seminal study from 1973 identified extravasation of contrast from the hypogastric arteries in 23 of 27 autopsy cases. Bleeding sources were bilateral in 63%,

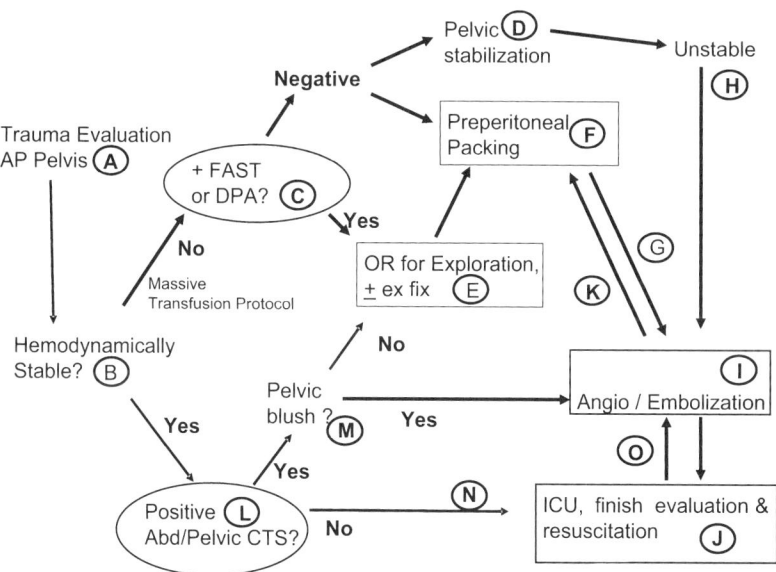

FIGURE 1.—Algorithm for management of pelvic fracture. Editor's Note: The essential aspects of this Western Trauma Association algorithm are identifying the hemodynamically unstable patient who requires blood products and rapid evaluation of the peritoneal cavity for bleeding associated with abdominal injuries. In 2009, this is best done with ultrasound. The unstable patient goes on to stabilization typically done with angiography. Authors in the Western Trauma Association have also recommended packing of the preperitoneal space to control bleeding. The stable patient (L) is evaluated in CT scan where a "blush" consistent with ongoing bleeding is sought. Angiography and embolization are used to control bleeding in this case. In some situations, internal iliac embolization is required with attendant risks of perineal ischemia. Ultimately, the patient completes resuscitation in the intensive care unit. (Courtesy of Davis JW, Moore FA, McIntyre RC Jr, et al. Western trauma association critical decisions in trauma: management of pelvic fracture with hemodynamic instability. *J Trauma.* 2008;65:1012-1015.)

and 61% had more than one bleeding site identified. Careful dissection revealed lesions to main arteries in only three specimens, and the authors noted that bleeding from cancellous bone and from vessels in adjacent soft tissue hampered identification of arterial injuries. They also stressed the significance of hemorrhage from the fracture sites. A more recent study reported that over 70% of unstable patients with pelvic fractures will have arterial bleeding.

Furthermore, blunt force injury severe enough to fracture the pelvic ring can cause concomitant intra-abdominal injuries. The frequency of abdominal injury, in association with pelvic fracture can range from 16% to 55%. Appropriate evaluation of the abdomen for associated intra-abdominal injuries cannot be overstressed.

Management of hemodynamically unstable patients with pelvic fracture requires a multidisciplinary team. In addition to the general trauma surgeon, an experienced orthopedic surgeon and a skilled interventional radiologist are needed for optimal care (Fig 1).

▶ A small fraction of patients sustaining massive pelvic trauma go on to die from uncontrolled bleeding or complications related to massive transfusion. Timely evaluation and aggressive resuscitation are the keys to optimal outcome. This document presents a consensus statement from the Western Trauma Association. Several facts are worth review. Abdominal injury in addition to pelvic fracture is seen in 16% to 55% of patients. Thus, abdominal evaluation must be included in assessment of the injured pelvis.

There are several keys to management of patients with massive hemorrhage in association with complex pelvic fractures. First is the early use of an effective massive transfusion protocol. This intervention must provide clotting factors and red blood cells in appropriate proportions. If executed correctly, overall blood usage will be reduced.[1-3] Second, bedside evaluation includes diagnostic peritoneal aspiration (DPA) or diagnostic peritoneal lavage (DPL) with Focused Abdominal Sonography for Trauma (FAST) examination. DPA or DPL are rarely used today in the setting of trauma and while they have theoretical attractiveness in the management of pelvic fracture, the practitioner unfamiliar with these techniques is best left to use ultrasound.[4,5]

Two other modalities, which see complimentary use, are preperitoneal packing and angiography. Preperitoneal packing has been introduced in the United States by authors from the Western Trauma Association. Frequently, even in the setting of preperitoneal packing, retroperitoneal bleeding associated with pelvic fractures is not controlled and angiography is still required. I consider the recommendation for preperitoneal packing to be beyond routine practice of most trauma centers.[6] Angiography remains the "gold standard" for diagnosis and intervention with pelvic trauma.[7] In the stable patient, angiography can be focused if prestudy computed tomography discloses hematoma with an associated blush of vascular injury.

The role of reduction in pelvic volume by orthopedic intervention such as external fixation is dependent on availability of practitioners for these techniques at the trauma center. These authors appropriately mention the simple bed sheet wrap as a means to reduce pelvic volume. This intervention may have greater short-term relevance than more elaborate but time-consuming ortho-pedic techniques.

D. J. Dries, MSE, MD

References

1. Sperry JL, Ochoa JB, Gunn SR, et al. An FFP: PRBC transfusion ratio >/= 1:1.5 is associated with a lower risk of mortality after massive transfusion. *J Trauma.* 2008;65:986-993.
2. Borgman MA, Spinella PC, Perkins JG, et al. The ratio of blood products trans-fused affects mortality in patients receiving massive transfusions at a combat support hospital. *J Taruma.* 2007;63:805-813.
3. O'Keeffe T, Refaai M, Tchorz K, Forestner JE, Sarode R. A massive transfusion protocol to decrease blood component use and costs. *Arch Surg.* 2008;143:686-691.
4. Breitkreutz R, Walcher F, Seeger FH. Focused echocardiographic evaluation in resuscitation management: concept of an advanced life support-conformed algo-rithm. *Crit Care Med.* 2007;35:S150-S161.
5. Mendez C, Gubler KD, Maier RV. Diagnostic accuracy of peritoneal lavage in patients with pelvic fractures. *Arch Surg.* 1994;129:477-482.
6. Cothren CC, Osborn PM, Moore EE, Morgan SJ, Johnson JL, Smith WR. Preper-itoneal pelvic packing for hemodynamically unstable pelvic fractures: a paradigm shift. *J Trauma.* 2007;62:834-839.
7. Routt ML, Falicov A Jr, Woodhouse E, Schildhauer TA. Circumferential pelvic antishock sheeting: a temporary resuscitation aid. *J Orthop Trauma.* 2002;16:45-48.

Impact of the 80-Hour Work Week on Mortality and Morbidity in Trauma Patients: An Analysis of the National Trauma Data Bank
Morrison CA, Wyatt MM, Carrick MM (Baylor College of Medicine, Houston, TX)
J Surg Res 154:157-162, 2009

Introduction.—The implementation of the 80-h work week restrictions implemented by the Accreditation Council for Graduate Medical Educa-tion (ACGME) in July 2003 were intended, in part, to improve patient outcomes by reducing fatigue-related resident errors. Although concerns were raised regarding the possibility for increased error due to decreased continuity of patient care, recent studies have shown no significant change in mortality or complication rates since the onset of these new restrictions. This study is the first to examine the effects of the 80-h work week on mortality in trauma patients on a national level.

Methods.—Data were obtained from the National Trauma Data Bank (NTDB) version 6.2 from 1994 to 2005. Data were then divided into two groups: "pre-80-h work week" (2001–2002) and "post-80-h work week" (2004–2005). Because the ACGME's guidelines were implemented mid-year in 2003, and because the NTDB classifies admission date only by year, all patients admitted during 2003 were excluded from the analysis. Information regarding patient demographics and hospital type (teaching

298 / Critical Care Medicine

TABLE 2.—Overall Clinical Outcomes Before and After Implementation of the 80-h Work Week

	Pre-80-h work week (2001–2002)	Post-80-h work week (2004–2005)	P value
Mortality rate	4.64%	4.46%	<.0001
LOS days	6	5.8	0.0003
ICU days	6.2	6.1	0.014
Vent days	7.6	7.5	0.047

versus nonteaching) was collected. Our primary outcome measure was mortality. Secondary outcomes included length of mechanical ventilation, length of ICU stay, and length of hospitalization.

Results.—The overall mortality rate decreased from 4.64% in the pre-80-h work week to 4.46% in the post-80-h work week (P < 0.0001). Of particular interest were the differences in outcomes observed in academic *versus* nonacademic institutions. In university hospitals, the mortality decreased from 5.16% to 5.03% (P = 0.03), whereas in nonteaching hospitals, mortality increased from 3.37% to 3.85% (P < 0.001). There were also small but statistically significant improvements seen in secondary outcomes during the post-80-h work week.

Discussion.—Despite the great deal of controversy surrounding the 80-h work week, few papers exist that specifically examine patient mortality within the field of trauma surgery. This large retrospective analysis demonstrates slightly decreased mortality and morbidity among trauma patients in university hospitals nationwide after implementation of the 80-h work week, even when controlling for possible confounders. Although these differences are not likely to be clinically important, the data are statistically very significant. Therefore, we conclude that the 80-h work week has not resulted in any significant deterioration in patient outcomes in this particular population (Table 2).

▶ I am relieved to see that introduction of the 80-hour work week has not affected outcome as measured in this large dataset obtained from the massive National Trauma Data Bank. A more interesting question is the impact of the 80-hour work week on early career performance in surgeons finished with reduced hours of acute surgery experience. Academic centers, which had slightly improved outcomes, typically have in-house faculty members. Thus, reduced impact of participating residents is buffered by staff surgeons and mid-level providers. What will happen when residents trained under a reduced work hour week are the staff surgeons?[1,2]

The dataset provided has all the limitations of a large retrospective review. Further, as the authors admit, the statistical observations are probably not clinically relevant. Outcomes specific to patients of particular types are not reported.

We wait to see the career choices, clinical work, and academic output of this new generation of surgeons. My hope is that the 80-hour work week will make us all respectful of personal needs, more efficient, and safer in the inevitable process of "hand-offs" that are part of trauma care and acute surgery.

D. J. Dries, MSE, MD

References

1. Ferguson CM, Kellogg KC, Hutter MM, Warshaw AL. Effect of work-hour reforms on operative case volume of surgical residents. *Curr Surg.* 2005;62: 535-538.
2. Mendoza KA, Britt LD. Resident operative experience during the transition to work-hour reform. *Arch Surg.* 2005;140:137-145.

Cirrhosis and Trauma Are a Lethal Combination

Georgiou C, Inaba K, Teixeira PGR, et al (Univ of Southern California, Los Angeles; et al)
World J Surg 33:1087-1092, 2009

Background.—The objective of this study was to evaluate the risk of mortality and complications associated with cirrhosis in trauma patients.

Methods.—This is an IRB-approved retrospective trauma registry study of patients admitted to an academic level 1 trauma center from 1997 to 2006. The following parameters were abstracted for analysis: age, gender, mechanism of injury, Abbreviated Injury Score, Injury Severity Score, Glasgow Coma Scale, mortality, and complications (ARDS, acute renal failure, pneumonia, intra-abdominal abscess, trauma-associated coagulopathy). Multivariable analysis was utilized to compare the mortality and complication rates between cirrhotic and noncirrhotic trauma patients. The subgroup of patients who underwent laparotomy was also analyzed.

Results.—During the 10-year study period there were 36,038 trauma registry patients, of which 468 (1.3%) had a diagnosis of cirrhosis. The mortality in the cirrhotic group was 12% vs. 6% in the noncirrhotic group [adjusted odds ratio = 5.65 (95% CI = 3.72 – 8.41, $p < 0.0001$)]. ARDS, trauma-associated coagulopathy, and septic complications were significantly more common in the cirrhotic group. The overall severe complication rate in the two groups was 10 and 4%, respectively [adjusted odds ratio = 2.05 (95% CI = 1.45 – 2.84, $p < 0.0001$)]. For the subgroup of patients who underwent emergent abdominal exploration, the mortality rate increased to 40% compared with that of noncirrhotics at 15% [adjusted odds ratio = 4.35 (95% CI = 2.00 – 9.18, $p = 0.0002$)].

Conclusion.—Cirrhosis is an independent risk factor for increased mortality and higher complication rate following trauma. Injured patients who undergo laparotomy are significantly more likely to die than noncirrhotic patients. Injured patients with cirrhosis warrant aggressive monitoring and treatment.

▶ This is one of series of articles identifying factors contributing to excess morbidity and mortality in a large group of trauma patients managed at a major Southern California trauma center over an extended period of time. This collection of nearly 500 cirrhotic patients is larger than any previously reported. We are given convincing evidence that cirrhosis is a marker for poor outcome.[1]

Unfortunately, despite a consistent incidence of cirrhosis and laparotomy in patients with cirrhosis over the study interval in this retrospective trial, factors associated with poor outcome are not well identified. These authors have described evolution in mechanical ventilation, blood transfusion, and crystalloid resuscitation strategies over the time interval discussed in this article.[2] Thus, patients with cirrhosis should have seen an evolving approach to pulmonary support, blood product administration, and quantities of clear fluids provided. Did these factors have any impact on the outcome of cirrhotic patients? We are not provided a temporal course of outcome in these patients.

Because the authors have data available, I hope that we will see a report indicating the impact of conservative transfusion, lung protective mechanical ventilation, and reduced crystalloid administration on the morbidity and mortality associated with trauma in cirrhotic patients. Another clear shortcoming of this trial is inability to stratify cirrhotic patients based on severity of underlying disease. A consistent laboratory approach for assessment is not available. Use of scoring systems such as the Childs-Pugh classification was not possible in this retrospective review.

Therefore, we can be reassured that cirrhosis is a marker for poor outcome. Whether contemporary resuscitation and critical care management strategies have affected the dismal results associated with cirrhosis remains unclear.

D. J. Dries, MSE, MD

References

1. Christmas AB, Wilson AK, Franklin GA, Miller FB, Richardson JD, Rodriguez JL. Cirrhosis and trauma: a deadly duo. *Am Surg.* 2005;71:996-1000.
2. Plurad D, Martin M, Green D, et al. The decreasing incidence of late posttraumatic acute respiratory distress syndrome: the potential role of lung protective ventilation and conservative transfusion practice. *J Trauma.* 2007;63:1-8.

The OPTICC trial: a multi-institutional study of occult pneumothoraces in critical care
Ouellet JF, Trottier V, Kmet L, et al (Centre Hospitalier Affilie Universitaire De Quebec, Canada; Grady Memorial Hosp, Atlanta, GA; et al)
Am J Surg 197:581-586, 2009

Background.—The management of pneumothoraces detected on CT but not on supine chest radiographs remains controversial, especially in those undergoing positive pressure ventilation (PPV) who are at risk for complications with both observation and treatment. Previous limited study yielded confusion regarding the need for routine drainage of these occult pneumothoraces (OPTXs). We conducted a pilot study at 2 trauma centers to address the feasibility and safety of randomizing traumatized patients undergoing PPV to drainage or observation.

Methods.—Stable mechanically ventilated (or en route to surgery) adults with OPTXs were identified at 2 centers (Calgary and Quebec). Patients were randomized to observation (unless drainage became clinically indicated) or to chest drainage. Episodes of respiratory distress (need for thoracostomy tube, acute/sustained increase in oxygen requirements, difficulty in achieving adequate ventilation and self-reported distress) and subsequent imaging abnormalities were recorded until discharge.

Results.—From August 2006 to April 2008, 24 trauma patients were enrolled (17 Calgary and 7 Quebec), with 2 later exclusions (final CT found no OPTX). Thirteen patients (59%) were randomized to observation, 9 to drainage (41%). Four observed (31%) later had chest tubes placed nonurgently for worsening OPTXs/effusions; none with increased morbidity. Overall rates of respiratory distress (drainage: 33%, observation: 41%) and mortality (drainage: 22%, observation: 15%) were similar across groups, as were median intensive care unit (drainage: 3, observation: 4) and in-hospital days (drainage: 10, observation: 16).

Conclusions.—With no important differences in morbidity, the OPTICC pilot lays the foundation for a future definitive trial comparing drainage or observation in posttraumatic OPTXs requiring PPV.

▶ The 2 widely cited articles from the American trauma literature discussing the management of occult pneumothorax present divergent views.[1,2] Brasel and coworkers from my institution argue that occult pneumothorax can be safely observed.[2] I have found this clinical impression to be true in my practice and this is the approach at our trauma center. I am not aware of any adverse consequences of observation for occult pneumothoraces. Enderson and colleagues, however, raise the appropriate concern that progression to tension pneumothorax may occur and is associated with a risk of sudden decompensation.[1] If it were not for the morbidity of tube thoracostomy, it would be easy to advocate placement of chest drains whenever a pneumothorax is identified.

Several valuable pieces of data are missing in this preliminary report. First, I note that the authors report that occult pneumothorax is a common phenomenon. I agree. Why did it take 2 years for 2 trauma centers to enroll approximately 20 patients? How many patients declined participation? How many patients were candidates for this study? Is it possible that this patient population is a selected group and the less aggressive approach to occult pneumothorax was safe due to the patient selection process?

With caution, recognizing limitations of present literature, I believe that occult pneumothorax can be safely observed even in patients receiving positive pressure ventilation. Where pulmonary reserve is limited and patients are hemodynamically unstable or where monitoring is difficult (lengthy operating room procedures), tube thoracostomy is clearly appropriate.

D. J. Dries, MSE, MD

References

1. Enderson BL, Abdalla R, Frame SB, Casey MT, Gould H, Maull KI. Tube thoracostomy for occult pneumothorax: a prospective randomized study of its use. *J Trauma.* 1993;35:726-730.
2. Brasel KJ, Stafford RE, Weigelt JA, Tenquist JE, Borgstrom DC. Treatment of occult pneumothoraces from blunt trauma. *J Trauma.* 1999;46:987-991.

Severity of injury does not have any impact on posttraumatic stress symptoms in severely injured patients
Quale AJ, Schanke A-K, Frøslie KF, et al (Sunnaas Rehabilitation Hosp, Nesoddtangen, Norway; Rikshospitalet-Radiumhospitalet Med Ctr, Oslo, Norway; et al)
Injury 40:498-505, 2009

Background.—Due to improved surgical techniques and more efficient decision making in treating severely injured patients, survival rates have increased over the years. This study was initiated to evaluate the incidence and identify risk factors for developing posttraumatic stress symptoms, using both extensive trauma-related data and data assessing the psychological trauma, in a population of severely injured patients.

Patients and Methods.—79 patients admitted to the Department of Multitrauma and Spinal Cord Injury at Sunnaas Rehabilitation Hospital from 2003 to 2005, prospectively completed semistructured psychological interviews and questionnaires, such as Impact of Event Scale-Revised. In addition, extensive injury-related data, such as injury severity score (ISS), new injury severity score (NISS), and probability of survival (PS) were collected.

Results.—39% had multiple trauma, 34% had multiple injuries including spinal cord injuries, and 27% had isolated spinal cord injuries. Mean NISS was 31.5 (S.D. 13.7). 6% met diagnostic criteria for posttraumatic stress disorder (PTSD) and 9% met the criteria for subsyndromal PTSD. Injury-related data did not influence the prevalence of posttraumatic stress symptoms, however, some psychosocial variables did have a significant impact.

Conclusions.—We found a low incidence of PTSD and subsyndromal PTSD. No significant differences were found between the patients suffering from posttraumatic stress symptoms and the non-symptoms group in relation to injury-related data such as ISS/NISS, PS, or multiple trauma versus spinal cord injury. The most evident risk factors for developing posttraumatic stress symptoms were symptoms of anxiety, female gender and negative attitudes toward emotional expression.

▶ This work combines retrospective trauma center experience with prospective detailed psychological testing for posttraumatic stress syndromes (PTSS) and formal posttraumatic stress disorder (PTSD). Perhaps the greatest limitation of this study is the small sample set, which limits implications that can be drawn. Nonetheless, the discrepancy identified between physiological and psychological outcomes of trauma is important.[1]

The authors identify a small number of psychological predictors, which they relate to PTSS and PTSD. One predictor that is poorly explained is female gender. As females represent 25% of this study population, they are a minority in a subject group typically involved in high-risk behavior. Other factors identified in this analysis are consistent with other work from Scandinavia suggesting that emotional and psychological factors present before injury had a greater impact on this form of outcome than mechanical forces involved.

Several paragraphs are spent discussing the low overall rates of PTSD and PTSS in this Norwegian study population. I note that there were several sets of patients excluded, which may contribute to the low incidence of PTSD and PTSS reported. Another factor is outstanding support for patients coming from a small socially sophisticated and relatively homogeneous society. Work from larger heterogeneous populations in the United States and United Kingdom show similar patterns of outcome at a higher absolute rate of PTSD.[1-3]

D. J. Dries, MSE, MD

References

1. Michaels AJ, Michaels CE, Moon CH, et al. Posttraumatic stress disorder after injury: impact on general health outcome and early risk assessment. *J Trauma.* 1999;47:460-467.
2. Chang D, Cornwell EE 3rd, Phillips J, Baker D, Yonas M, Campbell K. Community characteristics and demographic information as determinants for a hospital-based injury prevention outreach program. *Arch Surg.* 2003;138:1344-1346.
3. Holtslag HR, van Beeck EF, Lindeman E, Leenen LP. Determinants of long-term functional consequences after major trauma. *J Trauma.* 2007;62:919-927.

Battlefield extremity injuries in Operation Iraqi Freedom
Dougherty AL, Mohrle CR, Galarneau MR, et al (Science Applications International Corporation, San Diego, CA; Naval Health Res Ctr, San Diego, CA)
Injury 40:772-777, 2009

Objective.—Extremity injuries account for the majority of wounds incurred during US armed conflicts. Information regarding the severity and short-term outcomes of patients with extremity wounds, however, is limited. The aim of the present study was to describe patients with battlefield extremity injuries in Operation Iraqi Freedom (OIF) and to compare characteristics of extremity injury patients with other combat wounded.

Patients and Methods.—Data were obtained from the United States Navy-Marine Corps Combat Trauma Registry (CTR) for patients who received treatment for combat wounds at Navy-Marine Corps facilities in Iraq between September 2004 and February 2005. Battlefield extremity injuries were classified according to type, location, and severity; patient demographic, injury-specific, and short-term outcome data were analysed. Upper and lower extremity injuries were also compared.

Results.—A total of 935 combat wounded patients were identified; 665 (71%) sustained extremity injury. Overall, multiple wounding was common (an average of 3 wounds per patient), though more prevalent amongst patients with extremity injury than those with other injury (75% vs. 56%, $P < .001$). Amongst the 665 extremity injury patients, 261 (39%) sustained injury to the upper extremities, 223 (34%) to the lower extremities, and 181 (27%) to both the upper and lower extremities. Though the total number of *patients* with upper extremity injury was higher than lower extremity injury, the total number of extremity *wounds* ($n = 1654$) was evenly distributed amongst the upper and lower extremities (827 and 827 wounds, respectively). Further, lower extremity injuries were more likely than the upper extremity injuries to be coded as serious to fatal (AIS > 2, $P < .001$).

Conclusions.—Extremity injuries continue to account for the majority of combat wounds. Compared with other conflicts, OIF has seen increased prevalence of patients with upper extremity injuries. Wounds to the lower extremities, however, are more serious. Further research on the risks and outcomes associated with extremity injury is necessary to enhance the planning and delivery of combat casualty medical care.

▶ These epidemiologic data are important from the standpoint that priorities for care of the military in specific situations, ie, combat and convoy work, can be clarified. However, there are significant limitations in the sources of data used, which are not emphasized in the title or the abstract. These authors focus on injury involving the Marines and casualties treated in Navy and Marine medical facilities. Army injuries and care provided in frontline Army facilities are not reflected in this data.

Extremity injury can have lifelong limitations for the rehabilitation and ultimate reintegration of involved soldiers into society. Because of the importance of extremity injury in rehabilitation of combatants, these data warrant careful examination. However, for reasons stated, the data cannot stand alone as indicative of the pattern of injuries seen throughout the Middle East Theater without collection of comparable data from units in other services serving in Operation Iraqi Freedom.

We need a balanced delivery of data to optimize planning and delivery of combat casualty care and to better identify protective strategies.[1,2]

D. J. Dries, MSE, MD

References

1. Champion HR, Holcomb JB, Young LA. Injuries from explosives: physics, biophysics, pathology, and required research focus. *J Trauma*. 2009;66: 1468-1477.
2. Brown KV, Ramasamy A, McLeod J, Stapley S, Clasper JC. Predicting the need for early amputation in ballistic mangled extremity injuries. *J Trauma*. 2009;66: S93-S98.

The impact of uncross-matched blood transfusion on the need for massive transfusion and mortality: analysis of 5,166 uncross-matched units
Inaba K, Teixeira PG, Shulman I, et al (Univ of Southern California, Los Angeles)
J Trauma 65:1222-1226, 2008

Background.—The objective of this study was to analyze the outcomes associated with uncross-matched blood transfusion during trauma resuscitation. Our hypothesis was that uncross-matched blood transfusion is a predictor of the need for massive transfusion and mortality.

Methods.—All injured patients receiving packed red blood cell (PRBC) transfusion during a 6-year period ending December 2005 were identified from the blood bank database at a level I trauma center. Uncross-matched red blood cell (URBC) and cross-matched red blood cells, plasma and platelet utilization, and injury demographics were abstracted for each patient.

Results.—Of 25,599 trauma patients, 4,241 (16.6%) patients received 29,375 units of PRBC and 1,236 (29.1%) of the transfused patients received 5,166 units of URBC during their resuscitation. Patients requiring URBC had a higher mortality (39.6% vs. 11.9%, $p < 0.001$) and were more likely to require massive (> or $= 10$ PRBC during 12 hours) transfusion (29.3% vs. 1.8%, $p < 0.001$). There was a stepwise increase in mortality with increasing URBC transfusion. After adjusting for age, gender, mechanism, hypotension at admission, emergency department intubation, initial hemoglobin, Glasgow Coma Scale, Abbreviated Injury Scale, Injury Severity Score, and amount of blood products received; URBC remained an independent predictor of mortality (adjusted odds ratio 2.15; 95% confidence interval 1.58-2.94; $p < 0.001$) and massive transfusion (adjusted odds ratio, 11.87; 95% confidence interval, 8.43-16.7; $p < 0.001$). Patients receiving URBC also utilized more blood components (11.9 +/- 12.7 vs. 4.9 +/- 5.8 units of PRBC, $p < 0.001$; 5.1 +/- 8.9 vs. 2.0 +/- 4.8 units of plasma, $p < 0.001$; and 1.1 +/- 2.5 vs. 0.4 +/- 1.6 units of platelets, $p < 0.001$).

Conclusion.—The requirement for uncross-matched blood during the acute resuscitation of trauma patients is an independent predictor of mortality and the need for massive transfusion. A URBC request during resuscitation should be considered by the blood bank as a potential trigger to prepare for massive transfusion.

▶ These data come from the extensive trauma experience at the Los Angeles County Medical Center. Use of uncross-matched blood is a predictor of massive transfusion and is associated with incremental increase in mortality based on the number of uncross-matched products used. While a number of statistical tests are performed and multivariate analysis suggests that the use of uncross-matched blood is an independent predictor of poorer outcome, one can read between the lines and see that patients receiving the uncross-matched products were a more severely injured group.

It would be interesting to examine patients receiving a comparable amount of cross-matched blood to patients receiving uncross-matched products. To undertake this comparison, a larger data set than this retrospective analysis may be required. While the patient group receiving uncross-matched blood transfusion had poorer outcome, there were no data provided to suggest that the incidence of complications specific to transfusion such as Transfusion-Related Acute Lung Injury (TRALI) or transfusion reaction leading to other organ injury such as renal failure were specifically increased.[1]

We are left with the important observation that the clinical decision to use uncross-matched blood should carry the realization that the patient faces a significant increase in risk for bad outcome.[1]

D. J. Dries, MSE, MD

Reference

1. Marik PE, Corwin HL. Acute lung injury following blood transfusion: expanding the definition. *Crit Care Med*. 2008;36:3080-3084.

The evaluation of pneumomediastinum in blunt trauma patients
Dissanaike S, Shalhub S, Jurkovich GJ (Univ of Washington, Seattle)
J Trauma 65:1340-1345, 2008

Background.—Pneumomediastinum occurs in up to 10% of patients with blunt thoracic and cervical trauma. Mandatory evaluation of all patients with bronchoscopy and esophageal imaging to exclude a major injury has been recommended. There is little data on the safety or efficacy of this approach. We evaluated the incidence of major injuries associated with pneumomediastinum, the accuracy of diagnostic modalities, and the results of observation versus aggressive evaluation.

Methods.—Medical records of all blunt trauma patients diagnosed with pneumomediastinum and/or aerodigestive tract injury between 1998 and 2005 were reviewed. The patient's hospital course was reviewed for demographic data, admission diagnoses, diagnostic imaging and procedures, operations, missed injuries, length of stay, and mortality.

Results.—The review identified a total of 136 patients with pneumomediastinum, and an additional 22 patients with thoracic aerodigestive tract injuries but without pneumomediastinum. Only patients with pneumomediastinum were considered in subsequent analysis. Pneumomediastinum was detected by CT scan in all 136 (100%) patients, although identified on plain radiograph in only 20 (15%) patients. Computed tomography findings were suspicious for a major aerodigestive tract injury in 27 (20%) patients. Ten (37%) of these 27 patients had an injury requiring operative intervention: five (4%) laryngeal injuries, three (2%) tracheal disruptions, and two (1%) esophageal perforations. Eighty-one patients (60%) never had endoscopic evaluation. There were no delayed diagnoses, missed injuries, or complications in the observation-only cohort. The overall sensitivity and specificity of CT scan for major aerodigestive tract injury was 100% and 85%, respectively.

Conclusion.—Major airway or esophageal injury is an uncommon cause of pneumomediastinum. CT scan was able to identify patients at high risk for aerodigestive injury in all cases, and should be the preferred screening tool for airway injury in patients with pneumomediastinum.

▶ This is a helpful observation from a leading academic trauma group that allows clinicians having access to CT imaging to use this technology rather than expensive and time-consuming protocols previously employed. In the past, patients with a suspicious mediastinum were evaluated with bronchoscopy and esophagoscopy. New-generation CT scanning allows these tests to be eliminated unless focal intervention for a particular injury is necessary.[1,2]

A number of observations must be made from these data. First, the authors searched the trauma registry based on identified injury. We could learn more by looking at the number of patients with CT imaging of the chest done for trauma and identifying pneumomediastinum. As we have learned from vascular injury, with increased quality of imaging and frequency of its use, minimal injuries are more readily detected. Thus, the incidence of injury in this series is probably overstated.

Second, charts are reviewed between 1998 and 2005. I suspect that there has been evolution in scanning technology at the trauma center during this interval. It would be interesting to examine changes in CT scanning and its use during the period of this trial. I suspect that there has been a change in the use of bronchoscopy, esophagoscopy, and other secondary studies by the Harborview group. As we become more and more comfortable with CT imaging, the need for secondary studies is reduced.

An additional, important observation is the frequent appearance of the Macklin effect caused by air dissecting medially along bronchovascular sheaths after alveolar rupture.[3] This is a common mechanism in blunt trauma and should always be considered in the patient with pneumomediastinum after blunt injury. The authors note that criteria for follow-up endoscopy were not consistent in this series. Perhaps future studies can better identify the patient needing more than CT imaging when the potential for significant injury is great and initial findings subtle.

D. J. Dries, MSE, MD

References

1. Miller PR, Meredith JW. Tracheal and tracheobronchial tree injuries. In: Asensio JA, Trunkey DD, eds. *Current Therapy of Trauma and Surgical Critical Care.* Philadelphia: Elsevier; 2008:278-281.
2. Karmy-Jones R, Wood DE, Jurkovich GJ. Esophagus, trachea, and bronchus. In: Feliciano DV, Mattox KL, Moore EE, eds. *Trauma.* Sixth Edition. New York: McGraw Hill; 2008:553-567.
3. Wintermark M, Schnyder P. The Macklin effect: a frequent etiology for pneumomediastinum in severe blunt chest trauma. *Chest.* 2001;120:543-547.

Theraputic anticoagulation in the trauma patient: Is it safe?
Golob JF Jr, Sando MJ, Kan JC, et al (Case Western Reserve Univ School of Medicine, Cleveland, OH)
Surgery 144:591-596, 2008

Purpose.—Trauma patients who require therapeutic anticoagulation pose a difficult treatment problem. The purpose of this study was to determine: (1) the incidence of complications using therapeutic anticoagulation in trauma patients, and (2) if any patient factors are associated with these complications.

Methods.—An 18-month retrospective review was performed on trauma patients $\geq$ 15 years old who received therapeutic anticoagulation using unfractionated heparin (UH) and/or fractionated heparin (FH). Forty different pre-treatment and treatment patient characteristics were recorded. Complications of anticoagulation were documented and defined as any unanticipated discontinuation of the anticoagulant for bleeding or other adverse events.

Results.—One-hundred-fourteen trauma patients were initiated on therapeutic anticoagulation. The most common indication for anticoagulation was deep venous thrombosis (46%). Twenty-four patients (21%) had at least 1 anticoagulation complication. The most common complication was a sudden drop in hemoglobin concentration requiring blood transfusion (11 patients). Five patients died (4%), 3 of whom had significant hemorrhage attributed to anticoagulation. Bivariate followed by logistic regression analysis identified chronic obstructive pulmonary disease (OR = 9.2, 95%CI = 1.5–54.7), UH use (OR = 3.8, 95%CI = 1.1–13.0), and lower initial platelet count (OR = 1.004, 95%CI = 1.000–1.008) as being associated with complications. Patients receiving UH vs. FH differed in several characteristics including laboratory values and anticoagulation indications.

Conclusion.—Trauma patients have a significant complication rate related to anticoagulation therapy, and predicting which patients will develop a complication remains unclear. Prospective studies are needed to determine which treatment regimen, if any, is appropriate to safely anticoagulate this high risk population.

▶ The role of anticoagulation in routine management of injury is frequently debated, particularly in the setting of head trauma. These authors explore a slightly different patient group; that cleared to receive therapeutic anticoagulation. The most common complication was bleeding, but traumatic or operative triggers could not be identified. Unfractionated heparin use was associated with the majority of complications. When discussion of the data is examined, the activated partial thromboplastin time (aPTT) during unfractionated heparin use was significantly higher in patients with complications than in those without complications.

Five patients in this review died. We are not given additional detail regarding mortality. No difference was identified in intensive care unit length of stay, hospital length of stay, and duration of anticoagulation therapy for patients with and without complications. The most feared complication, intracranial hemorrhage, is not specifically discussed. When final analysis is concluded, we are left with COPD, use of unfractionated heparin, and thrombocytopenia as risk factors. (Risk with thrombocytopenia is similar to use of activated protein C where thrombocytopenia is a risk factor for bleeding complications.[1])

These authors provide a warning and some background data regarding the risk of therapeutic anticoagulation in the setting of injury. Unfortunately, details regarding injury and operative therapy, which might serve to better inform us, are not provided. In particular, the pattern of mortality seen and presentation may be invaluable data. The injured patient remains an anticoagulation challenge in part because of heterogeneity in presentation and lack of solid prospective data specific to this group.

D. J. Dries, MSE, MD

Reference

1. Bernard GR, Vincent JL, Laterre PF, et al. Efficacy and safety of recombinant human activated protein C for severe sepsis. *N Engl J Med.* 2001;344:699-709.

The risk factors and management of posttraumatic empyema in trauma patients
Eren S, Esme H, Sehitogullari A, et al (Dicle Univ, Diyarbakir, Turkey; Kocatepe Univ, Afyon, Turkey; Gen Hosp, Van, Turkey)
Injury 39:44-49, 2008

Background.—Posttraumatic empyema increases patient morbidity, mortality and length of hospital stay, and the cost of treatment. The aim of this study was to identify the risk factors for posttraumatic empyema and to review our treatment outcomes in patients with this condition.

Methods.—A total of 2261 patients who were admitted with thoracic traumas and underwent tube thoracostomy between January 1989 and January 2006 were investigated retrospectively. Posttraumatic empyema developed in 71 patients. Logistic regression was used to assess the association between potential risk factors for posttraumatic empyema. All values were expressed as the mean ± S.D.

Results.—Eight hundred and thirty-six (37%) of the patients had penetrating type trauma, while 1425 (63%) had blunt type trauma. The rate of posttraumatic empyema development was 3.1% for all patients. Pulmonary contusion was seen in 221 (9.8%) patients and fractures of more than two ribs were seen in 191 (8.4%) patients. Tube thoracostomy placement was performed in the emergency room in 1728 (76.4%) patients, in the hospital ward in 197 (8.7%), in the intensive care unit in 182 (8.0%), and in the operating room in 154 (6.8%). The duration of tube thoracostomy was 6.11 ± 2.99 (1–21) days. Retained haemothorax was seen in 175 (7.7%) patients. The mean lengths of hospital and intensive care unit stay were 6.42 ± 3.45 and 2.36 ± 2.66 days, respectively. The analysis showed that duration of tube thoracostomy (OR, 2.49, $p < 0.001$), length of intensive care unit stay (OR, 4.21, $p < 0.001$), and presence of contusion (OR, 3.06, $p < 0.001$), retained haemothorax (OR, 5.55, $p < 0.001$), and exploratory laparotomy (OR, 2.46, $p < 0.001$) were independent predictors of posttraumatic empyema. The relative risk of posttraumatic empyema was higher than 1 for each of the following risk factors: penetrating trauma (OR, 1.59, $p = 0.055$), associated injuries (OR, 1.12, $p = 0.628$) and fractures of more than two ribs (OR, 1.60, $p = 0.197$).

Conclusion.—Prolonged duration of tube thoracostomy and length of intensive care unit stay, and the presence of contusion, laparotomy and retained haemothorax are independent predictors of posttraumatic empyema. Use of prophylactic antibiotics may be recommended in patients with these risk factors.

▶ The role of antibiotic prophylaxis in various forms of trauma is a matter of ongoing discussion. To speak strictly, trauma patients cannot receive prophylactic antibiotics, as the injurious insult has already occurred. However, antibiotic prophylaxis can be provided for surgical procedures. The role of antibiotic prophylaxis for tube thoracostomy after trauma is a controversial subject.

These authors indicate a number of risk factors for posttraumatic empyema. Most important, in my view, is limitation in chest tube technique and failure to clear hemothorax after various forms of blunt and penetrating injury. In the age of thoracoscopy, retained hemothorax is a clear indication for early and aggressive use of minimally invasive technologies to reduce clot burden. Failure to do so increases the risk of empyema regardless of late administration of antibiotics.

If antibiotics are to be used with tube thoracostomy, the most appropriate application of this therapy is as a single dose associated with the procedure itself. Long-term use of antibiotics increases the risk of emergence for multidrug-resistant organisms. Antibiotic penetration of clot sitting in the chest must be dismal. In my practice, the EAST Practice Management Guidelines cited by the authors are accepted.[1] This consensus statement concludes that there are insufficient data available to recommend routine antibiotic prophylaxis for management of tube thoracostomy in traumatic hemothorax.

D. J. Dries, MSE, MD

Reference

1. Luchette FA, Barrie PS, Oswanski MF, et al. Practice management guidelines for prophylactic antibiotic use in tube thoracostomy for traumatic hemopneumo-thorax: the EAST Practice Management Guidelines Work Group. Eastern Association for Trauma. *J Trauma*. 2000;48:753-757.

Enterocutaneous Fistula Complicating Trauma Laparotomy: A Major Resource Burden

Teixeira PGR, Inaba K, Dubose J, et al (Univ of Southern California, Los Angeles; et al)
Am Surg 75:30-32, 2009

Enterocutaneous fistula (ECF) is an uncommon and poorly studied post-operative complication. The objective of this study was to analyze the incidence and resource utilization of patients who developed an ECF after trauma laparotomy. All patients with an ECF occurring after trauma laparotomy at a Level I trauma center were identified through a review of both the Trauma Registry and the Morbidity and Mortality reports for a 9-year period ending in December 2006. Each ECF case was matched with a control (non-ECF) that did not develop this complication after laparotomy. The matching criteria were: age, gender, mechanism of injury, Injury Severity Score, Abbreviated Injury Score, and damage control laparotomy requiring an open abdomen. Outcomes analyzed were intensive care unit (ICU) and hospital length of stay, mortality, and total hospital charges. During the 9-year period, of 2373 acute trauma laparotomies performed, 36 (1.5%) patients developed an enterocutaneous fistula, and were matched to 36 controls. Patients with an ECF were 31 ± 12 years of age, were 97 per cent male, had a mean Injury Severity Score of 21 ± 10, and 75 per cent were penetrating. Eighty-nine per cent of the ECF patients had a hollow viscus injury. The most common was colon (69%), followed by small bowel (53%), duodenum (36%), and stomach (19%). Fifty-six per cent of the ECF patients had multiple hollow viscus injuries. The development of an ECF was associated with significantly increased ICU length of stay (28.5 ± 30.5 *vs* 7.6 ± 9.3 days, $P = 0.004$), hospital length of stay (82.1 ± 100.8 *vs* 16.2 ± 17.3 days, $P < 0.001$), and hospital charges ($539,309 *vs* $126,996, $P < 0.001$). In conclusion, the development of an enterocutaneous fistula after laparotomy for trauma resulted in a significant impact on resource utilization including longer ICU and hospital length of stay and higher hospital charges. Further investigation into the prevention and treatment of this costly complication is warranted.

▶ At first glance, this article appropriately demonstrates the importance of enterocutaneous fistula as a source of morbidity and increased resource consumption after injury. Concealed in the data are 2 important facts. With present resuscitation techniques and nutrition support strategies, the early loss of life associated with fistulas has been virtually eliminated.[1] Total parenteral nutrition (TPN) allows repletion of electrolytes and nutrition support.[2] Infection control is much better than indicated on initial reports where high early mortality after fistulas was noted due to metabolic failure and uncontrolled infection. The second important observation is related to the changing character of enterocutaneous fistulas. We now see a growing number of fistulas complicating patients managed with the open abdomen.

In these data, 61% of fistulas reported follow the management of patients with an open abdomen. Unfortunately, technical details of operation used, segment of intestine injured, and management details for the open abdomen are not provided. Thus, the result we can safely glean from this article is the increased resource consumption associated with the fistula occurring in exposed bowel from an open abdomen now described as the enteroatmospheric fistula.

We clearly need better data on the operative management and ICU support of patients with the open abdomen as part of staged operative care for abdominal injury. Failure to close the fascia in a timely manner regardless of internal injury seems to be a marker of poor outcome. While it is inappropriate to close the fascia in many circumstances, a suitable strategy to optimally protect the bowel has not been identified. I suspect that new synthetic materials and a new pattern of use for local tissue flaps may provide part of the answer.

D. J. Dries, MSE, MD

References

1. Schecter WP, Hirshberg A, Chang DS, et al. Enteric fistulas: principles of management. *J Am Coll Surg.* 2009;209:484-491.
2. Dudrick SJ, Wilmore DW, Vars HM, Rhoads JE. Can intravenous feedings as the sole means of nutrition support growth in the child and restore weight loss in an adult? An affirmative answer. *Ann Surg.* 1969;169:974-984.

The Changing Face of Trauma: New Orleans Before and After Hurricane Katrina
Wahl GM, Marr AB, Brevard SB, et al (Tulane School of Medicine, New Orleans, LA; Louisiana State Univ Health Science Ctr, New Orleans)
Am Surg 75:284-286, 2009

Charity Hospital (CH) was devastated by Hurricane Katrina and remains closed. Design and staffing of a new, temporary dedicated trauma hospital relied on data from prior experience at CH, updated census information, and a changed trauma demographic. The study objective was to analyze the new trauma program and evaluate changes in demographics, injury patterns, and outcomes between pre- (PK) and post-Katrina (POK) trauma populations. A retrospective review of trauma patients' demographics, anatomical variables, and physiological variables 6 months PK and POK was performed under an approved Institutional Review Board protocol. Trauma activation triage criteria between study periods were also analyzed. Continuous data comparisons between the two time periods were made with Student's t test. Dichotomous data were analyzed using χ^2 test. The demographic of trauma patients is different in the POK interval, reflecting changes in the New Orleans population. Modification of triage criteria by the exclusion of mechanism as an activation criterion resulted in an increase of patients with higher acuity and Injury Severity Score, lower initial Glasgow Coma Score, and a higher proportion of penetrating mechanism. Outcome measures reflect longer length of stay (4.4 *vs* 6.8 days, $P < 0.0001$) without a significant difference in mortality (6.0 *vs* 7.5, $P = 0.227$). Hospital data demonstrates that the POK trauma system was stressed by the increased acuity, penetrating injury, and number of procedures per patient (1.7 *vs* 3.4). Resources should be directed toward patients requiring multidisciplinary care by increasing intensive care unit beds and operating room capacity. Future resource planning in the recovery phases of large-scale natural disasters should take into account these observations.

▶ The authors describe changing demographics in trauma as reflected by activity of the center that replaced Charity Hospital, the legendary trauma center in New Orleans. An increased volume of penetrating trauma and ICU admission is seen in the post-Hurricane Katrina practice. Reasons for this change in

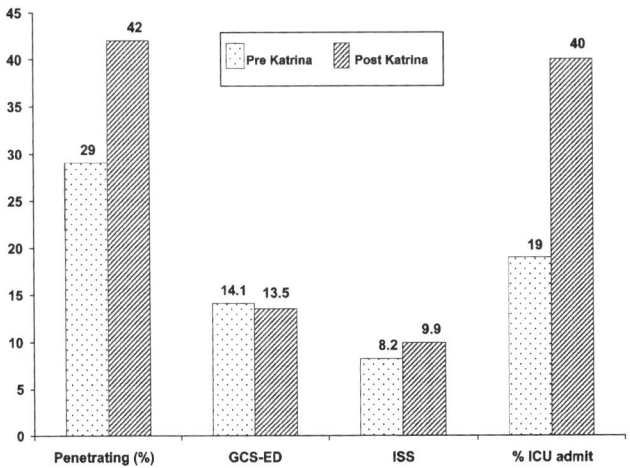

FIGURE 1.—Injury characteristics of trauma activations based on anatomic and physiological criteria only. (Reprinted from Wahl GM, Marr AB, Brevard SB, et al. The changing face of trauma: New Orleans before and after Hurricane Katrina. *Am Surg.* 2009;75:284-286.)

practice are unclear. Admission criteria for the trauma center but not the ICU are provided. Another fundamental concern in this study is the changing admission pool for trauma patients to the trauma center. The authors have reduced the catchment area and note an increasing injury severity score (ISS) and a lower initial Glasgow Coma Score in the patients from the post-Katrina catchment area. In fact, this may reflect location of high-risk patients from pre-Katrina New Orleans. Thus, a constant referral population cannot be assumed.

The authors have nicely compensated for reduced hospital resources by providing an increasingly efficient trauma service. Perhaps Elmwood Trauma Hospital, the hospital used to replace Charity Hospital, though smaller, may be a more efficient replacement. Possibly, the most important and saddest reflection in this article is the inconsistency between plans and realities in New Orleans after Katrina (Fig 1).

D. J. Dries, MSE, MD

Early evaluation of acute traumatic coagulopathy by thrombelastography
Carroll RC, Craft RM, Langdon RJ, et al (Univ of Tennessee Graduate School of Medicine, Knoxville)
Transl Res 154:34-39, 2009

Posttraumatic coagulopathy is a major cause of morbidity. This prospective study evaluated the thrombelastography (TEG) system and Platelet-Mapping (Haemoscope Corporation, Niles, Ill) values posttrauma, and it correlated those values with transfusions and fatalities. After institutional review board approval, assays were performed on 161 trauma patients. One citrated blood sample was collected onsite (OS), and 1 citrate and 1 heparinized sample were collected within 1 h of arrival to the emergency department (ED). Paired and unpaired *t*-testing was performed for nominal data with chi square testing for categorical values. Except for a slight increase in clot strength (maximal amplitude [MA]), there were no significant changes from OS to the ED. None of the TEG parameters

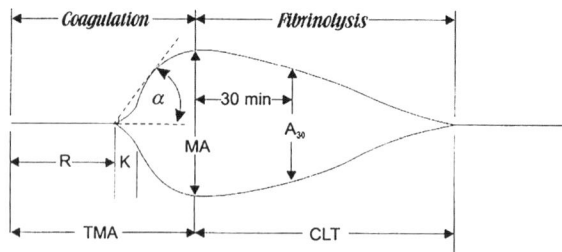

FIGURE 1.—Standard TEG parameters (used with permission of Haemoscope Corporation). Reaction (R) time, clot formation (K) time, clotting rate (angle = α), strength of clot (maximal amplitude [MA]), and percent fibrinolysis at 30 min (A30) and at 60 min (LY60) not shown. (Reprinted from Carroll RC, Craft RM, Langdon RJ, et al. Early evaluation of acute traumatic coagulopathy by thrombelastography. *Transl Res.* 2009;154:34-39, with permission from Elsevier.)

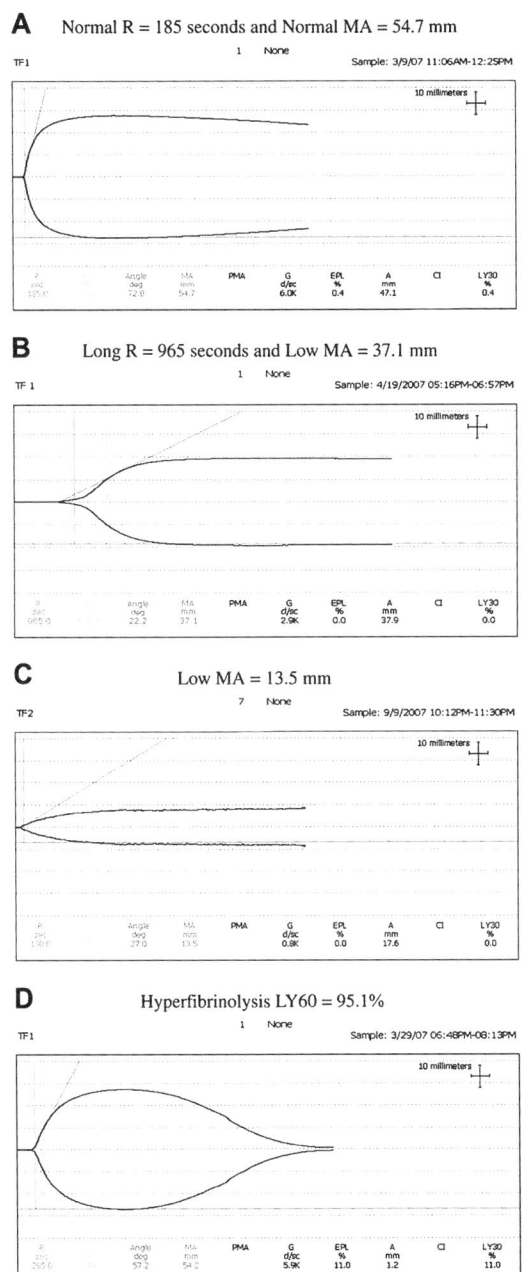

FIGURE 2.—Representative patient TEG tracings. A, Normal R = 185 s and normal MA = 54.7 mm. B, Long R = 965 s and Low MA = 37.1 mm. C, Low MA = 13.5 mm. D, Hyperfibrinolysis LY60 = 95.1%. (Color version of figure is available online.) (Reprinted from Carroll RC, Craft RM, Langdon RJ, et al. Early evaluation of acute traumatic coagulopathy by thrombelastography. *Transl Res.* 2009;154:34-39, with permission from Elsevier.)

were significantly different for the 22 patients who required transfusion. PlateletMapping showed lower platelet adenosine diphosphate (ADP) responsiveness in patients who needed transfusions (MA = 22.7 ± 17.1 vs MA = 35.7 ± 19.3, $P = 0.004$) and a correlation of fibrinogen < 100 mg/dL with fatalities ($P = 0.013$). For the 14 fatalities, TEG reaction (R) time was 3703 ± 11,618 versus 270 ± 393 s ($P = <0.001$), and MA was 46.4 ± 22.4 versus 64.7 ± 9.8 mm ($P < 0.001$). Hyperfibrinolysis (percent fibrinolysis after 60 min [LY60] > 15%) was observed in 3 patients in the ED with a 67% fatality rate ($P = <0.001$ by chi-square testing). PlateletMapping assays correlated with the need for blood transfusion. The abnormal TEG System parameters correlated with fatality. These coagulopathies were already evident OS. The TEG assays can assess coagulopathy, platelet dysfunction, and hyperfibrinolysis at an early stage posttrauma and suggest more effective interventions.

▶ Thrombelastography is receiving significant attention as an improved means to evaluate coagulopathy occurring as a function of tissue ischemia and vascular bed injury after trauma (Figs 1 and 2). Thrombelastography has the advantages of rapidity and provision of an integrated evaluation of the coagulation response from the injured patient.[1-3] However, this technique is extremely operator sensitive and requires a technical commitment on the part of institutions considering employment of this modality.

The authors nicely identify correspondence between coagulopathy and adverse outcomes in the setting of trauma. This is not surprising given other literature that is available on the coagulopathy of trauma. In this study, we are given no details regarding injury other than the presence or absence of mortality. Thus, the correlation of coagulopathy with specific injury patterns cannot be investigated. In addition, virtually every patient is coagulopathic as evaluated by thrombelastography. Thrombelastography, in the hands of these investigators, appears to be an extremely sensitive indicator of injury. Unfortunately, the specificity of TEG appears to be low.

The authors demonstrate that coagulation changes may be detected in the field though we are not given convincing evidence that field management can impact this assay. It does appear that evaluation in the emergency department will provide a sensitive evaluation of patient outcome. For thrombelastography to gain broad acceptance in the trauma community, reproducible assays that are simple to execute must be developed. The effectiveness of this technology would be enhanced by studies linking thrombelastography data to the physiology of differing injuries and demonstration that thrombelastography can direct blood component therapy, particularly in the setting of patients receiving massive transfusion.

D. J. Dries, MSE, MD

References

1. Kashuk JL, Moore EE, Le T, et al. Noncitrated whole blood is optimal for evaluation of postinjury coagulation with point-of-care rapid thrombelastography. *J Surg Res.* 2009;156:133-138.
2. Jeger V, Zimmermann H, Exadaktylos AK. Can rapid TEG accelerate the search for coagulopathies in the patient with multiple injuries? *J Trauma.* 2009;66: 1253-1257.
3. Park MS, Martini WZ, Dubick MA, et al. Thromboelastography as a better indicator of hypercoagulable state after injury than prothrombin time or activated partial thromboplastin time. *J Trauma.* 2009;67:266-276.

Surgical Response to Multiple Casualty Incidents Following Single Explosive Events

Propper BW, Rasmussen TE, Davidson SB, et al (The 332nd Expeditionary Med Group/Air Force Theater Hosp Balad Air Base, Iraq; Wilford Hall United States Air Force Med Ctr, Lackland Air Force Base, TX; Bronson Methodist Hosp, Kalamazoo, MI)
Ann Surg 250:311-315, 2009

Background.—Modern publications on response to single explosive events are from non-US hospitals, predate current resuscitation guidelines and lack detail on surgical and intensive care unit (ICU) requirements. The objective of this study is to provide a contemporary account of surge response to multiple casualty incidences following explosive events managed at a US trauma hospital in Iraq.

Methods.—Observational study and retrospective chart review of 72-hour transfusion, operating room, and ICU resource utilization from 3 multiple casualty incidences managed at the US Air Force Theater Hospital, Balad AB, Iraq between February and April 2008.

Results.—Fifty patients were treated with a mean injury severity score of 19. Forty-eight percent (n = 24) of casualties required blood transfusion with 4 patients receiving 43% (N = 74 units) of the packed red blood cells (pRBC). An average of 3.5 and 3.8 units of pRBC and plasma, respectively, was transfused per casualty (pRBC:plasma ratio of 1:1.1). Seventy-six percent (n = 38) of patients required immediate operation upon initial presentation. A total of 191 procedures were performed in parallel during 75 operations (3.8 procedures per casualty). Fifty percent (n = 25) of patients required ICU admission with nearly the same number (n = 24) requiring mechanical ventilator support beyond that required for operation. All cause, in-hospital mortality was 8% (n = 4).

Conclusions.—Results from this study provide a contemporary assessment of transfusion, surgical, and intensive care resource requirements after a single explosive event. Data from this experience may translate into useful guidelines for emergency planners worldwide.

▶ The authors present a military hospital experience with individual explosive events in an attempt to provide a model for civilian trauma hospitals facing similar problems in the United States. There are a number of inconsistencies, however. We have no scene data in this article. Thus, the type of explosive device and initial response, which can have a significant impact on hospital effectiveness, is not provided.

There are a number of simple and important messages. Patients sustaining blast injury have a significant likelihood of requiring surgery on an urgent basis. Over 50% of injured patients are likely to require some form of critical care. Perhaps the most important critical care resource is mechanical ventilation, which many patients will require even after initial operative procedures. Transfusion is also extremely likely with most products provided within the first day after injury (Fig 2 in the original article).

In comparison with events reported on an international stage, these 3 bombing incidents appear relatively small. Only single hospital response is reported. Nonetheless, it is clear that patients involved in terrorist events will require far higher resource consumption than the typical trauma patient seen in civilian practice. Thus, resources of the overcrowded, designated trauma centers may be insufficient to manage a large multicasualty situation in civilian practice. In many communities, therefore, the trauma center will attract the most severely injured patients while serving as a guide for distribution of less severely injured individuals to neighboring facilities.[1,2]

D. J. Dries, MSE, MD

References

1. Kashuk JL, Halperin P, Caspi G, Colwell C, Moore EE. Bomb explosions in acts of terrorism: evil creativity challenges our trauma systems. *J Am Coll Surg.* 2009;209: 134-140.
2. Peleg K, Kellermann AL. Enhancing hospital surge capacity for mass casualty events. *JAMA.* 2009;302:565-567.

A 6-year review of total parenteral nutrition use and association with late-onset acute respiratory distress syndrome among ventilated trauma victims

Plurad D, Green D, Inaba K, et al (Univ of Southern California and Los Angeles County Hosp Division of Trauma/Surgical Critical Care)
Injury 40:511-515, 2009

Aim.—To establish whether total parenteral nutrition (TPN) for ventilated trauma victims is associated with late-onset acute respiratory distress syndrome (ARDS) independent of ventilation and transfusion parameters.

Method.—Intensive care unit data over 6 years from a level I centre regarding all trauma victims ≥16 years old who underwent mechanical

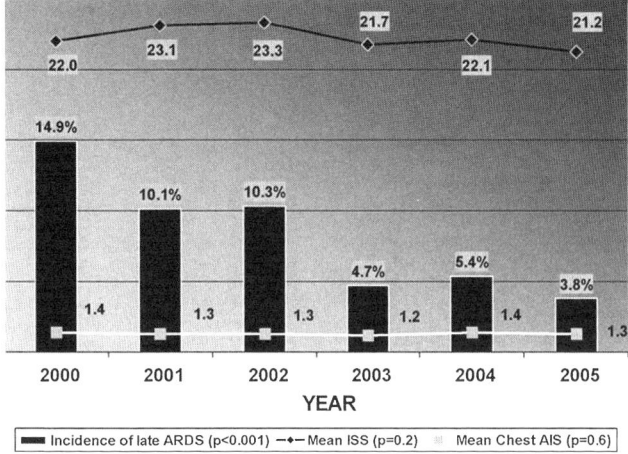

FIGURE 1.—Late ARDS, mean Injury Severity Score (ISS) and mean Chest Abbreviated Injury Score (Chest AIS) by year of admission. (Reprinted from Plurad D, Green D, Inaba K, et al. A 6-year review of total parenteral nutrition use and association with late-onset acute respiratory distress syndrome among ventilated trauma victims. *Injury.* 2009;40:511-515, with permission from Elsevier.)

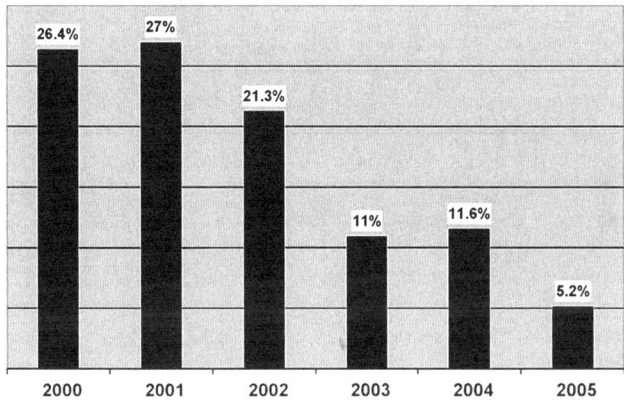

FIGURE 2.—Percentage of study population exposed to total parenteral nutrition by year of study. (Reprinted from Plurad D, Green D, Inaba K, et al. A 6-year review of total parenteral nutrition use and association with late-onset acute respiratory distress syndrome among ventilated trauma victims. *Injury.* 2009;40:511-515, with permission from Elsevier.)

ventilation within the first 48 h of admission were examined. Patients were prospectively followed for late ARDS. Variables were examined for significant changes over time and independent associations with late ARDS were determined.

Results.—Of 2346 eligible patients among whom 404 (17.2%) were exposed to TPN, 192 (8.2%) met criteria for late ARDS. The incidence of late ARDS among those exposed to TPN was 28.7% (116/404) compared with 3.9% (76/1942) among those not so exposed. Adjustments for potential confounding associated risk factors were made.

Conclusions.—TPN administration is independently associated with late ARDS, and its use among critically ill trauma victims should be carefully scrutinised.

▶ The authors build on analysis previously published in *The Journal of Trauma* and with a large database from a busy American trauma center to examine relationships between good and bad outcome, particularly with respect to pulmonary dysfunction.[1] Traditional definitions for acute respiratory distress syndrome (ARDS) are employed. Standard statistical methods, including multivariate logistic regression, are appropriately used. With over 2000 patients to study, a high frequency of associations will be seen.

Conservative resuscitation strategies, including reduced use of blood, decreased crystalloid volumes, and lung protective ventilator strategies, reduce the incidence of acute lung injury and ARDS.[1] ARDS in the setting of trauma typically is related to extrapulmonary causes. The predominant extrapulmonary cause in the setting of injury is resuscitation. Thus, the improved outcomes after injury with respect to pulmonary dysfunction correspond directly to changes in the resuscitation practice in this busy trauma center.

The impact of total parenteral nutrition on outcome is also examined.[2,3] Total parenteral nutrition (TPN) use is associated with an increased incidence of ARDS. We are not given data, however, regarding factors that contributed to TPN use.[4,5] I note that patients receiving TPN also received higher fluid volumes; therefore, an increased risk of extrapulmonary ARDS can be anticipated. A critical piece of data, which is unavailable in this retrospective review, is the abdominal abbreviated injury score (AIS), which could shed light on the need for TPN in these patients. In all, this work reinforces the need to provide nutrient support in the injured patient using the gut, if possible. The high rate of adverse outcomes associated with TPN in this patient population is not matched in other studies where metabolic complications of parenteral nutrition are carefully controlled.[6,7] To summarize, I do not doubt the association of TPN with poorer outcome in this population but note that may other factors, which are not completely described, may be associated with poor outcome in the TPN group (Figs 1 and 2).

D. J. Dries, MSE, MD

References

1. Plurad D, Martin M, Green D, et al. The decreasing incidence of late posttraumatic acute respiratory distress syndrome: the potential role of lung protective ventilation and conservative transfusion practice. *J Trauma.* 2007;63:1-8.
2. Perioperative total parenteral nutrition in surgical patients: the Veterans Affairs Total Parenteral Nutrition Cooperative Study Group. *N Engl J Med.* 1991;325:525-532.
3. Rapp RP, Young B, Twyman D, et al. The favorable effect of early parenteral feeding on survival in head-injured patients. *J Neurosurg.* 1983;58:906-912.
4. Elke G, Schadler D, Engel C, et al. Current practice in nutritional support and its association with mortality in septic patients-results from a national, prospective, multicenter study. *Crit Care Med.* 2008;36:1762-1767.

5. Sena MJ, Utter GH, Cuschieri J, et al. Early supplemental parenteral nutrition is associated with increased infectious complications in critically ill trauma patients. *J Am Coll Surg.* 2008;207:459-467.
6. Ahrens CL, Barletta JF, Kanji S, et al. Effect of low-calorie parenteral nutrition on the incidence and severity of hyperglycemia in surgical patients: A randomized, controlled trial. *Crit Care Med.* 2005;33:2507-2512.
7. Peter JV, Moran JL, Phillips-Hughes J. A metaanalysis of treatment outcomes of early enteral versus early parenteral nutrition in hospitalized patients. *Crit Care Med.* 2005;33:213-220.

American College of Surgeons trauma centre designation and mechanical ventilation outcomes

DuBose JJ, Teixeira PGR, Shiflett A, et al (Los Angeles County Hosp/Univ of Southern California School of Medicine)
Injury 40:708-712, 2009

Objective.—The association between hospital volume and outcomes following mechanical ventilation has been previously examined in diverse patient populations. The American College of Surgeons (ACS) Committee on Trauma has outlined criteria for trauma centre level designations with specific requirements for both specialty capabilities and hospital volume. Our objective is to determine the relationship between ACS centre designation and outcomes for trauma patients undergoing mechanical ventilation.

Methods.—We conducted a retrospective cohort study using the National Trauma Databank (NTDB), identifying 13,933 adult (age ≥ 18) trauma patients receiving mechanical ventilation for greater than 48 h from 2000 to 2004 who were admitted to either an ACS Level I or Level II trauma centre. The primary endpoints examined were mortality, pneumonia and Acute Respiratory Distress Syndrome (ARDS). Univariate analysis defined differences between those patients admitted to ACS Level I and Level II facilities. Logistic regression analysis was used to identify if ACS level designation was an independent risk factor for the goal outcomes.

Results.—Patients admitted to a Level I facility and mechanically ventilated for greater than 48 h were more commonly greater than age 55 (71.3% vs. 67.9%, $p < 0.01$), hypotensive (SBP < 90) (16.1% vs. 12.8%, $p < 0.01$), and likely to have sustained injury due to penetrating mechanism (11.1% vs. 5.1%, $p < 0.01$). On univariate analysis, mortality and the incidence of pneumonia did not differ between the two groups. Level I admission was, however, less commonly associated with the development of ARDS (5.8% vs. 7.7%, $p < 0.01$) and patients admitted to Level I facilities were significantly more likely to be discharged to home than Level II counterparts (29.7% vs. 22.9%, $p < 0.01$). Logistic regression revealed that, while ACS Level designation was not a predictive factor for mortality or the development of pneumonia, admission to an ACS Level II facility was an independent predictor for the development of ARDS [$p < 0.01$, odds ratio, 95% CI: 1.35 (1.18–1.59)].

Conclusion.—For trauma patients requiring mechanical ventilation for >48 h, ACS trauma centre designation had no effect on overall mortality or the incidence of pneumonia. Compared to Level I counterparts, however, patients admitted to an ACS Level II facility were significantly more likely to develop ARDS following trauma. This finding needs further investigation in a large, prospective analysis.

▶ These data come from the massive outcome databank from the American College of Surgeons and the American trauma community, the National Trauma Databank. With multiple comparisons made between level I and level II centers, it is not surprising that some are statistically significant. It is not clear how many of these observations are clinically significant even where statistical differences exist. However, from my experience in level I and level II centers a number of observations can be made.[1] The typical level I center sees a patient with greater physiologic derangement as reflected by hypotension on admission and a higher fraction of penetrating trauma. Level I centers tend to see not only the older patient population but also more penetrating trauma. Of the 4 major complications reported, death, acute respiratory distress syndrome (ARDS), pneumonia, and renal failure, level I centers provide superior outcome with respect to death and ARDS. However, when multivariate analysis takes place, only the difference in ARDS remains.

Why is this? Recent clinical data suggest that the likelihood of ARDS is driven by practice patterns including ventilator prescriptions, crystalloid use, and blood transfusion.[2] Where the risk of ARDS has been reduced, a coincident reduction in crystalloid use, blood transfusion, and airway pressures has been realized. I am not surprised that academic centers, which tend to be level I centers, are leading the way in this evolution in critical care of the injured patient. These data, in my opinion, reflect the learning curve in surgical critical care units.

D. J. Dries, MSE, MD

References

1. American College of Surgeons, Committee on Trauma. *Resources for Optimal Care of the Injured Patient.* Chicago, IL: American College of Surgeons; 2006.
2. Plurad D, Martin M, Green D, et al. The decreasing incidence of late posttraumatic acute respiratory distress syndrome: the potential role for lung protective ventilation and conservative transfusion practice. *J Trauma.* 2007;63:1-8.

Association of Preexisting Medical Conditions with In-Hospital Mortality in Multiple-Trauma Patients

Wutzler S, Trauma Registry of the German Society for Trauma Surgery (Univ of Witten/Herdecke, Cologne, Germany; et al)

J Am Coll Surg 209:75-81, 2009

Background.—Mortality after trauma has been shown to be influenced by host factors, such as age and preexisting medical conditions (PMCs). The independent predictive value of specific PMCs for in-hospital mortality after adjustment for injury severity, injury pattern, age, and presence of other PMCs has not been fully elucidated.

Study Design.—Records of 11,142 trauma patients (18 years of age or older, Injury Severity Score ≥ 16, years 2002 to 2007) documented in the Trauma Registry of the German Society for Trauma Surgery were analyzed to assess the association of PMCs with in-hospital mortality. Multiple logistic regression models were used for this analysis.

Results.—PMCs were affirmed for 3,836 of the 11,142 patients studied (34.4%). An independent statistical association with increased in-hospital mortality was found for 6 of 14 analyzed PMCs after adjustment for age and the Revised Injury Severity Classification score, respectively, ie, heart disease, obesity, hepatitis/liver cirrhosis, malignancies, coagulation disorder, and peripheral arterial occlusive disease stage IV. The association with mortality varied with different injury patterns.

Conclusion.—Specific PMCs were associated with increased mortality after trauma independent from injury severity and age. Knowledge of the identified relevant PMCs could help the medical team to be able to assess the mortality risk profile of trauma patients in a more detailed and quantifiable way.

▶ This is a nicely performed study from the German Trauma Registry identifying factors associated with adverse outcome in older trauma patients. As we age, the likelihood is 1 in 3 that one of these preexisting medical conditions will be present. There are no real surprises here. Cardiovascular disease, cirrhosis, coagulopathy, and malignancy are likely predictors of poor outcome either by primary effects or by secondary weakening of critical organ systems.

The role of obesity is particularly difficult to assess.[1,2] Obesity is associated with multiple organ system complications, including cardiovascular disease and metabolic disorders. As the authors point out, it is not clear whether obesity or associated organ dysfunction is the greatest problem.

This study raises a number of interesting questions. For example, for important preexisting medical conditions, what are true age thresholds for adverse outcomes?[3-5] When should we screen for preexisting medical conditions in the setting of injury? What is the most cost-effective and timely way to screen for these conditions in the setting of multiple trauma? Perhaps, there are tests that can be eliminated in younger trauma patients unless stigmata of preexisting disease are present (Fig 2).

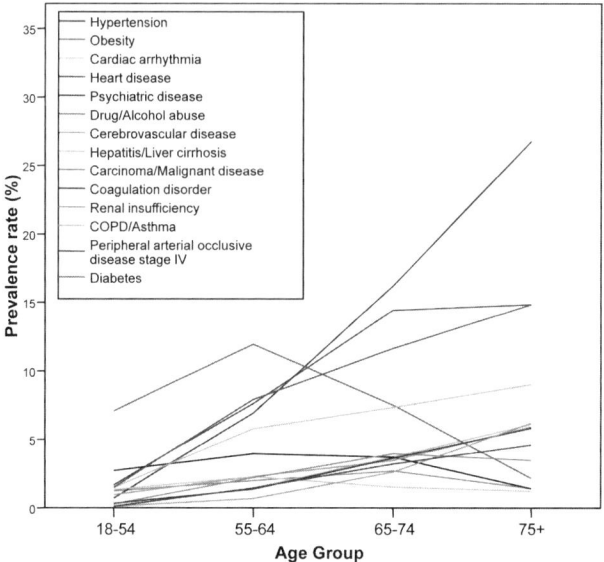

FIGURE 2.—Frequency of different preexisting medical conditions in multiple trauma patients with increasing age: n = 7,579 (18 to 54 years); n = 1,314 (55 to 64 years); n = 1,185 (65 to 74); n = 1,064 (75 years and older). (Reprinted from Wutzler S, Trauma Registry of the German Society for Trauma Surgery. Association of preexisting medical conditions with in-hospital mortality in multiple-trauma patients. *J Am Coll Surg.* 2009;209:75-81, with permission from American College of Surgeons.)

The typical trauma patient is depicted as young and healthy. As our society ages, we will need more work such as this, because the impact of comorbid conditions will continue to grow. This study also begins the sensitive analysis of combined effects of preexisting conditions and examines impact on outcome. There is much work to be done.

D. J. Dries, MSE, MD

References

1. Dossett LA, Dageforde LA, Swenson BR, et al. Obesity and site-specific nosocomial infection risk in the intensive care unit. *Surg Infect.* 2009;10:137-142.
2. Newell MA, Bard MR, Goettler CE, et al. Body mass index and outcomes in critically injured blunt trauma patients: weighing the impact. *J Am Coll Surg.* 2007; 204:1056-1064.
3. Sampalis JS, Nathanson R, Vaillancourt J, et al. Assessment of mortality in older trauma patients sustaining injuries from falls or motor vehicle collisions treated in regional level I trauma centers. *Ann Surg.* 2009;249:488-495.
4. Tepas JJ, Veldenz HC, Lottenberg L, et al. Elderly injury: a profile of trauma experience in the sunshine (retirement) state. *J Trauma.* 2000;48:581-586.
5. McGwin G Jr, Melton SM, May AK, Rue LW. Long-term survival in the elderly after trauma. *J Trauma.* 2000;49:470-476.

11 Neurologic: Traumatic and Non-traumatic

Early Venous Thromboembolism Prophylaxis With Enoxaparin in Patients With Blunt Traumatic Brain Injury
Norwood SH, Berne JD, Rowe SA, et al (East Texas Med Ctr, Tyler)
J Trauma 65:1021-1026, 2008

Objective.—To determine the safety of early enoxaparin for venous thromboembolism (VTE) prophylaxis in patients with blunt traumatic brain injury (TBI).

Methods.—Prospective observational study of patients with TBI who received enoxaparin within 48 hours after admission. Brain computed tomography (CT) scans were obtained at the time of admission, at 24 hours, and at variable intervals thereafter based on clinical course. Patients were excluded from the study for intracerebral contusions ≥2 cm, multiple contusions within one brain region, subdural or epidural hematomas ≥8 mm, increased size or number of lesions on follow-up CT, persistent intracranial pressure >20 mm Hg, or neurosurgeon or trauma surgeon reluctance to initiate early pharmacologic VTE prophylaxis. Bleeding complications were defined as CT progression of hemorrhage by Marshall CT Classification or radiologists' report, regardless of any neurologic deterioration. Main outcomes measured were intracranial bleeding complications, discharge Glasgow Outcome Score, and hospital mortality.

Results.—Five hundred twenty-five patients were studied. Eighteen patients (3.4%) had progressive hemorrhagic CT changes after receiving enoxaparin, 12 of whom had no change in treatment, neurologic status, or outcome. Six patients (1.1%) had a change in treatment or potential outcome, including three who required subsequent craniotomy. Twenty-one patients (4.0%) died, and pharmacologic prophylaxis may have contributed to one death (0.2%). Discharge Glasgow Outcome Scores were 445 (84.8%) good recovery, 19 (3.6%) moderate disability, 36 (6.8%) severe disability, 4 (0.8%) persistent vegetative state, and 21 (4.0%) dead.

Conclusion.—Enoxaparin should be considered as an option for early VTE prophylaxis in selected patients with blunt TBI. Early enoxaparin should be strongly considered in those patients with TBI with additional high risk traumatic injuries.

▶ Few subjects generate more discussion in my trauma intensive care unit than the timing of venous thromboembolism (VTE) prophylaxis after head injury.[1] Practices of trauma surgeons and neurosurgeons vary widely. Many neurosurgeons prefer to wait at least 3 weeks to initiate chemical VTE prophylaxis even through mechanical methods offer incomplete protection at best.[2,3] Norwood and associates provide additional data expanding on work published previously in the *Archives of Surgery*.[4]

In a study of over 500 patients from a single center, 18 individuals had evolution of hemorrhagic changes on CT scanning after initiation of enoxaparin therapy. Twelve of these individuals had no subsequent change in treatment, neurologic status, or outcome. Six patients (1.1%) required a change in treatment including 3 individuals with subsequent craniotomy. It is unclear that enoxaparin had any adverse effect on outcomes observed.

Treated patients received enoxaparin sodium (30 mg subcutaneously every 12 hours) "early after admission" in all individuals considered at risk for VTE. Surveillance Doppler studies were not performed unless VTE prophylaxis was delayed for 5 or more days. Thus, rigorous data on the impact of this enoxaparin program on VTE outcome are incomplete at best.[5-7]

Enoxaparin was not offered to all patients suffering traumatic brain injury (TBI). The following patients were excluded from early prophylaxis by agreement of the neurosurgeons and trauma service:

- Intracerebral contusions or hematomas > 2 cm in diameter.
- Multiple smaller contusions within one region of the brain.
- Subdural or epidural hematomas > 8 mm in thickness.
- Persistent intracranial pressure > 20 mm Hg.
- Increased size or number of brain lesions on follow-up CT scan at 24 hours after admission.

A significant number of patients with TBI (1330) were not entered into the study for a number of reasons. Trauma registry data demonstrate no difference in VTE rate between patients not entered into this study and TBI patients in the study group. Remarkably, the authors report 10 cases of pulmonary embolism and 26 cases of deep vein thrombosis (DVT) in the entire trauma patient population of over 6000 patients during the period of this study. I suspect that more aggressive screening for these complications could have significantly affected this outcome.[5,6]

Progressive hemorrhagic injury was documented in 3.4% of patients after starting enoxaparin. Interestingly, progression of head injury on subsequent CT scans has been previously reported in up to 12% of patients with head injury.[8] Thus, it is unclear that enoxaparin contributed in any significant way to progression of changes on CT of TBI patients.

Clearly, to effectively answer the question of a role for early VTE chemical prophylaxis, prospective rather than observational data are needed. Many patients who are eligible for this study were excluded for various reasons. Most important was surgeon preference in nearly 25% of cases. Obviously a risk of bias was present. If anything, this large body of observational data supports safety but not efficacy of early chemical VTE prophylaxis in selected patients sustaining TBI.

D. J. Dries, MSE, MD

References

1. Geerts WH, Code KI, Jay RM, Chen E, Szalai JP. A prospective study of venous thromboembolism after major trauma. *N Engl J Med*. 1994;331:1601-1606.
2. Rogers FB, Cipolle MD, Velmahos G, Rozycki G, Luchette FA. Practice management guidelines for the prevention of venous thromboembolism in trauma patients: The EAST Practice Management Guidelines Work Group. *J Trauma*. 2002;53:142-164.
3. Bratton SL, Chestnut RM, Ghajar J, et al. Guidelines for the management of severe traumatic brain injury. V. Deep vein thrombosis prophylaxis. *J Neurotrauma*. 2007;24:S32-S36.
4. Norwood SH, McAuley CE, Berne JD, et al. Prospective evaluation of the safety of enoxaparin prophylaxis for venous thromboembolism in patients with intracranial hemorrhagic injuries. *Arch Surg*. 2002;137:696-702.
5. Pierce CA, Haut ER, Kardooni S, et al. Surveillance bias and deep vein thrombosis in the National Trauma Data Bank: The more we look, the more we find. *J Trauma*. 2008;64:932-937.
6. Schultz DJ, Brasel KJ, Washington L, et al. Incidence of asymptomatic pulmonary embolism in moderately to severely injured trauma patients. *J Trauma*. 2004;56: 727-733.
7. Menaker J, Stein DM, Scalea TM. Incidence of early pulmonary embolism after injury. *J Trauma*. 2007;63:620-624.
8. Patel NY, Hoyt DB, Nakaji P, et al. Traumatic brain injury: patterns of failure of nonoperative management. *J Trauma*. 2000;48:367-375.

Combined Neuroprotective Modalities Coupled with Thrombolysis in Acute Ischemic Stroke: A Pilot Study of Caffeinol and Mild Hypothermia
Martin-Schild S, Hallevi H, Shaltoni H, et al (Univ of Texas-Houston Med School)
J Stroke Cerebrovasc Dis 18:86-96, 2009

Background.—Both caffeinol and hypothermia are neuroprotective in preclinical models of transient middle cerebral artery occlusion. We tested whether combining caffeinol and hypothermia with tissue plasminogen activator (t-PA) in patients with acute stroke is safe and feasible.

Methods.—Twenty patients with acute ischemic stroke were treated with caffeinol (caffeine 8-9 mg/kg + ethanol 0.4 g/kg intravenously [IV] × 2 hours, started by 4 hours after symptom onset) and hypothermia (started by 5 hours and continued for 24 hours [target temperature 33-35°C] followed by 12 hours of rewarming). IV t-PA was given to eligible patients. Meperidine and buspirone were used to suppress shivering.

Results.—All patients received caffeinol, and most reached target blood levels. Cooling was attempted in 18 patients via endovascular (n = 8) or surface (n = 10) approaches. Two patients were not cooled due to catheter or machine failure. Thirteen patients reached target temperature; average time from symptom onset was 9 hours and 43 minutes. The last 5 hypothermia patients received surface cooling with iced saline induction and larger doses of meperidine; all patients reached target temperature, on average within 2 hours and 30 minutes from induction and 6 hours and 21 minutes from symptom onset. Three patients died: one from symptomatic hemorrhage, one from malignant cerebral edema, and one from unrelated medical complications. No adverse events were attributed to caffeinol. One patient had reduced respiratory drive due to meperidine, requiring BiPAP.

Discussion.—Combining caffeinol with hypothermia in patients with acute stroke given IV t-PA is feasible. A prospective placebo-controlled randomized study is needed to further assess safety and to test the efficacy of caffeinol, hypothermia, or both.

▶ The relentless search for the optimal neuroprotective therapy for stroke victims continues. Nevertheless, all neuroprotective agents that were found to be beneficial in animal models have failed in human stroke trials. Hypothermia has received international recognition after multiple randomized trials showing improved mortality and long-term outcome benefit in out-of-hospital, ventricular fibrillation cardiac arrest survivors.[1,2] After numerous experimental preclinical studies revealing the association between fever/hyperthermia and poor outcome after ischemic stroke, now there are human data regarding the effect of hyperthermia on ischemic stroke. The data are consistent with the previous experimental studies in that the hyperthermia is associated with a poor functional outcome.[3] The obvious question has been whether the hypothermia for ischemic stroke would pan out to be neuroprotective and beneficial in long-term neurological outcome. The safety and feasibility data are being reported, such as this present article, and further investigation may be needed—perhaps as a combined therapy or multimodal approach—to enhance the true neuroprotective effect.

K. Lee, MD

References

1. Bernard SA, Gray TW, Buist MD, et al. Treatment of comatose survivors of out-of-hospital cardiac arrest with induced hypothermia. *N Engl J Med.* 2002;346:557-563.
2. Bernard SA. Hypothermia improves outcome from cardiac arrest. *Crit Care Resusc.* 2005;7:325-327.
3. Saini M, Saqqur M, Kamruzzaman A, Lees KR, Shuaib A, VISTA Investigators. Effect of hyperthermia on prognosis after acute ischemic stroke. *Stroke.* 2009; 40:3051-3059.

Get With the Guidelines–Stroke Is Associated With Sustained Improvement in Care for Patients Hospitalized With Acute Stroke or Transient Ischemic Attack

Schwamm LH, Fonarow GC, Reeves MJ, et al (Massachusetts General Hosp, Boston, MA; UCLA Med Ctr, Los Angeles, CA; Michigan State Univ, East Lansing; et al)
Circulation 119:107-115, 2009

Background.—Adherence to evidence-based guidelines for treatment of stroke or transient ischemic attack is suboptimal. We sought to establish whether participation in Get With the Guidelines–Stroke was associated with improvements in adherence.

Methods and Results.—This prospective, nonrandomized, national quality improvement program measured adherence to guideline recommendations in 322 847 hospitalized patients discharged with a diagnosis of ischemic stroke or transient ischemic attack. A volunteer sample of 790 US academic and community hospitals participated from 2003 through 2007. The main outcome measures were change in adherence over time to 7 prespecified performance measures and a composite measure (total number of interventions provided in eligible patients divided by total number of care opportunities among eligible patients). Generalized estimating equations were used to identify factors associated with improvement. Participation in Get With the Guidelines–Stroke was associated with improvements in the 7 individual and 1 composite measures from baseline to the fifth year: intravenous thrombolytics (42.09% versus 72.84%), early antithrombotics (91.46% versus 97.04%), deep vein thrombosis prophylaxis (73.79% versus 89.54%), discharge antithrombotics (95.68% versus 98.88%), anticoagulation for atrial fibrillation (95.03% versus 98.39%), lipid treatment for low-density lipoprotein > 100 mg/dL (73.63% versus 88.29%), smoking cessation (65.21% versus 93.61%), and composite (83.52% versus 93.97%) ($P < 0.0001$ for all comparisons). Multivariate analysis showed that time in Get With the Guidelines–Stroke was associated with a 1.18-fold yearly increase in the odds of fulfilling care opportunities that was independent of secular trends.

Conclusions.—Get With the Guidelines–Stroke participation was associated with increased adherence to all stroke performance measures. Markedly improved stroke care was seen in all hospitals regardless of size, geography, and teaching status.

▶ Acute stroke (AS) protocols are institution based, and the practice pattern may be significantly different among hospitals. The current multidisciplinary group guideline for AS[1] is based on solid evidence, and the adherence to evidence-based guidelines for AS is shown in this article to be correlating with improved stroke care, including not only for the acute care involving the use of thrombolysis, but also variables that are important for secondary stroke prevention. Increasing the rate of use of thrombolytic therapy and improved secondary stroke prevention may lead to even greater positive impact beyond what was found in this 4-year observation period, further signifying the importance. As it was mentioned in the article, a drawback of this study was that the study population was based on voluntary participation, making the observed data not applicable to the centers that chose not to participate in the survey.

K. Lee, MD

Reference

1. Adams HP Jr, Del Zoppo G, Alberts MJ, et al. Guidelines for the early management of adults with ischemic stroke: a guideline from the American Heart Association/American Stroke Association Stroke Council, Clinical Cardiology Council, Cardiovascular Radiology and Intervention Council, and the Atherosclerotic Peripheral Vascular Disease and Quality of Care Outcomes in Research Interdisciplinary Working Groups: the American Academy of Neurology affirms the value of this guideline as an educational tool for neurologists. *Circulation.* 2007;115: e478-e534.

Off-Hour Admission and In-Hospital Stroke Case Fatality in the Get With The Guidelines-Stroke Program

Reeves MJ, on behalf of the GWTG-Stroke Steering Committee & Investigators (Michigan State Univ, East Lansing; et al)
Stroke 40:569-576, 2009

Background and Purpose.—Previous reports have shown higher in-hospital mortality for patients with acute stroke who arrived on weekends compared with regular workdays. We analyzed the effect of presenting during off-hours, defined as weekends and weeknights (versus weekdays), on in-hospital mortality and on quality of care in the Get With The Guidelines (GWTG)-Stroke program.

Methods.—We analyzed data from 187 669 acute ischemic stroke and 34 845 acute hemorrhagic stroke admissions who presented to the emergency departments of 857 hospitals that participated in the GWTG-Stroke program during the 4-year period 2003 to 2007. Off-hour presentation was defined as presentation anytime outside of 7:00 AM to 6:00 PM on weekdays. Quality of care was measured using standard GWTG quality indicators covering acute, subacute, and discharge measures. The relationship between off-hour presentation and in-hospital case fatality was examined using generalized estimating equation logistic regression adjusting for demographics, risk factors, arrival mode, and hospital characteristics.

Results.—Half of ischemic stroke admissions and 57% of hemorrhagic stroke admissions presented during off-hours. Among ischemic stroke admissions, the in-hospital case fatality rate was 5.8% for off-hour presentation compared with 5.2% for on-hour presentation ($P < 0.001$). For hemorrhagic stroke admissions, in-hospital case fatality was 27.2% for off-hour presentation compared with 24.1% for on-hour presentation

($P < 0.001$). After adjusting for patient-level and hospital-level factors, presentation during off-hours was significantly associated with higher in-hospital mortality for both ischemic stroke (adjusted OR, 1.09; 95% CI, 1.03 to 1.14) and hemorrhagic stroke admissions (adjusted OR, 1.19; 95% CI, 1.12 to 1.27). No differences were observed between off-hour presentation and any of the quality of care measures.

Conclusions.—Off-hour presentation was associated with an increased risk of dying in-hospital, although the absolute effect was small for ischemic stroke admissions (0.6% difference; number needed to harm = 166) and moderate for hemorrhagic stroke (3.1% difference; number needed to harm = 32). Reducing the disparity in hospital-based outcomes for admissions that present during off-hours represents a potential target for quality improvement efforts, although evidence of differences in the quality of care by time of presentation was lacking.

▶ A few large well-designed studies have been published in recent years suggesting that day of the week and time of day are independent risk factors relating to patient mortality. One of these studies reported increased mortality in 23 out of 100 conditions and delay in the timing of critical procedures.[1] Two studies have also reported increased mortality risk in patients admitted to the hospital due to myocardial infarction.[2,3] The authors analyzed 187 699 acute ischemic stroke and 34 845 hemorrhagic stroke admissions who presented to the emergency departments of 857 participating hospitals in Canada. Off-hour admissions were defined as those occurring outside of the time period between 7:00 AM and 6:00 PM or during weekends. In-hospital case-fatality rate in ischemic stroke admissions was higher for off-hour presentation at 5.8% compared with 5.2% for on-hour presentation ($P < .001$). In hemorrhagic stroke admissions case fatality was 24.1 for on-hour presentation and 27.2 for off-hour presentation ($P < .001$). Adjusting for confounding did not eliminate this association.

This article brings to our attention statistical evidence of something that has been intuitively assumed by clinicians for years. The effect of off-hour admission on patient mortality is less pronounced than others have hypothesized with a number needed to harm of 166 off-hour admissions. Characteristics inherent to the Canadian National Health System may make the results of this trial difficult to generalize. Previous studies performed in California have failed to find a similar association, but further research is needed into the topic.[4] Eliminating the difference between outcomes during on and off-hours will surely be the focus of further attention as we continue to debate on the allocation of resources and the improvement of cost-effective medical interventions.

K. Lee, MD

References

1. Bell CM, Redelmeier DA. Waiting for urgent procedures on the weekend among emergently hospitalized patients. *Am J Med.* 2004;117:175-181.
2. Kostis WJ, Demissie K, Marcella SW, et al, Myocardial Infarction Data Acquisition System (MIDAS 10) Study Group. Weekend versus weekday admission and mortality from myocardial infarction. *N Engl J Med.* 2007;356:1099-1109.

3. Magid DJ, Wang Y, Herrin J, et al. Relationship between time of day, day of week, timeliness of reperfusion, and in-hospital mortality for patients with acute ST-segment elevation myocardial infarction. *JAMA*. 2005;294:803-812.
4. Cram P, Hillis SL, Barnett M, Rosenthal GE. Effects of weekend admission and hospital teaching status on in-hospital mortality. *Am J Med*. 2004;117:151-157.

Patients with Acute Stroke Treated with Intravenous tPA 3–6 Hours after Stroke Onset: Correlations between MR Angiography Findings and Perfusion- and Diffusion-weighted Imaging in the DEFUSE Study

Marks MP, On behalf of the DEFUSE investigators (Stanford Univ Med Ctr, CA; et al)

Radiology 249:614-623, 2008

Purpose.—To study magnetic resonance (MR) angiography findings in patients with acute stroke treated with intravenous tissue plasminogen activator (tPA) in relationship to perfusion- and diffusion-weighted imaging changes and clinical outcome.

Materials and Methods.—Patients treated with intravenous tPA 3–6 hours after stroke onset (with informed consent) were evaluated in a HIPAA-compliant multicenter prospective study approved by all institutional review boards. MR imaging and MR angiography studies were performed before and 3–6 hours after treatment. MR angiography studies that were technically adequate at both time points were evaluated for occlusion, decreased flow, any early recanalization, and degree of recanalization. These results were compared with favorable clinical response (an improvement in National Institutes of Health Stroke Scale score of ≥ 8 points at 30 days or a modified Rankin scale score of 0 or 1 at 30 days) in patients with and those without mismatch between perfusion- and diffusion- weighted imaging at baseline.

Results.—Seventy-four patients were enrolled in the initial investigation; pre-and posttreatment MR angiography studies were both technically adequate in 62 patients. MR angiography demonstrated occlusion or decreased flow in 46 patients. Patients with isolated middle cerebral artery (MCA) occlusion and early recanalization at MR angiography had higher rates of favorable clinical response than those with tandem internal carotid artery–MCA occlusion and early recanalization ($P = .05$). Any early recanalization was not associated with favorable clinical response, but degree of recanalization did correlate with favorable clinical response ($P = .048$). Favorable clinical response was more frequently seen in patients with mismatch between perfusion- and diffusion-weighted imaging findings at baseline who experienced early recanalization than in those who did not have early recanalization (odds ratio = 6.2; 95% confidence interval: 1.3, 30.2; $P = .021$). No relationship between early recanalization and favorable clinical response was seen in patients without mismatch.

Conclusion.—Early recanalization seen at MR angiography before and after treatment coupled with diffusion- and perfusion-weighted imaging data may predict clinical outcome in patients with stroke treated with tPA 3–6 hours after symptom onset.

▶ The intra-arterial intervention—whether thrombolytic or mechanical thrombectomy—has shown some promising results in recanalization rate in acute ischemic patients. Among investigators, efforts have been made to identify useful clinical or radiographic predictors for long outcome after the use of these advanced interventional techniques. The notion of "mismatch" between diffusion-weighted image and perfusion-weighted image (either by CT or MR perfusion studies) may provide valuable information in terms of the presence and magnitude of the brain regions at risk, so called ischemic penumbra.[1] The danger zone defined by the ischemic penumbra is at risk for turning into an irreversible damage and the intervention to achieve vessel recanalization is geared toward salvaging this area at risk. As the advancement in interventional technique and more innovative devices and thrombolytic therapies become available, it appears to be equally important to be able to stratify the stroke patient population into different categories. Depending on each category's need, appropriate adjustments in intervention may lead to better results, especially in salvaging the tissue at risk.

K. Lee, MD

Reference

1. Cho TH, Hermier M, Alawneh JA, et al. Total mismatch: negative diffusion-weighted imaging but extensive perfusion defect in acute stroke. *Stroke*. 2009; 40:3400-3402.

Strokes After Cardiac Surgery and Relationship to Carotid Stenosis
Li Y, Walicki D, Mathiesen C, et al (Lehigh Valley Hosp and Health Network, Allentown, PA)
Arch Neurol 66:1091-1096, 2009

Objective.—To critically examine the role of significant carotid stenosis in the pathogenesis of postoperative stroke following cardiac operations.

Design.—Retrospective cohort study.

Setting.—Single tertiary care hospital.

Participants.—A total of 4335 patients undergoing coronary artery bypass grafting, aortic valve replacement, or both.

Main Outcome Measures.—Incidence, subtype, and arterial distribution of stroke.

Results.—Clinically definite stroke was detected in 1.8% of patients undergoing cardiac operations during the same admission. Only 5.3% of these strokes were of the large-vessel type, and most strokes (76.3%) occurred without significant carotid stenosis. In 60.0% of cases, strokes identified via computed tomographic head scans were not confined to a single carotid artery territory. According to clinical data, in 94.7% of patients, stroke occurred without direct correlation to significant carotid stenosis. Undergoing combined carotid and cardiac operations increases the risk of postoperative stroke compared with patients with a similar degree of carotid stenosis but who underwent cardiac surgery alone (15.1% vs 0%; $P = .004$).

Conclusions.—There is no direct causal relationship between significant carotid stenosis and postoperative stroke in patients undergoing cardiac operations. Combining carotid and cardiac procedures is neither necessary nor effective in reducing postoperative stroke in patients with asymptomatic carotid stenosis.

▶ Li and colleagues report on a retrospective cohort assessing the association between severe carotid stenosis and postoperative, clinically defined stroke. They found 1.8% (76) of the 4335 patients were diagnosed with a clinically evident stroke. Only 5% of these postoperative strokes in the cohort were judged as "large vessel type" using the Trial of Org 10172 in Acute Stroke Treatment (TOAST) classification.[1] A large artery lesion was defined by (a) cortical or cerebellar lesions, subcortical or brainstem lesions of more that 1.5 cm; and (b) ≥50% stenosis in the internal carotid or basilar artery. Of note, >76% of the strokes developed in the absence of significant (defined as ≥50% stenosis) carotid artery narrowing, and 77.8% occurred outside the territory of the diseased carotid artery. Despite the limitations inherent to this retrospective trial, namely that they only captured clinically apparent strokes (ie, patients were not systematically assessed in a standardized fashion for perioperative stroke), this article reraises the very important question about the value of preoperative carotid assessment in asymptomatic patients. Importantly, even if this test exhibited better performance (positive predictive value <10%), it is uncertain what is the best way to approach patients who have even the most severe disease. In this cohort, although the numbers were small, 15% of the 53 patients who underwent a combined carotid and cardiac operation suffered a clinically evident stroke, compared with 0 out of 16 with a staged operation, 1 out of 5 that had preoperative carotid stenting, and 0 out of 16 patients with ≥80% stenosis and no perioperative intervention. There are no convincing data to tell us whether a combined carotid-cardiac procedure or a staged procedure would be the optimal approach for patients with even the most severe disease, eg, patients presenting with neurological and cardiac symptomatology. This study suggests that the risk of a combined procedure results in a significantly higher incidence of stroke and should be avoided and that there seems to be no correlation between the site of stroke and the site of carotid disease. There remains a need for a randomized trial to ascertain the best intervention for the highest-risk patients. With the increasing use of carotid stenting for occlusive disease, this question will only be able to be answered conclusively if less invasive approaches are included in such a trial.

E. A. Martinez, MD, MHS

Reference

1. Adams HP Jr, Bendixen BH, Kappelle LJ, et al. Classification of subtype of acute ischemic stroke. Definitions for use in a multicenter clinical trial. TOAST. Trial of Org 10172 in Acute Stroke Treatment. *Stroke*. 1993;24:35-41.

Sonographic monitoring of mass effect in stroke patients treated with hypothermia. Correlation with intracranial pressure and matrix metalloproteinase 2 and 9 expression

Horstmann S, Koziol JA, Martinez-Torres F, et al (Univ of Heidelberg, Germany; The Scripps Res Inst, La Jolla, CA; et al)
J Neurol Sci 276:75-78, 2009

Severe stroke leads to subsequent cerebral oedema. Patients with severe stroke develop midline shift (MLS) which can be measured by transcranial duplex sonography (TCD). We measured MLS with TCD in 30 patients with large infarction in the territory of the middle cerebral artery (MCA). All of the examined patients had intracranial pressure (ICP) measure devices and the ICP at the time of the TCD was recorded. MLS was also determined on CT scan on day 4. Ten of the 30 patients were treated with hypothermia. We also determined matrix metalloproteinase 2 (MMP2) and matrix metalloproteinase 9 (MMP9) in serum by zymography.

MLS measured by TCD correlated significantly with MLS on CT. In addition there was a strong correlation between the ICP measured at the time of TCD and MLS. In patients treated with hypothermia MLS was less pronounced. MMP9 and MMP2 showed a characteristic time course and had strong associations with MLS. We confirm earlier reports that TCD is a reliable noninvasive method for serially monitoring patients with intracranial lesions. Hypothermia reduces MMP9 activity as well as MLS. TCD may reduce the need for repetitive CT scans in neurological critically ill patients.

▶ Monitoring of patients with large hemispheric infarction often requires frequent neuroradiological follow-up to promptly identify neurological worsening. However, it is often hampered by the patient's unstable condition; hence, this raises a need for less invasive but comparably accurate diagnostic tools including radiological or biophysical markers. Transcranial duplex sonography (TCD) is a noninvasive tool with a fairly good correlation with brain CT in measuring midline shift (MLS),[1] and matrix metalloproteinase 9 (MMP-9) is reported to reflex ischemic stroke burdens in animals and patients.[2,3]

This article focuses on the predictability of MLS using bedside monitoring with TCD in patients with large hemispheric stroke. It is notable that MLS assessed by CT and TCD showed a good correlation, and intracranial pressure also was well correlated with MLS on TCD. It suggests the possibility of TCD as a bedside monitoring tool for patients with hemispheric infarction. The authors tried to prove the beneficial effect of hypothermia; however, they did not find any significant change with regard to the level of MMP9.

K. Lee, MD

References

1. Stolz E, Gerriets T, Fiss I, Babacan SS, Seidel G, Kaps M. Comparison of transcranial color-coded duplex sonography and cranial CT measurements for determining third ventricle midline shift in space-occupying stroke. *AJNR Am J Neuroradiol.* 1999;20:1567-1571.
2. Koh SH, Chang DI, Kim HT, et al. Effect of 3-aminobenzamide, PARP inhibitor, on matrix metalloproteinase-9 level in plasma and brain of ischemic stroke model. *Toxicology.* 2005;214:131-139.
3. Park KP, Rosell A, Foerch C, et al. Plasma and brain matrix metalloproteinase-9 after acute focal cerebral ischemia in rats. *Stroke.* 2009;40:2836-2842.

IV t-PA therapy in acute stroke patients with atrial fibrillation

Kimura K, Iguchi Y, Shibazaki K, et al (Kawasaki Med School, Okayama, Japan)
J Neurol Sci 276:6-8, 2009

Background and Purpose.—Atrial fibrillation (AF) is a predictor for severe stroke. Intravenous administration of tissue plasminogen activator (t-PA) can improve clinical outcomes in patients with acute ischemic stroke. We investigated clinical characteristics and patient outcome in patients with and without AF after t-PA therapy.

Methods.—Consecutive ischemic stroke patients treated with t-PA within 3 h of stroke onset were studied prospectively. MRI examinations, including diffusion weighted imaging and MRA, were performed before t-PA thrombolysis. NIHSS scores were obtained before and 7 days after t-PA infusion. The patients were divided into two groups (AF group and Non-AF group). Their clinical characteristics and outcome 7 days and 3 months after t-PA therapy were compared.

Results.—85 patients (56 males, mean age, 73.4 ± 11.5 years) were enrolled in the present study. The AF-group had 44 patients, and the Non-AF group had 41 patients. Fewer patients with AF had dramatic improvement at 7 days and favorable outcome (mRS 0–1) at 3 months after t-PA therapy than patients without AF (31.8% vs. 61.0%, $P = 0.007$, and 15.9% vs. 46.3%, $P = 0.002$). On the other hand, worsening at 7 days and poor outcome (mRS > 3 and death) at 3 months after t-PA therapy were more frequently observed in AF group than Non-AF group (22.7% vs. 9.8%, $P = 0.107$, and 70.5% vs. 41.5%, $P = 0.007$). After adjusting age and gender, patients with AF more frequently had worsening and poor outcome than those without AF (adjusted OR; 4.54, 95% CI 1.04–19.75, $P = 0.044$, and adjusted OR; 2.8, 95% CI 1.10–7.28, $P = 0.032$).

Conclusion.—The present study found that acute ischemic stroke patients with AF more frequently had poor outcome after IV-t-PA therapy compared with those without AF.

▶ It has been suggested that the early recanalization achieved during thrombolytic therapy after acute ischemic stroke is associated with improved outcome.[1] In the past years, intravenous and intra-arterial thrombolytic therapy and thrombectomy intervention have been used increasingly with various recanalization rates and long-term outcome results. Despite some promising results in terms of reopening of the occluded vessels, the intra-arterial intervention has not been shown to improve the long-term outcome as of yet. Stroke remains a heterogeneous disease, not only in terms of the etiology but also in terms of the nature of the clot. As the authors of this article point out, there are multiple factors contributing to the long-term outcome, one of which includes the density and the texture of the clot. In case of the cardioembolic stroke due to atrial fibrillation, the densities of some of the "old" clots are found to be well organized with tremendously increased density. These calcified, well-organized clots are known to be resistant to conventional thrombolytic agents, therefore leading to poor recanalization rates. Different technologies and pharmacotherapies are needed depending on the type of the clot and the likely etiology of the stroke subtypes in order to improve the success rate defined by the recanalization and possibly even long-term outcome.

K. Lee, MD

Reference

1. Molina CA, Alexandrov AV, Demchuk AM, et al, CLOTBUST Investigators. Improving the predictive accuracy of recanalization on stroke outcome in patients treated with tissue plasminogen activator. *Stroke.* 2004;35:151-156.

Prognostic Value of Brain Diffusion-Weighted Imaging after Cardiac Arrest
Wijman CAC, Mlynash M, Caulfield AF, et al (Stanford Univ, Palo Alto, CA; et al)
Ann Neurol 65:394-402, 2009

Objective.—Outcome prediction is challenging in comatose postcardiac arrest survivors. We assessed the feasibility and prognostic utility of brain diffusion-weighted magnetic resonance imaging (DWI) during the first week.

Methods.—Consecutive comatose postcardiac arrest patients were prospectively enrolled. AWI data of patients who met predefined specific prognostic criteria were used to determine distinguishing apparent diffusion coefficient (ADC) thresholds. Group 1 criteria were death at 6 months *and* absent motor response or absent pupillary reflexes *or* bilateral absent cortical responses at 72 hours *or* vegetative at 1 month. Group 2 criterion was survival at 6 months with a Glasgow Outcome Scale score of 4 or 5 (group 2A) or 3 (group 2B). The percentage of voxels below different ADC thresholds was calculated at 50×10^{-6} mm^2/sec intervals.

Results.—Overall, 86% of patients underwent DWI. Fifty-one patients with 62 brain DWIs were included. Forty patients met the specific prognostic criteria. The percentage of brain volume with an ADC value less than 650 to 700×10^{-6} mm^2/sec best differentiated between Group 1 and Groups 2A and 2B combined ($p < 0.001$), whereas the 400 to 450×10^{-6} mm^2/sec threshold best differentiated between Groups 2A and 2B ($p = 0.003$). The ideal time window for prognostication using DWI was between 49 and 108 hours after the arrest. When comparing DWI in this time window with the 72-hour neurological examination, DWI improved the sensitivity for predicting poor outcome by 38% while maintaining 100% specificity ($p = 0.021$).

Interpretation.—Quantitative DWI in comatose postcardiac arrest survivors holds promise as a prognostic adjunct.

▶ The ability to predict brain death or severe neurologic impairment after an arrest is an important aspect of care provided for the patient and their family. Presently, neurologic exam along with ancillary testing such as somatosensory-evoked potentials (SSEPs) and electroencephalogram (EEG) are used. Prognosis is most commonly not made in the first 72 hours and may not be made until a week or later after the event. The financial cost of care may thus be elevated while providing limited value to the patient and family. The family's emotional stress may be increased as well during these time frames. Access to a bed may also be inhibited during this time frame in units with high occupancy and high demand rates. Thus, the ability to accurately prognosticate sooner would be of great value in this population. These authors evaluated diffusion-weighted imaging by MRI as a possible tool. Although they indeed found an improvement in sensitivity for predicting bad outcomes as compared with clinical exam (Table 2), the positive predictive value was unchanged. In addition, SSEPs were also found to be predictive if there were no recordable evoked potentials bilaterally. Thus, the MRI seemed to offer little advantage over presently used methodologies, and the data showed that the diffusion imaging was still demonstrating changes through the first 72 hours, thus not

TABLE 2.—Comparison of the Prognostic Value of the Neurological Examination and Quantitative Diffusion-Weighted Magnetic Resonance Imaging in 32 Patients with Diffusion-Weighted Magnetic Resonance Imaging Obtained between 49 and 108 Hours after the Arrest

Test Type	Poor Outcome (n)	FP	FN	TP	TN	Sensitivity	Specificity	PPV	NPV
Neurological examination	21	0	12	9	11	43%	100%	100%	48%
MRI	21	0	4	17	11	81%	100%	100%	73%

FP = number of patients with a false-positive test result; FN = number of patients with a false-negative test result; TP = number of patients with a true positive test result; TN = number of patients with a true negative test result; PPV = positive predictive value; NPV = negative predictive value. MRI = Magnetic Resonance Imaging.

making it a useful early predictor. The fact that the negative predictive value was significantly better than neurologic exam is intriguing and needs further study. Maybe if the cut value is altered, this value could be improved to the high 90%, which is where it would be needed to be truly clinically useful.

T. Dorman, MD

Scandinavian clinical practice guidelines for therapeutic hypothermia and post-resuscitation care after cardiac arrest
Castrén M, Silfvast T, Rubertsson S, et al (Karolinska Ins, Stockholm, Sweden; Helsinki Univ Central Hosp, Finland; Uppsala Univ Hosp, Sweden; et al)
Acta Anaesthesiol Scand 53:280 288, 2009

Background and Aim.—Sudden cardiac arrest survivors suffer from ischaemic brain injury that may lead to poor neurological outcome and death. The reperfusion injury that occurs is associated with damaging biochemical reactions, which are suppressed by mild therapeutic hypothermia (MTH). In several studies MTH has been proven to be safe, with few complications and improved survival, and is recommended by the International Liaison of Committee on Resuscitation. The aim of this paper is to recommend clinical practice guidelines for MTH treatment after cardiac arrest from the Scandinavian Society of Anaesthesiology and Intensive Care Medicine (SSAI).

Methods.—Relevant studies were identified after two consensus meetings of the SSAI Task Force on Therapeutic Hypothermia (SSAITFTH) and via literature search of the Cochrane Central Register of Controlled Trials and Medline. Evidence was assessed and consensus opinion was used when high-grade evidence (Grade of Recommendation, GOR) was unavailable. A management strategy was developed as a consensus from the evidence and the protocols in the participating countries.

Results and Conclusion.—Although proven beneficial only for patients with initial ventricular fibrillation (GOR A), the SSAITFTH also recommend MTH after restored spontaneous circulation, if active treatment is chosen, in patients with initial pulseless electrical activity and asystole (GOR D). Normal ethical considerations, premorbid status, total anoxia time and general condition should decide whether active treatment is required or not. MTH should be part of a standardized treatment protocol, and initiated as early as possible after indication and treatment have been decided (GOR E). There is insufficient evidence to make definitive recommendations among techniques to induce MTH, and we do not know the optimal target temperature, duration of cooling and rewarming time. New studies are needed to address the question as to how MTH affects, for example, prognostic factors.

▶ There are multiple randomized controlled trials showing improved outcomes for patients who received therapeutic hypothermia after surviving cardiac arrest.[1,2] It still remains unknown whether the initiating time of the cooling makes any difference in outcome. It is also not clear whether the speed of cooling makes any difference. For practitioners who treat patients with cardiac arrest, these are valid and yet difficult-to-answer questions. Considering the fact that there is now an increasing body of literature on the beneficial effect on outcomes on rapid treatment (eg, thrombolytic therapy for acute ischemic stroke), it makes logical sense to provide faster onset with more rapid cooling for all cardiac arrest survivors in an attempt to reduce disability and improve outcomes. Such a conclusion, however, can only be made after further investigations.

K. Lee, MD

References

1. The Hypothermia After Cardiac Arrest (HACA) Study Group. Mild therapeutic hypothermia to improve the neurologic outcome after cardiac arrest. *N Engl J Med.* 2002;346:549-556.
2. Bernard SA, Gray TW, Buist MD, et al. Treatment of comatose survivors of out-of-hospital cardiac arrest with induced hypothermia. *N Engl J Med.* 2002;346: 557-563.

Early achievement of mild therapeutic hypothermia and the neurologic outcome after cardiac arrest
Wolff B, Machill K, Schumacher D, et al (HELIOS Kliniken Schwerin, Germany)
Int J Cardiol 133:223-228, 2009

Background.—Mild therapeutic hypothermia (MTH) achieved by endovascular cooling has emerged as a new treatment strategy to reduce hypoxic brain injury after cardiac arrest (CA). It remains to be established how the time interval between CA and MTH impacts the neurologic outcome. We hypothesized that a more rapid achievement of MTH (time to target temperature [TTT], time to coldest temperature [TCT]) improves the outcome after CA.

Methods.—Forty-nine consecutive patients successfully resuscitated from CA were enrolled. MTH with a body core temperature between 32.0 and 34.0°C (target temperature: 33.0°C) over 24 h was achieved using a closed-loop endovascular system. Based on the neurologic outcome at discharge, the patient group was dichotomized into good (no/mild cerebral disability) and poor (severe disability, coma/vegetative state, brain death) outcomes. Serum neurone specific enolase (NSE) as biochemical marker of brain damage was sampled at 24, 48, and 72 h after CA.

Results.—Twenty-eight patients were discharged with a good outcome. Multivariate stepwise regression showed TTT (odds ratio for every h TTT: 0.69 [95% confidence interval: 0.51–0.98]) or, if entered into the model, TCT (odds ratio for every h TCT: 0.72 [95% confidence interval: 0.56–0.94]) to be independent predictors for good outcome. Further independent determinants were age, BMI, asystole as presenting rhythm, and thrombolysis during resuscitation. However, TCT was the only variable to correlate with maximum NSE values after CA ($r = 0.32$, $P < 0.05$).

Conclusions.—Early achievement of MTH by endovascular cooling appears to reduce hypoxic brain injury and to favour a good neurologic outcome after CA.

▶ Several trials have established mild therapeutic hypothermia as an effective neuroprotective agent in patients after cardiac arrest.[1,2] New protocols using external cooling devices,[3] intravascular cooling devices,[4] and ice-cold saline infusions[5] have been developed to bring core body temperature down quickly, safely, and reliably. Studies now need to focus on methods of inducing hypothermia and implementation in broad clinical settings.[6]

This study implemented an endovascular cooling system and focused on the time interval between cardiac arrest and induced hypothermia. The results show patients with good neurologic outcomes had on average lower body temperature after 1 hour of cooling and a shorter time interval between cardiac arrest and the lowest body temperature. They also found an association between the time to lowest temperature and neuron-specific enolase (NSE) levels, a marker of neuronal damage. The quicker patients were cooled, the lower the maximum NSE level. This is a preliminary attempt at addressing important questions regarding the ideal rate of induction of hypothermia and its effects on outcome, as well as correlations with serum markers of neuronal damage.

K. Lee, MD

References

1. Hypothermia after Cardiac Arrest Study Group. Mild therapeutic hypothermia to improve the neurologic outcome after cardiac arrest. *N Engl J Med*. 2002;346: 549-556.
2. Bernard SA, Gray TW, Buist MD, et al. Treatment of comatose survivors of out-of-hospital cardiac arrest with induced hypothermia. *N Engl J Med*. 2002;346: 557-563.
3. Mayer SA, Kowalski BS, Presciutti M, et al. Clinical trial of a novel surface cooling system for fever control in neurocritical care patients. *Crit Care Med*. 2004;32: 2508-2515.
4. Al-Senani FM, Graffagnino C, Grotta JC, et al. A prospective, multicenter pilot study to evaluate the feasibility and safety of using the coolgard system and icy catheter following cardiac arrest. *Resuscitation*. 2004;62:143-150.
5. Kim F, Olsufka M, Longstreth WT Jr, et al. Pilot randomized clinical trial of prehospital induction of mild hypothermia in out-of-hospital cardiac arrest patients with a rapid infusion of 4 degrees C normal saline. *Circulation*. 2007;115: 3064-3070.
6. Oddo M, Schaller MD, Feihl F, Ribordy V, Liaudet L. From evidence to clinical practice: effective implementation of therapeutic hypothermia to improve patient outcome after cardiac arrest. *Crit Care Med*. 2006;34:1865-1873.

The Early Evolution of Spinal Cord Lesions on MR Imaging Following Traumatic Spinal Cord Injury

Leypold BG, Klanders AE, Burns AS (Thomas Jefferson Univ Hosp, Philadelphia, PA)
AJNR Am J Neuroradiol 29:1012-1016, 2008

Background and Purpose.—How early spinal cord injury (SCI) lesions evolve in patients after injury is unknown. The purpose of this study was to characterize the early evolution of spinal cord edema and hemorrhage on MR imaging after acute traumatic SCI.

Materials and Methods.—We performed a retrospective analysis of 48 patients with clinically complete cervical spine injury. Inclusion criteria were the clear documentation of the time of injury and MR imaging before surgical intervention within 72 hours of injury. The length of intramedullary spinal cord edema and hemorrhage was assessed. The correlation between time to imaging and lesion size was determined by multiple regression analysis. Short-interval follow-up MR imaging was also available for a few patients ($n = 5$), which allowed the direct visualization of changes in spinal cord edema.

Results.—MR imaging demonstrated cord edema in 100% of patients and cord hemorrhage in 67% of patients. The mean longitudinal length of cord edema was 10.3 ± 4.0 U, and the mean length of cord hemorrhage was 2.6 ± 2.0 U. Increased time to MR imaging correlated to increased spinal cord edema length ($P = .002$), even after accounting for the influence of other variables. A difference in time to MR imaging of 1.2 days corresponded to an average increase in cord edema by 1 full vertebral level. Hemorrhage length was not affected by time to imaging ($P = .825$). A temporal increase in the length of spinal cord edema was confirmed in patients with short-interval follow-up MR imaging ($P = .003$).

Conclusion.—Spinal cord edema increases significantly during the early time period after injury, whereas intramedullary hemorrhage is comparatively static.

▶ Using regression analysis, the authors note evolution of edema in cervical spinal cord injuries, which is directly related to time from initial traumatic insult. The changes in spinal cord hemorrhage with cervical injury do not evolve similarly over time. These changes support the clinical observation that functional level of patients with spinal cord injury can evolve over the initial hours to days after trauma occurs ("secondary damage").[1,2]

Despite the attractive data for evolution of cord edema, the authors fail to provide coincident physical examination data. We can be reassured, however, that the likelihood of increasing spinal cord hemorrhage is low following this variety of injuries. The authors do not indicate the frequency with which decompressive neurosurgical interventions are required. Since the likelihood of increased bleeding is low, I suspect that the need for neurosurgeons based on spinal cord hemorrhage changes is also reduced.

Although limited by its retrospective nature, this clever study design provides information that cannot be obtained in any prospective format. My only question is why a dataset obtained several years before the publication was used in this work.

D. J. Dries, MSE, MD

References

1. Lindsey RW, Gugala Z, Pneumaticos SG. Injury to the vertebrae and spinal cord. In: Feliciano DV, Mattox KL, Moore EE, eds. *Trauma*. Sixth Edition. New York: McGraw Hill; 2008:479-512.
2. Chiles BW, Cooper PR. Acute spinal injury. *N Engl J Med*. 1996;334:514-520.

The relationship between the intracranial pressure–volume index and cerebral autoregulation

Lavinio A, Rasulo FA, De Peri E, et al (Univ of Brescia, Italy; et al)
Intensive Care Med 35:546-549, 2009

Objective.—The pressure–volume index (PVI) can be used to assess the cerebrospinal fluid dynamics and intracranial elastance in critically ill brain injured patients.

The dependency of PVI on the state of cerebral autoregulation within the physiologic range of cerebral perfusion pressure (CPP) can be described by mathematical models that account for changes in cerebral blood volume during PVI testing. This relationship has never been verified clinically using direct PVI measurement and independent cerebral autoregulation assessment.

Design, Setting, and Patients.—PVI and cerebral autoregulation were prospectively assessed in a cohort of 19 comatose patients admitted to an academic intensive care unit in Brescia, Italy.

Intervention.—None.

Methods.—PVI was measured injecting a fixed volume of 2 ml of 0.9% sodium chloride solution into the cerebral ventricles through an intraventricular catheter. Cerebral autoregulation was assessed using transcranial Doppler transient hyperaemic response (THR) test.

Measurements and Results.—Fifty-nine PVI assessments and 59 THR tests were performed. Mean PVI was 20.0 (SD 10.2) millilitres in sessions when autoregulation was intact (THR test ≥ 1.1) and 31.6 (8.8) millilitres in sessions with defective autoregulation (THR test < 1.1) ($\Delta PVI = 11.7$ ml, 95% $CI = 4.7$–19.3 ml; $P = 0.002$). Intracranial pressure, CPP and brain CT findings were not significantly different between the measurements with intact and disturbed autoregulation.

Conclusions.—Cerebral autoregulation status can affect PVI estimation despite a normal CPP. PVI measurement may overestimate the tolerance of the intracranial system to volume loads in patients with disturbed cerebral autoregulation.

▶ A cerebral pressure-volume index (PVI) can be calculated by observing intracranial pressure (ICP) and the ICP waveform after an intraventricular bolus injection in patients with an intraventricular catheter. The PVI can help identify subjects with exhausted intracranial buffering capacity before intracranial hypertension is evident. Autoregulation is the ability to maintain a constant cerebral blood flow across a range of cerebral perfusion pressures and can be tested using transcranial Doppler ultrasound.[1] Because blood represents an important part of the intracranial volume, it stands to reason that the status of autoregulation will affect the PVI. It is possible to describe the relationship of PVI and autoregulation via mathematical models. Fifty-nine measurements were obtained in 19 patients. Mean PVI was found to be 20.0 (SD 10.2) in cases of intact autoregulation and 31.6 (8.8) in cases of impaired autoregulation. This difference proved to be statistically significant with a $P = .002$.

This article highlights the importance of determining cerebral autoregulatory status for the understanding of a patient's pathophysiological state. Noninvasive and simple bedside measurements can be used to assess autoregulatory status. In critically ill patients necessitating placement of an intraventricular catheter, it is possible to identify PVI autoregulatory relationships.[2] Knowledge of this relationship may aid clinicians in compensating for the tendency of the PVI to overestimate the tolerance of the intracranial system in the face of impaired autoregulation.

K. Lee, MD

References

1. Giller CA. A bedside test for cerebral autoregulation using transcranial Doppler ultrasound. *Acta Neurochir (Wien).* 1991;108:7-14.
2. Andrews PJ, Citerio G. Intracranial pressure. Part one: historical overview and basic concepts. *Intensive Care Med.* 2004;30:1730-1733.

Inter-observer variability of the EEG diagnosis of seizures in comatose patients
Ronner HE, Ponten SC, Stam CJ, et al (VU Univ Med Ctr, Amsterdam, The Netherlands)
Seizure 18:257-263, 2009

Objective.—To assess the inter-observer agreement of the electroencephalogram (EEG) diagnosis of (non-convulsive) seizures in comatose patients.

Design/Setting/Patients.—Nine clinicians with different levels of experience in clinical neurophysiology were asked to evaluate in a strictly controlled way 90 epochs (10 s each) of 30 EEG's of 23 comatose patients admitted to the intensive care unit (ICU). For each EEG clinicians had to decide whether there was an electrographic seizure or not. Furthermore,

TABLE 2.—Kappa Scores for the Diagnosis Seizure and Proportion of Complete or Nearly Complete Consensus for Experienced and Inexperienced Observers

	Experienced Raters ($n = 5$)	Inexperienced Raters ($n = 4$)
Overall kappa score for diagnosis seizure	0.50	0.29
Consensus between all raters on presence or absence of seizure	15/30	12/30
Consensus in $n - 1$ raters on presence or absence of seizure	22/30	22/30

Young's EEG criteria for (non-convulsive) seizures were scored in detail for all EEG's. Agreement was determined by calculating kappa values.

Results.—The inter-observer agreement of an EEG diagnosis of seizure was limited. The overall kappa score for the five experienced raters was 0.5, and the kappa score for less experienced raters was 0.29. Kappa values for the individual Young's criteria were highly variable, indicating discrepancies in the interpretation of specific phenomena. Especially, some types of periodic discharges gave rise to different interpretations.

Conclusions.—The EEG diagnosis of (non-convulsive) seizures in ICU patients is not very reliable, even when strict criteria such as proposed by Young are applied. There is a need for less ambiguous EEG criteria for (non-convulsive) seizures and status epilepticus.

▶ As the use of standard EEG and processed EEG grows in clinical medicine, this is an important study regarding the validity and reliability of interpretation of such data. Clinicians require a high positive and negative predictive value from tests. Clinicians cannot be expected to interpret all tests and are highly reliant on the interpretation of a test that requires special skills like the reading of an EEG. Therapeutic interventions that have associated toxicity are at stake or the continuation of subclinical status. In addition, use of costly ICU/monitored bed resources are often dictated by findings from this test and as such accurate and reliable interpretations are required. As can be seen in Table 2, the overall kappa score ranged from 0.29 to 0.50. For those less familiar with kappa scoring, a value between 0.21 and 0.40 is considered only fair and a value between 0.41 and 0.60 is considered only moderate. Thus this study disturbingly shows a lack of correlation between interpretations of standard EEG. Limitations in this study include that the interpreters were trained for knowledge not competency and not all segments of the EEG were shown to them, but only representative samples.

T. Dorman, MD

Non-convulsive status epilepticus; the rate of occurrence in a general hospital

Alroughani R, Javidan M, Qasem A (Univ of British Columbia, Vancouver, Canada)
Seizure 18:38-42, 2009

Background.—Non-convulsive status epilepticus (NCSE) has been increasingly recognized as a cause of impaired level of consciousness in the ICU and emergency rooms. The diagnosis can be easily missed without an electroencephalogram (EEG) given the paucity of overt clinical signs in this condition. Recently few published data estimated the prevalence to be between 3% and 8%.

Objective.—To assess the rate of occurrence of NCSE among patients with various degrees of impaired consciousness referred to the Neurophysiology Laboratory at Vancouver General Hospital.

Method.—We conducted a retrospective analysis of 451 adult patients (>16 years of age) with a question of NCSE or with an unknown cause of impaired level of consciousness between the years 2002 and 2004. NCSE was defined according to the Young's criteria of electrographic status epilepticus. NCSE was categorized into focal and generalized epileptic activity based on the continuous EEG monitoring (CEEG). Further analysis of age, gender and etiology was performed.

Results.—Of 451 patients, EEG demonstrated electrographic status epilepticus with no overt clinical signs in 42 patients (9.3%). Median age was 61.8 years (range 21–94). According to etiology, 38.1% of patients with NCSE had hypoxic–anoxic injury, 19% had intracerebral hemorrhage (including trauma), 11.9% had the diagnosis of idiopathic or cryptogenic epilepsy, 7.1% had ischemic stroke, 4.8% were secondary to tumors and 4.8% to viral encephalitis.

Conclusion.—The rate of occurrence of NCSE in patients with decreased level of consciousness was 9.3%. The cohort represented a group of patients who were comatose and required assisted ventilation or had altered level of consciousness. Hypoxic brain injury was the most responsible etiology of NCSE in the cohort studied.

▶ Nonconvulsive status epilepticus (NCSE) is an important etiology to consider for any practicing intensivist due to (1) its proven existence in the critically ill patient population, and (2) its absent clinical signs of seizure despite being a true seizure activity. While there are conflicting data as to whether having NCSE is always an independent risk factor that leads to worse long-term outcome, emerging radiographic and neuropsychological testing data indicate that NCSE may lead to both neuronal damage as well as cognitive and behavioral problems.[1] From the functional MRI, SPECT, and PET studies, it has been shown that the seizure activities lead to cerebral hypermetabolism.[2] In ICU settings, elevated intracranial pressure (ICP), hypermetabolism with high demand of oxygen extraction can lead to significant brain damage. Normal brains do not necessarily get damaged by high ICP and abnormal brain metabolism rate. However, critically ill patients with severe brain injury may be particularly vulnerable to the effects of continuous seizure activities. For comatose patients in any type of ICU, NCSE should be considered as part of the differential diagnosis. This article, along with other currently available data, strongly endorses the importance of availability of continuous EEG monitoring in critically ill patients.

K. Lee, MD

References

1. Sutula TP, Hagen J, Pitkanen A. Do epileptic seizures damage the brain? *Curr Opin Neurol.* 2003;16:189-195.
2. la Fougére C, Rominger A, Förster S, Geisler J, Bartenstein P. PET and SPECT in epilepsy: a critical review. *Epilepsy Behav.* 2009;15:50-55.

The use of dynamic CT surview for cervical spine clearance in comatose trauma patients: A pilot prospective study

Anekstein Y, Jeroukhimov I, Bar-Ziv Y, et al (Tel Aviv Univ, Israel)
Injury 39:339-346, 2008

Background.—Bedside flexion and extension fluoroscopy was proposed for detecting occult ligamentous instability in comatose trauma patients. Nevertheless, a recent study showed that the C7–T1 motion segment is rarely visualised by this technique. We propose a new method for clearing the cervical spine in comatose patients.

Methods.—We conducted a prospective clinical pilot study on 31 consecutive comatose trauma patients to evaluate a new dynamic imaging technique for cervical spine clearance in comatose trauma patients. All patients were examined by a fine-cut helical CT scan of the entire cervical spine (C-spine) and by four-stage flexion–extension examination using the surview function of the CT scanner. The mean range of motion between extension and full flexion, the lowest visualised vertebrae, complications, positive findings, and the time from arrival to clearance was recorded.

Results.—The mean range of motion of the subaxial cervical spine was 39°. The C7–T1 segment was fully visualised at the CTsurview in 15 patients. The C6–C7 segment was visualised in all patients. No complication directly related to the study protocol was observed. C-spine clearance was completed in less than 6 h from arrival in 26 patients.

Conclusion.—The CTsurview allows better visualisation of the C6–C7 and cervicothoracic junctions during flexion and extension. A short series of CT cuts can be used when visualisation is inadequate. Further studies are needed to assess the risks and benefits of the suggested protocol.

▶ This is a small but intriguing study using CT technology to provide elements of flexion/extension imaging and high-resolution static CT images in patients with significant trauma such that clinical clearance of the cervical spine is impossible.[1,2] As noted by the authors, clearance of the cervical spine in comatose patients is a controversial matter. Many trauma centers will clear the cervical spine with high-resolution static CT scan while others demand either fluoroscopy with flexion/extension evaluation or magnetic resonance imaging.[3-7] Ideally, the latter is obtained within 72 hours of injury. However, coexisting injury frequently makes collection of MRI images impossible until the second week of hospitalization. Nonetheless, leaders in the trauma community continue to advocate MRI as a complementary imaging modality to high-resolution CT scans in assessment of the cervical spine in the comatose patient.[5-7] Regardless of the approach taken to identify cervical injuries, the likelihood of positive findings is relatively small and a large number of patients must be studied to support or refute the use of a particular technique.

These authors use the surview function (we call them scout views) to assess the cervical spine in flexion and extension and detect changes in angulation or orientation of cervical vertebrae. This technique is not as effective as true flexion/extension imaging as the spine is moved without direct observation. Moving of the spine in this protocol takes place before imaging occurs. Thus, the risk of injury exists prior to the collection of surview images.

The greatest limitation of this study is the small dataset. Thirty-one cases were retrieved in 6 months. This is a small number of comatose patients for acute evaluation in a major trauma center. As waiver of consent was obtained, what happened to the other patients?

With improving technology, CT may permit static and dynamic evaluation of the cervical spine. As practiced by these authors, the use of surview images is fraught with risk.

D. J. Dries, MSE, MD

References

1. Chiles BW, Cooper PR. Acute spinal injury. *N Engl J Med.* 1996;334:514-520.
2. Bagley LJ. Imaging of spinal trauma. *Radiol Clin North Am.* 2006;44:1-12.
3. Stelfox HT, Velmahos GC, Gettings E, Bigatello CM, Schmidt U. Computed tomography for early and safe discontinuation of cervical spine immobilization in obtunded multiply injured patients. *J Trauma.* 2007;63:630-636.
4. Chiu WC, Haan JM, Cushing BM, Kramer ME, Scalea TM. Ligamentous injuries of the cervical spine in unreliable blunt trauma patients: incidence, evaluation, and outcome. *J Trauma.* 2001;50:457-464.
5. Stassen NA, Williams VA, Gestring ML, Cheng JD, Bankey PE. Magnetic resonance imaging in combination with helical computed tomography provides a safe and efficient method of cervical spine clearance in the obtunded trauma patient. *J Trauma.* 2006;60:171-177.
6. Ackland HM, Cooper DJ, Malham GM, Stuckey SL. Magnetic resonance imaging for clearing the cervical spine in unconscious intensive care trauma patients. *J Trauma.* 2006;60:668-673.
7. Tomycz ND, Chew BG, Chang YF, et al. MRI is unnecessary to clear the cervical spine in obtunded/comatose trauma patients: the four-year experience of a level I trauma center. *J Trauma.* 2008;64:1258-1263.

Surgical Management and Case-fatality Rates of Intracerebral Hemorrhage in 1988 and 2005

Adeoye O, Woo D, Haverbusch M, et al (Univ of Cincinnati, OH)
Neurosurgery 63:1113-1118, 2008

Objective.—To compare surgical management and case-fatality rates of intracerebral hemorrhage (ICH) in 1988 and 2005.

Methods.—We identified all adult residents (age, $\geq$ 18 years) from the 5-county Greater Cincinnati region who were hospitalized with ICH in 1988 and 2005. Demographics, severity of illness, ICH volume, ICH location, rates and timing of surgery, and 30-day case-fatality rate were compared between the groups.

Results.—In 1988, 171 ICH patients (67 lobar, 80 deep cerebral, 10 brainstem, and 14 cerebellar) met the study criteria; in 2005, 259 ICH patients (91 lobar, 123 deep cerebral, 19 brainstem, and 26 cerebellar) met the study criteria. In 1988, 16% of the patients had surgical removal of their ICH versus 7% in 2005 ($P = 0.003$). In both 1988 and 2005, patients treated with surgery were younger ($P < 0.001$) and had a higher percentage of cerebellar hemorrhages than nonsurgical patients. The timing of surgery was similar in 1988 and 2005. In 1988, the 30-day case-fatality rate was 32% in surgical patients versus 50% in nonsurgical patients ($P = 0.06$). In 2005, the 30-day case-fatality rate was 16% (surgical) versus 45% (nonsurgical) ($P = 0.02$).

Conclusion.—The frequency of surgery for ICH was lower in 2005 than in 1988, which may reflect the influence of recent clinical trial data showing no benefit for surgery rather than medical management. The ICH case-fatality rate was essentially the same in 1988 and 2005. Innovative clinical trials to improve ICH outcomes are warranted.

▶ This article addresses an important and ongoing discussion regarding the surgical versus medical management of the patients with acute intracerebral hemorrhage (ICH). Authors indicate that the lower incidence of surgery may be secondary to the lack of evidence for surgical benefit based on the Surgical Trial in ICH (STICH) trial.[1] Retrospective observational studies such as this study face inevitable biases and limitations as pointed out in the Discussion section of the article. Besides the statistical limitation, the mortality and neurological functional outcome after acute ICH is heavily influenced by the timing of the surgery. The article does include this as a variable, but it is only within 12 hours of a surgical evacuation time window. In the setting of the cerebral herniation, performing surgery up to 12 hours after symptom onset/diagnosis may or may not be fast enough to make any differences. For some patients, potential benefits from surgery may be seen even beyond 12 hours. However, 12 hours may be too late for some patients. This is the unfortunate fact of how human brains have absolutely different margins as to how much and how long each brain can tolerate the harmful effect of the acute ICH. Time is brain, and each brain requires different deadlines. This raises a concern for even randomized trials. One may argue that this issue may be ameliorated by including all patients with the same clinical status (ie, same degree of mental status, pupillary changes, etc), but even then human brains behave differently as the herniation continues. While evidence-based practice is crucial, it should be emphasized that individualized management might be even more important in the setting of cerebral herniation.

K. Lee, MD

Reference

1. Mendelow AD, Gregson BA, Fernandes HM, et al. Early surgery versus initial conservative treatment in patients with spontaneous supratentorial intracerebral haematomas in the International Surgical Trial in Intracerebral Haemorrhage (STICH): a randomised trial. *Lancet.* 2005;365:387-397.

Clinical predictors of mechanical ventilation in Fisher/Guillain–Barré overlap syndrome

Funakoshi K, Kuwabara S, Odaka M, et al (Dokkyo Med Univ, Tochigi, Japan; Chiba Univ School of Medicine, Japan; et al)
J Neurol Neurosurg Psychiatry 80:60-65, 2009

Background.—Some patients with Fisher syndrome (FS) developed subsequent descending tetraparesis (Fisher/Guillain–Barré overlapping syndrome: FS/GBS). The assumption is that such descending progression may frequently lead to respiratory failure.

Objective.—To investigate whether patients with FS/GBS more often require artificial ventilation than those with typical GBS and which clinical and serological findings are useful predictors.

Methods.—Medical records were reviewed of patients who had acute ophthalmoplegia, ataxia and areflexia, as well as subsequent tetraparesis with monophasic course. Forty-five patients fulfilled the FS/GBS criteria. Clinical and serological features were analysed, and clinical predictors of mechanical ventilation were investigated.

Results.—FS/GBS patients more frequently required mechanical ventilation than did GBS patients (24% vs 10%, p = 0.04). The former also needed artificial ventilation earlier than the latter (p = 0.03), but none of the FS patients required it. As the initial symptom, ventilated FS/GBS patients more frequently showed titubation than non-ventilated patients (55% vs 18%, p = 0.04). During the course of the illness, descending tetraparesis was more common in 11 ventilated FS/GBS patients than in the other 34 non-ventilated patients (64% vs 21%, p = 0.02). The need for artificial ventilation was not associated with anti-GO1b IgG antibodies, monospecific anti-GT1a IgG antibodies or IgG antibodies to various ganglioside complexes.

Conclusions.—FS/GBS patients significantly needed mechanical ventilation more often. Such patients showing titubation and descending tetraparesis need to be carefully monitored as the illness progresses because those clinical features are helpful predictors of respiratory failure.

▶ This retrospective chart review studied the clinical predictors of respiratory failure and the need for mechanical ventilation, comparing Miller Fisher Variant (MFV), typical Guillain-Barré syndrome (GBS), and the combination of both MFV and GBS—so-called Fisher-Guillain Barré overlapping syndrome (FS/GBS). The statistically significant differences in predicting the respiratory failure among different clinical features is noteworthy as the initial clinical features can help clinicians regarding the level of respiratory monitoring. Descending, as opposed to ascending paralysis, being associated with higher risk for respiratory failure, is a valuable piece of information in managing the airway for these patients. As Charles Miller Fisher originally described, MFV is likely related closely to GBS, and the observation of differences in clinical predictors of mechanical ventilation simply might be secondary to the disease severity.[1] Nevertheless, the distinction between typical GBS and MFV-GBS overlap syndrome can now have clinical implications, and this is helpful at the bedside.

K. Lee, MD

Reference

1. Fisher CM. Syndrome of ophthalmoplegia, ataxia and areflexia. *N Eng J Med.* 1956;255:57-65.

Disappearing hyperdense middle cerebral artery sign in ischaemic stroke patients treated with intravenous thrombolysis: clinical course and prognostic significance

Kharitonova T, for the SITS investigators (Karolinska Univ Hosp, Stockholm, Sweden; et al)

J Neurol Neurosurg Psychiatry 80:273-278, 2009

Background and Purpose.—Hyperdense middle cerebral artery sign (HMCAS) on CT is a well known indication of thromboembolic arterial occlusion. Its disappearance after thrombolytic therapy is poorly described. Taking the rate of HMCAS disappearance as a surrogate for MCA recanalisation, its prognostic value after intravenous thrombolysis was examined.

Methods.—1905 stroke patients with HMCAS on admission CT scan in the Safe Implementation of Treatment in Stroke-International Stroke Thrombolysis Register (SITS-ISTR) were studied. On follow-up CT scans 22–36 h after thrombolysis, HMCAS disappeared in 831 cases, persisted in 788 and was uncertain in 122; follow-up CT was not done in 164 cases.

Results.—Patients whose HMCAS disappeared were younger (median age 67 years vs 69 years for persistent; p = 0.03), with milder stroke (admission National Institute of Health Stroke Scale (NIHSS) score was

16 vs 17; p<0.005) and were less likely to have early infarct signs on admission CT (26% vs 33%; p<0.005). Patients with disappearing HMCAS were more likely to have early improvement in NIHSS score (median improvement 2 vs 0 at 2 h; 4 vs 1 at 24 h), be independent at 3 months (42% vs 19%), with fewer deaths (15% vs 30%) than those with persistent HMCAS. In multivariate analysis, HMCAS disappearance independently predicted functional independence and survival. Early NIHSS improvement independently predicted HMCAS disappearance.

Conclusions.—HMCAS disappeared after intravenous thrombolysis in about half of cases and these patients had twice as good outcomes compared with those with persistent HMCAS. The prognosis in patients with MCA occlusion that persists after intravenous thrombolysis is poor, which may indicate the need for an alternative treatment approach to this subgroup.

▶ Hyperdense middle cerebral artery (MCA) sign seen on brain computed tomography usually represents acute stroke due to thromboembolic mechanism, and often signifies severe stroke with poor prognosis.[1] The M1 (proximal MCA) and carotid T lesion (top of the internal carotid artery occlusion) have been associated with poor prognosis, and the recanalization rate of these lesions after intravenous recombinant tissue plasminogen activator (IV TPA) therapy has been low.[2] However, more recent literature has reported better recanalization rates and outcomes with these lesions, raising a possibility that there may be other factors that play an important role in long-term outcome.[3,4] It is likely that the location of the occlusion alone is not the only factor in determining the outcome, and there may be even metabolic confounders such as presence or absence of severe diabetes.[5]

This article focuses on better defining the predictors of outcome based on the presence or disappearance of hyperdense MCA signs after IV TPA therapy. The positive association between the disappeared sign and improved outcome is not surprising as the disappearance of the hyperdensity suggests effective or at least partially effective thrombolysis. It is important to note, however, that when the disappearance of the hyperdense MCA sign occurs, this could also be due to self-mobilization of the clot, which may or may not be secondary to the effect of TPA.

K. Lee, MD

References

1. Barber PA, Demchuk AM, Hudon ME, Pexman JH, Hill MD, Buchan AM. Hyperdense sylvian fissure MCA "dot" sign: a CT marker of acute ischemia. *Stroke.* 2001;32:84-88.
2. Raninstein AA, Wijdicks EF, Nichols DA. Complete recovery after early intraarterial recombinant tissue plasminogen activator thrombolysis of carotid T occlusion. *AJNR Am J Neuroradiol.* 2002;23:1596-1599.
3. Georgiadis D, Oehler J, Schwarz S, Rousson V, Hartmann M, Schwab S. Does acute occlusion of the carotid T invariably have a poor outcome? *Neurology.* 2004;63:22-26.

4. Wunderlich M, Stolz E, Seidel G, et al, Duplex Sonography in Acute Stroke Study Group. Conservative medical treatment and intravenous thrombolysis in acute stroke from carotid T occlusion. *Cerebrovasc Dis.* 2005;20:355-361.

5. Zangerle A, Kiechl S, Spiegel M, et al. Recanalization after thrombolysis in stroke patients: predictors and prognostic implications. *Neurology.* 2007;68:39-44.

Comparison of the calculated and measured osmolality in intracranial bleeding and head injury patients

Açikgöz S, Can M, Mungan AG, et al (Zonguldak Karaelmas Univ, Turkey)
J Emerg Med 36:217-219, 2009

Not all clinical laboratories have an osmometer, and calculations for osmolality are a frequently used method for determining osmolality. The purpose of this study was to evaluate the performance of four formulas for the estimation of osmolality, with cryoscopic measurement as the reference standard in intracranial hemorrhage (ICH) and head injury (HI) patients who were not treated with mannitol. Forty HI and 31 ICH patients treated in the Neurosurgery Department were included in the study. Every 6 h over a period of 24 h, serum samples were collected from patients and osmolality was measured. In conclusion, our study shows that only formulas F1 [Osmolality = 1.86(Na) + 1.86(K) + Glucose + Urea] and F4 [Osmolality = 1.86(Na) + Glucose + Urea + Ethanol + 9] can be used to evaluate osmolality in ICH patients who were not treated with mannitol. In HI patients, none of the formulas should be used to calculate osmolality.

▶ Clinicians rely on calculated serum osmolality, specifically the osmolar gap, to assess for the use of hyperosmolar therapy in patients with intracranial hemorrhage or head injury.[1] The lack of osmometers to reliably measure the osmolality necessitates an accurate method of calculating serum osmolality. Several methods of calculating serum osmolality have been used and validated, but significant controversy exists regarding the most accurate equation.[1-3]

In this article osmolality was calculated using 4 different equations and compared with the measured osmolality. In intracranial hemorrhage (ICH) patients the equations: Osmolality = 1.86(Na) + 1.86(K) + Glucose + Urea[2] and Osmolality = 1.86 (Na) + Urea + Glucose + Ethanol + 9[3] were found to show good correlation with measured serum osmolality concentrations. In patients with head injury, none of the equations were shown to accurately calculate the osmolality. The results caution against the use of the calculated serum osmolality to estimate true serum osmolality, especially in head-injured patients.

K. Lee, MD

References

1. García-Morales EJ, Cariappa R, Parvin CA, Scott MG, Diringer MN. Osmole gap in neurologic-neurosurgical intensive care unit: its normal value, calculation, and

relationship with mannitol serum concentrations. *Critical Care Med.* 2004;32: 986-991.

2. Puliyel JM. Osmotonicity of acetoacetate: possible implications for cerebral edema in diabetic ketoacidosis. *Med Sci Monit.* 2003;9:BR130-BR133.

3. Dorwart WV, Chalmers L. Comparison of methods for calculating serum osmolality from chemical concentrations, and the prognostic value of such calculations. *Clin Chem.* 1975;21:190-194.

Microembolic signals in subarachnoid hemorrhage
Azarpazhooh MR, Velayati A, Chambers BR, et al (Mashhad Univ of Med Science (MUMS), Iran; Univ of Melbourne, Victoria, Australia)
J Clin Neurosci 16:390-393, 2009

Microembolic signals (MES) detected by transcranial Doppler (TCD) have been reported in subarachnoid hemorrhage (SAH), although their origin and contribution to brain ischemia remain uncertain. We conducted a prospective study to evaluate the frequency of MES among patients with SAH and to determine their origin. Twenty-seven patients with SAH, comprising 15 aneurysmal and 12 non-aneurysmal patients, participated in the study. TCD evaluation was performed using a 2 MHz probe. Patients were studied three times per week during their in-patient stay to detect vasospasm, and then each middle cerebral artery (MCA) was monitored for 30 min using the Monolateral Multigate mode to detect MES. Using this method, MES were detected in 7 out of 15 patients (47%) with aneurysmal SAH and were not seen in non-aneurysmal patients ($p = 0.007$). Vasospasm occurred in 52% (14/27) of cases. However, clinical signs and symptoms of vasospasm were identified in only 18.5% (5/27). There was no significant relationship between MES and vasospasm ($p = 0.224$). Also, no relationship was found between MES and the location of the aneurysm ($p = 0.685$). Thus, in this study MES were only detected in aneurysmal SAH. However, we did not find a relationship between the location of the aneurysm and MES, or the presence of vasospasm and MES. Therefore, MES in patients with SAH may also originate from vascular pathology other than the aneurysm sac or vascular spasm.

▶ Since the description of microembolic signals (MES) using transcranial Doppler ultrasonography has been reported, an increased level of attention has been paid to MES in a variety of vascular diseases.[1,2] Moreover, a growing body of evidence suggests that MES are closely related with embolic or ischemic phenomenon. Interestingly, MES have been reported in patients with aneurysmal subarachnoid hemorrhage (SAH).[3,4] Although the exact mechanism of MES was not known in SAH patients, it appears to be unrelated to vasospasm regardless of the location of aneurysm.[3] However, it shows a close association between MES and cerebral ischemic symptoms,[4] which is not surprising considering the fact that MES are originated from the impedance change from the microparticles.

This article focuses on a relationship between MES and vasospasm in SAH patients with or without underlying aneurysm. The lack of association between MES and vasospasm is not surprising. However, this article reiterates the significance of daily bedside monitoring and raises a question about a common phenomenon that requires further investigation.

K. Lee, MD

References

1. Spencer MP, Thomas GI, Nicholls SC, Sauvage LR. Detection of middle cerebral artery emboli during carotid endarterectomy. *Stroke.* 1990;21:415-423.
2. Spencer MP. Detection of Cerebral Arterial Emboli with Transcranial Doppler. In: Newell DW, Aaslid R, eds. *Transcranial Doppler.* New York, NY: Raven Press Ltd; 1992:215-230.
3. Romano JG, Forteza AM, Concha M, et al. Detection of microemboli by transcranial doppler ultrasonography in aneurysmal subarachnoid hemorrhage. *Neurosurgery.* 2002;50:1026-1030.
4. Romano JG, Rabinstein AA, Arheart KL, et al. Microemboli in aneurysmal subarachnoid hemorrhage. *J Neuroimaging.* 2008;18:396-401.

Intraarterial Therapy for Acute Ischemic Strokes
Belisle JG, McCollom VE, Tytle TL, et al (Univ of Oklahoma College of Medicine; Mercy Health Ctr, OK)
J Vasc Interv Radiol 20:327-333, 2009

Purpose.—To determine the safety and feasibility of intraarterial stroke therapy for acute ischemic strokes at a community-based medical center.

Materials and Methods.—This is a retrospective analysis of data gathered from consecutive stroke patients treated between June 2004 and April 2007. The following therapies were used to treat acute ischemic stroke within 6 hours of symptom onset: intraarterial thrombolytic drugs, intraarterial vasodilators, mechanical clot retrieval, intravascular stents, and angioplasty. The outcomes measured included posttherapy National Institutes of Health Stroke Score (NIHSS), neurologic function at 90 days graded according to the modified Rankin Scale (mRS), recanalization, symptomatic intracranial hemorrhage, and 90-day mortality.

Results.—Eighty-three patients with a median baseline NIHSS of 17 (range, 3–30) were treated with intraarterial therapy. The median posttherapy NIHSS was 5 (range, 0–33). Forty-two patients (76%) had an mRS score of 2 or less at 90 days. The recanalization rate was 76%. Five patients (6%) had symptomatic intracranial hemorrhage, and the 90-day mortality was 22%.

Conclusions.—The results of this review showed that an intraarterial therapeutic approach to acute ischemic stroke was feasible at a community-based heath center and demonstrated encouraging data for outcome and safety.

▶ The occlusive nature of the brain vasculature in all acute ischemic stroke cases has a similar pathophysiology in that the occlusion (due to various etiologies) leads to decreased perfusion followed by an irreversible infarction. There has been a great deal of effort among the investigators and interventionalists in trying to recanalize the acute occlusion using intra-arterial therapy. These therapies have evolved over time, and now there are different methods addressing both thrombolytic[1] methods as well as thrombectomy as the ultimate goal.[2] Brains are not resilient organs against ischemic injury and the notion of "time is brain" has been accepted by many. The technologies for achieving a more rapid and improved recanalization rate for acute ischemic stroke continue to evolve and get better, but there may be more to it than just the absolute time elapsed after the onset of the stroke symptoms: each stroke patient may have a different cerebrovascular margin with a different threshold for irreversible damage. Likewise, the rate of recanalization may not directly translate into improved long-term outcome. These are the challenges in developing new devices and techniques as well as designing a new stroke trial.

K. Lee, MD

References

1. Furlan A, Higashida R, Wechsler L, et al. Intra-arterial prourokinase for acute ischemic stroke. The PROACT II study: a randomized controlled trial. Prolyse in acute cerebral thromboembolism. *JAMA.* 1999;282:2003-2011.
2. Smith WS, Sung G, Saver J, et al. Mechanical thrombectomy for acute ischemic stroke: final results of the multi MERCI trial. *Stroke.* 2008;39:1205-1212.

12 Ethics/Socioeconomic/ Administrative Issues

Quality of Life/End of Life/Outcome Prediction

Donation after cardiac death: a survey of university student opinions on death and donation

Joffe AR, Byrne R, Anton NR, et al (Univ of Alberta, Edmonton, Canada)
Intensive Care Med 35:240-247, 2009

Objective.—To determine if university students consider the donation after cardiac death donor as dead.

Design.—Survey.

Setting.—University students.

Participants.—Medical ($n = 142$) and nursing ($n = 76$) students in a medical ethics class and philosophy students ($n = 102$).

Intervention.—Survey during class time with four patient scenarios in which a decision was made to donate organs after 5 min of absent circulation.

Measurements and Results.—Half the surveys had brief background information, and half had more detailed background information. Responses between groups were compared using the Chi-square statistic. The response rate of 320 students was 100%. In each scenario, 42–51% of those given detailed information strongly agree or agree that the patient is 'definitely dead', versus 55–58% given brief information (ns). When asked in what state this patient is, 26–30% given detailed information chose "dead," versus 41–45% given brief information ($P < 0.025$). Thirty-six to 39% given detailed information strongly agree or agree that the physician was truthful informing the family that at 5 min of absent circulation the patient is definitely dead, versus 48–52% given brief information ($P < 0.01$). On at least one of the scenarios, 65% of those given detailed information, and 50% of those given brief information responded uncertain, disagree, or strongly disagree that the patient is definitely dead ($P < 0.01$). Medical students were significantly less likely to agree that the patients in the scenarios were "dead," or that the physicians were being truthful in describing the patients as dead.

Conclusions.—Most respondents were not confident that a donation after cardiac death donor was actually dead.

▶ The debate regarding how to define death in an organ donor is still ongoing 40 years after initial brain death criteria were developed. Recently there has been a push to adopt a policy of donation after cardiac death (DCD) as a means to increase the cadaveric organ donor population. The central principles defining cardiac death are apnea, asystole, and pulselessness for 5 minutes following the withdrawal of cardiopulmonary support.

The main ethical controversy regarding DCD is centered on the premise that patients may not be physiologically dead at the time of organ donation, thus violating the standard medical, ethical, and legal practice of the dead donor rule.[1] There are ethical concerns surrounding the potential reversibility of cardiac death extending beyond the time period that defines DCD. For example, there are several reported cases of the Lazarus phenomenon, whereby patients can spontaneously undergo autoresuscitation up to 10 minutes following the withdrawal of cardiopulmonary support.[2]

Despite these ethical concerns, there is some literature suggesting public support for organ donation following cardiac death. However, the authors of this article suggest the survey questions used to obtain the data are somewhat misleading due to the fact that the issue of the reversibility of cardiac death was not addressed. The authors of this article set out to investigate if a subset of university students agreed that patients undergoing DCD are in fact dead.

Results revealed inconsistent responses regarding the patient's state at the time of donation. Subjects given more information regarding the ethical controversies surrounding DCD were less likely to agree the patients were dead at the time of donation as compared with those given minimal information.

This study demonstrates that with greater education regarding the ethical implications of DCD, respondents are less likely to agree patients were actually dead at the time of organ donation.

Organ transplant is a proven and effective means to extend the life of patients with organ failure. However, currently the demand for organs is much larger than the donor population. To respond to this ever increasing need, it is necessary to explore ways to expand the donor population. Currently, opinions regarding DCD are widely variable. Further research and education are needed to clarify the multitude of ethical issues surrounding this topic as well as to further clarify the role of DCD in organ transplantation.

K. Robinson, BS

V. K. Rajput, MD

References

1. Truog RD, Miller FG. The dead donor rule and organ transplantation. *N Engl J Med*. 2008;359:674-675.
2. Maleck WH, Piper SN, Triem J, Boldt J, Zittel FU. Unexpected return of spontaneous circulation after cessation of resuscitation (Lazarus phenomenon). *Resuscitation*. 1998;39:125-128.

The End-of-Life Care Experiences of Relatives of Brain Dead Intensive Care Patients

Lloyd-Williams M, Morton J, Peters S (Univ of Liverpool, UK; Univ of Manchester, UK)
J Pain Symptom Manage 37:659-664, 2009

Brain death is a traumatic and sudden event following a severe injury to the brain. Most patients with brain death spend the last days of life in an intensive care unit (ICU), where some families will be approached to ask for organ donation. This qualitative study was carried out with relatives of patients who had died of brain death in an ICU; all relatives were interviewed six months after the death. Twenty ICUs were recruited for this study. The next of kin of 130 patients who died during the study period were approached, and 30 (22%) agreed to be interviewed; one later withdrew. This paper focuses on the perceived palliative care needs of the 29 families. Participants valued the physical care their relatives had received, but communication and breaking bad news was a cause for concern. The facilities on many ICUs, for example, cramped relatives' rooms and little privacy to be with the patients or to say the final goodbye, was a common theme to emerge. Bereavement follow-up did not routinely occur, and this was an identified factor noted by relatives. Families living through the period of brain death in a loved one may have particular needs in terms of end-of-life care and should be offered the support of a palliative care team through the last days of a patient's life and into the period of bereavement. Staff training on how to communicate bad news also should be implemented as a matter of urgency.

▶ An enormous amount of time and effort is devoted by families and health care professionals toward the final few days and hours in a patient's life in the intensive care unit (ICU). The great majority of this attention is directed at the patient as nurses and physicians strive to ensure that the patient's wishes are respected while preparing for a pain-free and dignified death. During this tumultuous time, the needs and psychological well-being of a patient's family are often overlooked. Many families are burdened with trying to understand the complexity of the medical illness, the uncertainty of prognosis, and the difficulty with making decisions such as the withdrawal of life-sustaining care, all while being under immense emotional duress. The American College of Critical Care Medicine Task Force in 2004 to 2005 recognized this and one of its recommendations stressed the importance of family support before, during, and after a loved one's death.[1]

This qualitative study focused on the events experienced by families of brain-dead patients in the ICU and the perception of the support and care the families received in the ICU. The families were identified from 20 ICUs in the northwest portion of England with a 22% response rate. Mostly, families were satisfied with the care that they and the patient received in the ICU. However, some family members noted a lack of sensitivity in communication by the hospital staff. This inability by health care professionals to acknowledge or address a family's emotions has been noted in ICU family conferences where end-of-life issues are discussed.[2] Family members also experienced a sense of abandonment after their loved one's death. It has been shown that a physician condolence telephone call or letter can help improve bereavement outcomes and that the support from an interdisciplinary team can help recommend actions or behaviors that will help families cope with their grief.[3]

In spite of the qualitative nature of the study, the retrospective recollection of events by family members, and the small sample size of participants, this study still addresses many common and important issues with the care of caregivers. Constant communication between family members and the ICU team is imperative to help caregivers cope with the difficult situation at hand. One solution could be the presence and participation of family members during ICU rounds with physicians and nurses.[1] Hospitals are also creating palliative care programs, which are instituted at the start of an ICU admission in order to provide caregivers psychosocial and bereavement support.

It is imperative that family support be given during the time before, during, and after a loved one's death. A multidisciplinary team including, but not limited to, physicians, nurses, and social workers is required to help family members cope during this very stressful time and prevent dangerous sequelae in caregivers, such as depression and suicide.

S. Patel, MD
V. K. Rajput, MD

References

1. Davidson J, Powers K, Hedayat K, et al. Clinical practice guidelines for support of the family in the patient-centered intensive care unit: American College of Critical Care Medicine Task Force 2004–2005. *Crit Care Med.* 2007;35:605-622.
2. Curtis J, Engelberg R, Wenrich M, Shannon SE, Treece PD, Rubenfeld GD. Missed opportunities during family conferences about end-of-life care in the intensive care unit. *Am J Respir Crit Care Med.* 2005;171:844-849.
3. Rabow M, Hauser J, Adams J. Supporting family caregivers at the end of life: "they don't know what they don't know". *JAMA.* 2004;291:483-491.

Going home to die from surgical intensive care units
Huang Y-C, Huang S-J, Ko W-J, et al (Natl Taiwan Univ Hosp, Taipei)
Intensive Care Med 35:810-815, 2009

Purpose.—To better understand events related to going home to die (GHTD) from the intensive care unit (ICU), with the hope that this information might improve the palliative care of ICU patients.

Methods.—This retrospective observational study was performed at a tertiary medical center—the National Taiwan University Hospital. All surgical ICU mortality cases between 1 January 2003 and 31 December 2007 were included in this study.

Results.—The rate of GHTD from the ICU declined annually, but has reached a plateau of around 25% in recent years. Multivariate logistic regression analysis found independently significant factors associated with GHTD, including older age (OR: 1.013; $P = 0.001$), married status (OR: 2.128; $P < 0.001$), lower educational level (OR: 1.799; $P = 0.001$), and lack of DNR consent (OR: 1.499; $P = 0.006$). When treatment intensity was compared on the date of death, GHTD patients in general received more treatments and diagnostic procedures than those who died in the ICU. Univariate analysis showed that GHTD patients received significantly more advanced antibiotics, more chest radiography, greater use of sedatives, greater use of analgesics, and more transfusions, but less FiO_2 and mechanical circulatory support than patients who died in the ICU.

Conclusion.—GHTD from the ICU is a special phenomenon in the Chinese cultural area, representing a cultural tradition rather than a form of palliative care.

▶ The primary purpose of this retrospective observational study is to better understand events associated with going home to die (GHTD) from the ICU compared with those who die in the ICU. Subjects included surgical ICU patients from a tertiary medical center in Taipei, Taiwan. When a patient's clinical status became irreversible, the physician discussed end-of-life care, which included do-not-resuscitate (DNR), organ/tissue donation, or taking the patient home. Taking a patient home included intravenous (IV) sedation, ventilator support, and vasopressive drugs during transport and a nurse accompanying the patient. While at home, the nurse withdraws the endotracheal tube and discontinues vasopressive drugs, but maintains sedatives and analgesics until the patient expires. Death commonly occurred within minutes to hours. Rates of GHTD ranged from 44% to 25% during the course of this study with the rate declining annually before reaching a plateau of 25%. Independent factors associated with GHTD included older, married, lower educational levels, and lack of DNR consent. Interestingly, GHTD patients received more treatments and diagnostic procedures on the day of discharge from the ICU compared with those who died in the ICU.

This study does present subjects within the Chinese culture and going home to die may not be a desire in all cultures. Transporting a patient home with supportive therapies may not be a reality due to complex arrangements. When a patient is nearing the end of life, we should recognize the unique spiritual needs and diversity in our patients and families. A policy to ensure that the patient's pain is managed, visiting is extended for family, and that staff supports family values and maintains privacy for religious customs/rites at the bedside is often the best care we can deliver in this critically ill patient population.

C. A. Schorr, RN, MSN

Value choices and considerations when limiting intensive care treatment: a qualitative study

Halvorsen K, Førde R, Nortvedt P (Akershus Univ College, Lillestrøm, Norway; Univ of Oslo, Norway)
Acta Anaesthesiol Scand 53:10-17, 2009

Background.—To shed light on the values and considerations that affect the decision-making processes and the decisions to limit intensive care treatment.

Method.—Qualitative methodology with participant observation and in-depth interviews, with an emphasis on eliciting the underlying rationale of the clinicians' actions and choices when limiting treatment.

Results.—Informants perceived over-treatment in intensive care medicine as a dilemma. One explanation was that the decision-making base was somewhat uncertain, complex and difficult. The informants claimed that those responsible for taking decisions from the admitting ward prolonged futile treatment because they may bear guilt or responsibility for something that had gone wrong during the course of treatment. The assessments of the patient's situation made by physicians from the admitting ward were often more organ-oriented and the expectations were less realistic than those of clinicians in the intensive care unit who frequently had a more balanced and overall perspective. Aspects such as the personality and the speciality of those involved, the culture of the unit and the degree of interdisciplinary cooperation were important issues in the decision-making processes.

Conclusion.—Under-communicated considerations jeopardise the principle of equal treatment. If intensive care patients are to be ensured equal treatment, strategies for interdisciplinary, transparent and appropriate decision-making processes must be developed in which open and hidden values are rendered visible, power structures disclosed, employees respected and the various perspectives of the treatment given their legitimate place.

▶ The recent advancements in medical practice and technology have enabled us to prolong the lives of the most critically ill patients lurking on the edge of death. A European study published in 2006 found that 75% of physicians agree to initiate meaningless or physiologically futile intensive care treatment.[1] This practice of overtreatment, simply because "we can," is a difficult ethical dilemma faced by all health care professionals in today's intensive care units (ICUs).

In an effort to understand what drives health care workers to prolong intensive care treatment, the investigators of this qualitative study worked with anesthesiologists and nurses from 3 different ICUs in Norway. It is important to note that in Norway, advanced directives have no formal and judicial status and are not standard practice. In the United States, all competent individuals are allowed to dictate in advance how they would like their medical care to be managed if they should become incompetent. Directives appoint a health care proxy or surrogate to act as an advocate and enforce the patient's wishes in the event of resistance from health care providers. In the absence of discernible patient preferences, the advocate is instructed by statute to act in the patient's best interests and make medical decisions accordingly. Some authors have argued that the values or preferences of previously competent patients should be negated once the individual has become gravely debilitated and cannot appreciate any deviation from his or her previous instructions.[2]

The findings of this study suggest that decisions to limit life-prolonging treatment are not purely based on objective professional criteria. The researchers identify 4 main elements that lead to difficulty in limiting intensive care. The first is the uncertainty of decision making. Uncertainty arises from the lack of a standard solution, poor documentation of the patients' previous functional level from previous visits, and being unaware of the patients' wishes concerning life-prolonging treatment. The second element consists of the individual aspects that influence decision makers. Some of these aspects include the physicians' unrealistic expectations regarding treatment, feelings of guilt due to delivery of suboptimal medical care before entering the ICU, and varying areas of focus among the subspecialties. The researchers identified patient factors such as age and lifestyle choices (eg, alcoholics or drug addicts) as the third element. The final element involves the dynamic of the decision-making process, including hierarchies among the different specialties and between physicians and nurses.

With these 4 elements present within the ICU, how can we limit intensive care treatment? The researchers mention that a protocol is currently being drawn up in Norway to alleviate some of the uncertainty by standardizing treatment. Further studies to determine the efficacy of such guidelines will be critical in the future. The major conclusion of this study is the need for multidisciplinary discussion during the decision-making process. Through effective communication the researchers believe individual values will be made apparent and ultimately limit intensive care treatment. The role of ethics committees has been expanding beyond complex ethical dilemmas and the authors suggest that this may be an additional means of creating open communication. The role of mandatory ethics consultations has been explored in some institutions in the United States.

One concern is that the conclusions of this study may not be applicable to countries outside of Norway where there may be a different culture and dynamic present within the ICUs. For example, the authors did not address the specific interest of family members as a factor in the physicians' decision-making process, implying that family has minimal impact in Norway. A study conducted in the United States by Hardart and Truog found that most physicians they surveyed believed that family interests should be considered in making decisions for incompetent patients. Less than 10% preferred the traditional model in which the physician-patient relationship is exclusive and family interests are excluded.[3] Thus, to fully understand what drives physicians to prolong or limit intensive care treatment universally, it is crucial to consider the role of family members.

A. A. Naik, BS

V. K. Rajput, MD

References

1. Moselli NM, Debernardi F, Piovano F. Forgoing life sustaining treatments: differences and similarities between North America and Europe. *Acta Anaesthesiol Scand.* 2006;50:1177-1186.
2. Dresser R. Confronting the near irrelevance of advance directives. *J Clin Ethics.* 1994;1:55-56.
3. Hardart GE, Truog RD. Attitudes and preferences of intensivists regarding the role of family interests in medical decision making for incompetent patients. *Crit Care Med.* 2003;31:1895-1900.

Surrogate Decision-Makers' Perspectives on Discussing Prognosis in the Face of Uncertainty
Evans LR, Boyd EA, Malvar G, et al (Univ of California, San Francisco)
Am J Respir Crit Care Med 179:48-53, 2009

Rationale.—Many physicians are reluctant to discuss a patient's prognosis when there is significant prognostic uncertainty.

Objectives.—We sought to understand surrogate decision makers' views regarding whether physicians should discuss prognosis in the face of uncertainty.

Methods.—We conducted semi-structured interviews with 179 surrogates for 142 incapacitated patients at high risk of death in four intensive care units at an academic medical center. The interviews explored surrogates' attitudes about whether physicians should discuss prognosis when they cannot be certain their prognostic estimates are correct. We used constant comparative methods to analyze the transcripts. Validation methods included triangulation by multidisciplinary analysis and member checking.

Measurements and Main Results.—Eighty-seven percent (155/179) of surrogates wanted physicians to discuss an uncertain prognosis. We identified five main reasons for this, including surrogates' belief that prognostic uncertainty is unavoidable, that physicians are their only source for prognostic information, and that discussing prognostic uncertainty leaves room for realistic hope, increases surrogates' trust in the physician, and signals a need to prepare for possible bereavement. Twelve percent (22/179) of surrogates felt that discussions about an uncertain prognosis should be avoided. The main explanation was that it is not worth the potential emotional distress if the prognostications are incorrect. Surrogates suggested that physicians should explicitly discuss uncertainty when prognosticating.

Conclusions.—The majority of surrogates of patients that are critically ill want physicians to disclose their prognostic estimates even if they cannot be certain they are correct. This stems from surrogates' belief that prognostic uncertainty is simultaneously unavoidable and acceptable.

▶ Surrogate decision makers may labor under a somewhat paradoxical scenario where they may feel empowered to have a decision-making authority and at the same time feel inadequate to make a clinically informed and morally optimal decision.[1] Close family and friends serving as surrogates are assumed to be the better judges of what patients would have wanted for themselves (substitutive judgment) or are emotionally invested to make decisions that maximize patients' best interest (best interest standard). The moral justification for surrogate decision making, whether under substitutive judgment or best interest standard, assumes that surrogates have a good understanding of the likely disease trajectory and outcomes for their loved ones.

With the movement toward patient-centered and outcome-oriented care, physicians have professional responsibility not only to diagnose and treat patients but also to predict the fate of an illness and likely patient outcomes. Despite considerable progress made in the prognostic science, prognostic uncertainty remains a clinical reality. As authors have pointed out, the task of prognostication is particularly challenging in critical care settings where time-sensitive decisions ought to be made in the face of high disease acuity and multiple comorbidities. In this scenario, the traditional science of disease-specific prognostication, which itself is fraught with limitations, may offer little help in improving providers' prognostic accuracy and consequently surrogate decision making.[2]

Nevertheless, it is not surprising that the majority of surrogates in this study wanted physicians to discuss prognoses even in the face of uncertainty. Prognostication may allow families to seek refuge in the knowledge that experts have offered their best assessment and that they acted on the best information available to them. In this sense the prognostic communication in the face of uncertainty may help surrogates in sharing their burden of decision making with providers, which in turn may have implications for decision satisfaction, closure, and bereavement outcomes.

From a methodological standpoint, it is interesting to note that the authors framed their interview question in terms of the provider concern for upsetting the family should their predictions turn out to be wrong. Because prognostic uncertainty is not dichotomous and the consequences go far beyond upsetting the family, it would be interesting to investigate if participant response structures would be different if the interview question is framed differently.

Future research must focus on the complex intersections among clinical epidemiology, decision science, and surrogate-provider communication. Moreover, research is needed to improve prognostic accuracy in patients with multiple comorbidities and compounded clinical problems and those in high acuity settings to allow for more informed patient/surrogate decision making.

S. H. Meghani, PhD, MBE, CRNP

V. K. Rajput, MD

References

1. Arnold RM, Kellum J. Moral justifications for surrogate decision making in the intensive care unit: implications and limitations. *Crit Care Med.* 2003;31: S347-S353.
2. Mayr VD, Dunser MW, Greil V, et al. Causes of death and determinants of outcome in critically ill patients. *Crit Care.* 2006;10:R154.

Paramedic and Emergency Medical Technicians Views on Opportunities and Challenges When Forgoing and Halting Resuscitation in the Field

Grudzen CR, Timmermans S, Koenig WJ, et al (Mount Sinai School of Medicine, NY; Univ of California at Los Angeles; Emergency Med Services Agency, Los Angeles, CA; et al)

Acad Emerg Med 16:532-538, 2009

Objectives.—The objective was to assess paramedic and emergency medical technicians (EMT) perspectives and decision-making after a policy change that allows forgoing or halting resuscitation in prehospital atraumatic cardiac arrest.

Methods.—Five semistructured focus groups were conducted with 34 paramedics and 2 EMTs from emergency medical services (EMS) agencies within Los Angeles County (LAC), 6 months after a policy change that allowed paramedics to forgo or halt resuscitation in the field under certain circumstances.

Results.—Participants had an overwhelmingly positive view of the policy; felt it empowered their decision-making abilities; and thought the benefits to patients, family, EMS, and the public outweighed the risks. Except under certain circumstances, such as when the body was in public view or when family members did not appear emotionally prepared to have the body left on scene, they felt the policy improved care. Assuming that certain patient characteristics were present, decisions by paramedics about implementing the policy in the field involve many factors, including knowledge and comfort with the new policy, family characteristics (e.g., agreement), and logistics regarding the place of arrest (e.g., size of space). Paramedic and EMT experiences with and attitudes toward forgoing resuscitation, as well as group dynamics among EMS leadership, providers, police, and ED staff, also play a role.

Conclusions.—Participants view the ability to forgo or halt resuscitation in the field as empowering and do not believe it presents harm to patients or families under most circumstances. Factors other than patient clinical characteristics, such as knowledge and attitudes toward the policy, family emotional preparedness, and location of arrest, affect whether paramedics will implement it.

▶ According to the American Heart Association, the incidence of hospital cardiac arrest in North America is 0.55 per 1000 people, which is about 160 000 cardiac arrests annually.[1] Sixty percent of these unexpected cardiac deaths are treated by emergency medical services (EMS) and paramedics. The median survival after a first recorded rhythm is a mere 6.4%. In 2007, Los Angeles County (LAC) EMS handled 9256 cardiac arrests, of which 94% were medical. Only 1.2% were expected to have full neurological recovery.

This first-of-its-kind qualitative study examined the policy that allowed paramedics to forgo or halt resuscitation and tried to understand the barriers and facilitators to the implementation of this new policy. After 6 months, it was found that the EMS system had halted 50% more resuscitations under the new policy. A similar observation was made in King County, Washington, in cases where family members requested verbally or provided documentation that resuscitation was not desired. In half of the cases, honoring the verbal request had resulted in withholding resuscitation.[2] In a cross-sectional survey conducted among 3800 emergency medical technicians (EMTs) across the United States in 2002 to 2003, most responders felt that the existing policy of a written DNAR (do not attempt resuscitation) was inadequate. Fewer than 10% said that they would withhold resuscitation in the presence of an unofficial document or verbal advance directive. However, many experienced providers would withhold resuscitation if it seemed futile or in the presence of unofficial directives.[3]

EMS and paramedics have to make their own judgment on forgoing or halting a resuscitation based on the resources available, family attitude, and their own personal views about each specific situation. There were multiple factors that affected the implementation of this policy. Even though there were several limitations of this study such as gender and selection bias of participants, it still brings forth the very important issue that forgoing the resuscitation of a cardiac arrest is a complex, challenging issue for EMS responders.

The findings of this study indicate that the use of the policy to withhold resuscitation by paramedics is based on their judgments about the resources available, family attitude, and perception of futility of care. This concept differs from the traditional standards that dictate the withholding of resuscitation such as patient advance directives, living wills, and surrogate decisions made by health care proxy. In the right setting, it is felt that EMS responders should be able to determine in which cases to forgo resuscitation.

U. Patel, MD

V. K. Rajput, MD

References

1. Rea TD, Eisenberg MS, Sinibaldi G, White RD. Incidence of EMS-treated out-of-hospital cardiac arrest in the United States. *Resuscitation*. 2004;63:17-24.
2. Feder S, Matheny RL, Loveless RS Jr, Rea TD. Withholding resuscitation: a new approach to prehospital end-of-life decisions. *Ann Intern Med*. 2006;144:634-640.
3. Marco CA, Schears RM. Prehospital resuscitation practices: a survey of prehospital providers. *J Emerg Med*. 2003;24:87-89.

The presence of a family witness impacts physician performance during simulated medical codes

Fernandez R, Compton S, Jones KA, et al (Wayne State Univ School of Medicine, Detroit, MI)
Crit Care Med 37:1956-1960, 2009

Objective.—To determine whether the presence and behavior of a family witness to cardiopulmonary resuscitation (CPR) impacts critical actions performed by physicians.

Design.—This was a randomized comparison study of physicians' performance during a simulated cardiac arrest with three different family witness states.

Setting.—This study was conducted at the Wayne State University Eugene Applebaum College of Pharmacy and Health Science's Center for Healthcare Simulation.

Subjects.—Second-year and third-year emergency medicine (EM) residents from the Wayne State University Department of Emergency Medicine–affiliated residency programs and Michigan State University–affiliated EM residency programs.

Intervention.—Thirty teams comprised of one second-year and one third-year EM resident were randomly assigned to one of the three groups: 1) no family witness; 2) a nonobstructive "quiet" family witness; and 3) a family witness displaying an overt grief reaction.

Measurements and Main Results.—Each pair was assessed for time to critical actions (e.g., minutes to CPR and drug administration) and for resuscitation-based performance outcomes (e.g., number of shocks) during a simulated cardiac arrest. The time to critical events was similar across groups with respect to initiating CPR, attempting to intubate the patient, and pronouncing the death of the patient. However, the time to deliver the first defibrillation shock was longer for the overt reaction witness group (2.57 minutes) as compared with the quiet (1.77 minutes) and no family witness (1.67 minutes) groups. Additionally, fewer total shocks were delivered in the overt reaction witness groups (4.0 minutes) vs. the quiet (6.5 minutes) and no family witness groups (6.0 minutes).

Conclusion.—The presence of a family witness may have a significant impact on physicians' ability to perform critical actions during simulated medical resuscitations. Further study is necessary to see if this effect crosses over into real clinical practice and if training ameliorates this effect.

▶ Family-witnessed codes (FWC) or cardiopulmonary resuscitation of patients in the presence of family members is a controversial and complex subject. Cardiopulmonary resuscitation without family members present is only successful around 10% of the time. This article has interesting evidence that the presence of family members can negatively impact these already poor outcomes of codes in a simulated environment. This is the first study that used a controlled environment to quantify the effect of family presence, but its generalizability is limited because of the artificial setting.

It is difficult to design a study of real codes that obtains consent from family witnesses without introducing bias. The studies cited in this article as proponents of FWC either did not examine a full code, only isolated procedures, or failed to present objective evidence of the benefit to the families.[1-4] However, there is evidence in the literature that families benefit from this option.[5,6]

There is a need for more research because there might be a conflict between maximizing patient care and helping the bereavement process of the family. Medicine has a humanistic responsibility to facilitate the grieving process for the patient's family in situations such as this with a high mortality rate. Efforts to improve clinical outcomes should not necessarily have absolute priority over efforts to help bereavement. Current debate over end-of-life issues has shown that medical care is becoming more responsive to the role of death in a patient's and family's life.[7] FWC should also be part of this groundswell toward family-oriented caregiving and research into this field is valuable.

N. Samras, BSE, MPH

V. K. Rajput, MD

References

1. Doyle CJ, Post H, Burney RE, Maino J, Keefe M, Rhee KJ. Family participation during resuscitation: an option. *Ann Emerg Med.* 1987;16:673-675.
2. Meyers T, Eichhorn D, Guzzetta C. Do families want to be present during CPR? A retrospective survey. *J Emerg Nurs.* 1998;24:400-405.
3. Powers KS, Rubenstein JS. Family presence during invasive procedures in the pediatric intensive care unit—a prospective study. *Arch Pediatr Adolesc Med.* 1999; 153:955-958.
4. Belanger M, Reed S. A rural community hospital's experience with family-witnessed resuscitation. *J Emerg Nurs.* 1997;23:238-239.
5. Tsai E. Should family members be present during cardiopulmonary resuscitation? *N Engl J Med.* 2002;346:1019-1021.
6. McClenathan BM, Torrington KG, Uyehara CF. Family member presence during cardiopulmonary resuscitation—a survey of US and international critical care professionals. *Chest.* 2002;122:2204-2211.
7. Verpoort C, Gastmans C, De Bal N, Dierckx de Casterlé B. Nurses' attitudes to euthanasia: a review of the literature. *Nurs Ethics.* 2004;11:349-365.

Surrogate Decision Makers' Responses to Physicians' Predictions of Medical Futility

Zier LS, Burack JH, Micco G, et al (Univ of California, San Francisco; et al)
Chest 136:110-117, 2009

Background.—Although physicians sometimes use the futility rationale to limit the use of life-sustaining treatments, little is known about how surrogate decision makers view this rationale. We sought to determine the attitudes of surrogates of patients who are critically ill toward whether physicians can predict futility and whether these attitudes predict surrogates' willingness to discontinue life support when faced with predictions of futility.

Methods.—This multicenter, mixed qualitative and quantitative study took place at three hospitals in California from 2006 to 2007. We conducted semistructured interviews with surrogate decision makers for 50 patients who were critically ill and incapacitated that addressed their beliefs about medical futility and inductively developed an organizing framework to describe these beliefs. We used a hypothetical scenario with a modified time–trade-off design to examine the relationship between a patient's prognosis and a surrogate's willingness to withdraw life support. We used a mixed-effects regression model to examine the association between surrogates' attitudes about futility and their willingness to limit life support in the face of a very poor prognosis. Validation methods included the use and integration of multiple data sources, multidisciplinary analysis, and member checking.

Results.—Sixty-four percent of surrogates (n = 32; 95% confidence interval [CI], 49 to 77%) expressed doubt about the accuracy of physicians' futility predictions, 32% of surrogates (n = 16; 95% CI, 20 to 47%) elected to continue life support with a <1% survival estimate, and 18% of surrogates (n = 9; 95% CI, 9 to 31%) elected to continue treatment when the physician believed that the patient had no chance of survival. Surrogates with religious objections to the futility rationale (n = 18) were more likely to request continued life support (odds ratio, 4; 95% CI, 1.2 to 14.0; p = 0.03) than those with secular or experiential objections (n = 15; odds ratio, 0.95; 95% CI, 0.3 to 3.4; p = 0.90).

Conclusions.—Doubt about physicians' ability to predict medical futility is common among surrogate decision makers. The nature of the doubt may have implications for responding to conflicts about futility in clinical practice.

▶ According to Merriam Webster's dictionary a surrogate is described as one who takes the place of another. Futile means incapable of producing any result, useless, and unsuccessful. In the medical arena the term "futility" is best understood relative to specified treatment goals.

In the health care system medical futility is a complex issue arousing considerable dispute among various medical professional societies. By some, it has been perceived as an ultimate limitation on what services a patient can demand. A physician has the authority to decide what possible steps to take during physiological treatments. The goal is attained when each step achieves utmost utility. If a physician decides to withhold treatment on conclusion of physiological futility, there are 2 constraints physicians need to overcome. First, the physician must meet a professional standard of skills in judging treatment effects. Secondly, the hospitalist ought to inform the patient or surrogate decision maker about the treatment modality and physician judgment of futility; this will give a patient an opportunity to obtain a second opinion.

If the issue of futility is based on appropriateness of sustaining a severely impaired quality of life, the scope of professional judgment is limited. Such a decision depends largely on a valued judgment of patient, family, and medical staff. This is not an area of unilateral medical judgment. One of the most significant developments in this debate has been the Houston Task Force's unilateral do-not-attempt-resuscitation policy, which is process-based and interdisciplinary. A physician in an institutional context can ask for an ethics consultation in the hope of clarifying the medical situation. A few legal cases have also raised considerable discussion on medical futility, adding to the debate. In summary, a physician can only hope to invoke the futility concept and overturn a conscientious surrogate's insistence on continued life support when the surrogate's choice is abusive.

Two other factors that further cause complexity around futility are uncertainty in prognosis and effectiveness of treatments. Uncertainty in prognosis makes both physicians and caretaker feel uncomfortable on limiting or withdrawing treatments. The difficulty for physicians to be able to determine prognosis varies between physicians from all specialties.[1] Where the nonintensivist deals with more chronic issues of determining life expectancy, the intensivist is pressured into forming a prognosis within minutes of seeing a critically ill patient. Developing a relationship over time creates trust. From the literature, the best way to gain a surrogate's trust is to keep them well informed of a course of illness and prognosis early on.[2-4]

In the critical care setting surrogates and families need time to come to grips with reality. In the essence of time, the health care team and surrogate need to decide goals of care based on current information and frequently readdress the goals of care. It seems that establishing set goals of care and keeping the surrogate well informed of the justification of medical intervention eases the burden of uncertainty from surrogates.[1] Ongoing real-time communication can help surrogates to focus their emotions on the future short- and long-term goals of care. This entails burial preparations, notifying family members, and pastoral services. It creates a transition period from a state of uncertainty to steps toward closure.[3]

In conclusion, the surrogate-physician relationship is based on developing trust and keeping the surrogate informed in real time. These basic tenets of medical care aid in clarifying the issue of futility in poor prognostic outcomes. In each case, physicians need to realize that closure is the essential key component when dealing with surrogates and family members.

I. Shariff, MD
V. K. Rajput, MD

References

1. Truog RD, Brett AS, Frader J. The problem with futility. *N Engl J Med.* 1992;326:1560-1564.
2. Apatira L, Boyd EA, Malvar G, et al. Hope, truth, and preparing for death: perspectives of surrogate decision makers. *Ann Intern Med.* 2008;149:861-868.
3. Evans LR, Boyd EA, Malvar G, et al. Surrogate decision-makers' perspectives on discussing prognosis in the face of uncertainty. *Am J Respir Crit Care Med.* 2009;179:48-53.
4. Zier LS, Burack JH, Micco G, et al. Doubt and belief in physicians' ability to prognosticate during critical illness: the perspective of surrogate decision makers. *Crit Care Med.* 2008;36:2341-2347.

Are Physicians' Recommendations to Limit Life Support Beneficial or Burdensome? Bringing Empirical Data to the Debate

White DB, Evans LR, Bautista CA, et al (Univ of California, San Francisco; et al)
Am J Respir Crit Care Med 180:320-325, 2009

Rationale.—Although there is a growing belief that physicians should routinely provide a recommendation to surrogates during deliberations about withdrawing life support, there is a paucity of empirical data on surrogates' perspectives on this topic.

Objectives.—To understand the attitudes of surrogate decision-makers toward receiving a physician's recommendation during deliberations about whether to limit life support for an incapacitated patient.

Methods.—We conducted a prospective, mixed methods study among 169 surrogate decision-makers for critically ill patients. Surrogates sequentially viewed two videos of simulated physician–surrogate discussions about whether to limit life support, which varied only by whether the physician gave a recommendation.

Measurements and Main Results.—The main quantitative outcome was whether surrogates preferred to receive a physicians' recommendation. Surrogates also participated in an in-depth, semistructured interview to explore the reasons for their preference. Fifty-six percent (95/169) of surrogates preferred to receive a recommendation, 42% (70/169) preferred not to receive a recommendation, and 2% (4/169) felt that both approaches were equally acceptable. We identified four main themes that explained surrogates' preferences, including surrogates' perceptions of physicians' appropriate role in life or death decisions and their perceptions of the positive or negative consequences of a recommendation on the physician–surrogate relationship, on the decision-making process, and on long-term regret for the family.

Conclusions.—There is no consensus among surrogates about whether physicians should routinely provide a recommendation regarding life support decisions for incapacitated patients. These findings suggest that physicians should ask surrogates whether they wish to receive a recommendation regarding life support decisions and should be flexible in their approach to decision-making.

▶ In the United States, all states allow competent persons to dictate in advance how they would like their medical care to be managed once they become incompetent. Despite this overriding respect for patient autonomy and federal legislation of The Patient Self-Determination Act of 1991 for advance directives in the United States, the reality is most of the ICU patients do not have previous advance directives and living wills for goals of care during hospitalization. Their decision-making capacity is reduced secondary to their medical condition and medications that affect their neurocognitive function. Thus in the ICU, it is common for a patient surrogate or health care proxy to make decisions on behalf of the patient. The health care proxy or surrogate decision maker is usually a close family member who is familiar with the patient's wishes, beliefs, and values. These decisions include end-of-life decisions and decisions regarding withholding or withdrawal of treatment. The health care proxy can also act as an advocate and enforcer of patients' wishes in the event of resistance from health care providers. In the absence of discernible patient preferences, the surrogate decision maker is generally instructed by statute to follow the patient's best interests.

The common ethical principles that create real-time ethical dilemmas are autonomy, beneficence, and nonmaleficence. There is a consensus that the decision made on behalf of a patient should be in the patient's best interest and should reflect the patient's values and beliefs. But there is still a lot of debate about who should make that decision and what is the physician's role in this process. The fifth International Consensus Conference in End-of-Life Decision Making in Critical Care[1] recommends a shared decision-making process. According to this consensus, it should be a dynamic process where responsibility for the decision is shared between the caregiver team and patient surrogates. Heyland et al[2] has shown that more than 80% of surrogate decision makers preferred some kind of shared decision making.

Physician recommendations about life support decisions are an important aspect of shared decision making. This study suggests that there is no consensus among surrogates as to whether physicians should routinely provide recommendations regarding life support decisions, and more than 40% of surrogates preferred not to receive recommendations. The author suggests that life support decisions largely hinge on patient values rather than medical facts. We believe that physician involvement and physician recommendations play a vital role in these situations, but this creates an ethical dilemma for physicians. Physicians do want to respect a patient's wishes, but at the same time, they do not want to provide futile care if there are no chances of meaningful recovery. After becoming familiar with a patient's values and beliefs, the physician should make recommendations about life support decisions that will help the surrogate to make a rational decision about goals of care based on the patient's values. As it will be a shared decision, the surrogate and family feel less burden about the decision of withdrawing support, thus helping to alleviate anxiety and depression among family members.

H. Shingala, MD

V. K Rajput, MD

References

1. Thompson BT, Cox PN, Antonelli M, et al. Challenges in end-of-life care in the ICU: statement of the 5th International Consensus Conference in Critical Care: Brussels, Belgium, April 2003: executive summary. *Crit Care Med.* 2004;32: 1781-1784.
2. Heyland DK, Cook DJ, Rocker GM, et al. Decision-making in the ICU: perspectives of the substitute decision-maker. *Intensive Care Med.* 2003;29:75-82.

TRIAD II: do living wills have an impact on pre-hospital lifesaving care?
Mirarchi FL, Kalantzis S, Hunter D, et al (Hamot Med Ctr, Erie, PA)
J Emerg Med 36:105-115, 2009

Background.—Living wills accompany patients who present for emergent care. To the best of our knowledge, no studies assess pre-hospital provider interpretations of these instructions.

Objectives.—Determine how a living will is interpreted and assess how interpretation impacts lifesaving care.

Design Setting.—Three-part survey administered at a regional emergency medical system educational symposium to 150 emergency medical technicians (EMTs) and paramedics. Part I assessed understanding of the living will and do-not-resuscitate (DNR) orders. Part II assessed the living will's impact in clinical situations of patients requiring lifesaving interventions. Part III was similar to part II except a code status designation (full code) was incorporated into the living will.

Results.—There were 127 surveys completed, yielding an 87% response rate. The majority were male (55%) and EMTs (74%). The average age was 44 years and the average duration of employment was 15 years. Ninety percent (95% confidence interval [CI] 84.6–95.4%) of respondents determined that, after review of the living will, the patient's code status was DNR, and 92% (95% CI 86.5–96.6%) defined their understanding of DNR as comfort care/end-of-life care. When the living will was applied to clinical situations, it resulted in a higher proportion of patients being classified as DNR as opposed to full code (Case A 78% [95% CI 71.2–85.6%] vs. 22% [95% CI 14.4–28.8%], respectively; Case B 67% [95% CI 58.4–74.9%] vs. 33% [95% CI 25.1–1.6%], respectively; Case C 63% [95% CI 55.1–71.9%] vs. 37% [95% CI 28.1–44.9%]), respectively. With the scenarios presented, this DNR classification resulted in a lack of or a delay in lifesaving interventions. Incorporating a code status into the living will produced statistically significant increases in the provision of lifesaving care. In Case A, intubation increased from 15% to 56% ($p < 0.0001$); Case B, defibrillation increased from 40% to 59% ($p < 0.0001$); and Case C, defibrillation increased from 36% to 65% ($p < 0.0001$).

Conclusions.—Significant confusion and concern for patient safety exists in the pre-hospital setting due to the understanding and implementation of living wills and DNR orders. This confusion can be corrected by implementing clearly defined code status into the living will.

▶ The Patient Self Determination Act of 1990 stipulated that hospitals ask patients at the time of admission whether they have advance directives or a living will. This led to an enormous use of resources by hospitals to comply with this mandate and, in turn, has increased the awareness of living wills in the patient population. Despite this vast effort, there has been confusion among patients, family members, and even physicians in understanding what are the true protections and implications of a living will.[1,2]

This study analyzed how prehospital personnel, such as emergency medical technicians (EMTs) and paramedics, interpreted a living will and how this interpretation impacted lifesaving care. Of the respondents, there was a significantly higher number of EMTs than paramedics. Generally paramedics, in comparison with EMTs, have a longer training time, are able to use more advanced airway devices, and can give a much wider number of medications than EMTs (although the scope of practice of EMTs does vary from state to state).

The study demonstrated that both EMTs and paramedics were confused by the terminology in living wills, which made them either delay or withhold life-saving treatment in simulated clinical cases. In the simulated case slightly over 20% of the respondents correctly assigned a full code to the patient's code status, and surprisingly less than 50% of those making the correct full code decision would intubate the patient. This was likely due to the confusion in terminology from the living will stating life-sustaining treatment could be withheld if the patient was in a terminal condition or a state of persistent unconsciousness. When prehospital personnel were given a living will with a line written stating "Code Status Designation: FULL CODE," there was significant improvement in life-saving treatment indicating that clarity of the code status in the living will is required.

There were some limitations with this study. The participants were recruited from a single region, which may introduce a bias based on local sampling and hinder the ability for the study results to be generalized to other regions in the United States. A majority of the respondents in this study were EMTs and in some states EMTs are not allowed to intubate or defibrillate. This may skew the results, as EMTs may not have had a full understanding of the indications for those life-saving procedures in the simulated cases.

The findings in this study indicate that living wills need to be clearer about a patient's code status. The confusing terminology in a living will can lead prehospital personnel to withhold life-saving treatment at the detriment to the patient's life and wishes. A clearly defined code status in the living will or "Physician Orders for Life-Sustaining Treatment" (POLST), which some states have adopted to ensure that patient's wishes for life-saving treatments are honored, could be solutions to this dilemma.

S. Patel, MD

V. K. Rajput, MD

References

1. Thorevska N, Tilluckdharry L, Tickoo S, Havasi A, Amoateng-Adjepong Y, Manthous CA. Patients' understanding of advance directives and cardiopulmonary resuscitation. *J Crit Care*. 2005;20:26-34.
2. Upadya A, Muralidharan V, Thorevska N, Amoateng-Adjepong Y, Manthous CA. Patient, physician, and family member understanding of living wills. *Am J Respir Crit Care Med*. 2002;166:1430-1435.

Family members of critically ill cancer patients: assessing the symptoms of anxiety and depression

Fumis RRL, Deheinzelin D (Centro de Tratamento e Pesquisa Hosp A C Camargo, São Paulo, Brazil)
Intensive Care Med 35:899-902, 2009

Objective.—To determine prevalence and factors associated with symptoms of anxiety and depression in family members of critically ill cancer patients.

Design.—Prospective cohort study.

Setting.—A 23-bed intensive care unit in a tertiary cancer centre.

Patients and Participants.—Three hundred consecutive families of cancer patients with length of stay >72 h in ICU.

Intervention.—None.

Measurements and Main Results.—The Hospital Anxiety and Depression Scale questionnaire and critical care family needs inventory were completed by family members. Prevalence of anxiety and depression in family members was 71 and 50.3%, respectively. Regarding the patients' disease, family depression was correlated with presence of metastasis, whereas hematological malignancies correlated with family anxiety. Anxiety was independently associated with one patient-related factor (prolonged mechanical ventilation) and two family-related factors (catholic religion and gender). Factors associated with symptoms of depression included one patient-related factor (presence of metastasis) and one family-related factor (gender).

Conclusions.—Present findings demonstrated a high prevalence of anxiety and depression in critically ill cancer patients' family members during an intensive care unit stay.

▶ A terminal illness typically affects the entire family and not just the person with the terminal illness. As we care for patients with cancer and deal with end-of-life issues, it is easy to overlook the psychological impact it has on the family members and caregivers. Historically, hospice philosophy has been that "patient and family is the unit of care." This view has been endorsed by many national societies and accreditation organizations. Most hospice care programs emphasize treating both the patient and the family involved. We believe that communication with family is a crucial requirement to success in palliative care. The role of the physician's communication includes sharing information as well as responding appropriately to not only patient concerns but also issues and concerns of the family and caregiver. Any discussion of goals of end-of-life care is known to increase anxiety and depression in family and caregivers. However, communicating effectively helps clarify the prognosis and also dispels preconceived notions/myths about illness or treatment. In an ideal world, the goals of care need not remain the same but should evolve to meet the needs of patient and family after timely open communication.

Since the late 1990s approximately 18 studies have been done to evaluate symptoms experienced by the family members of critically ill.[1] This is the first prospective study done to determine the prevalence and the factors causing anxiety and/or depression in family members of critically ill cancer patients during the early course of the ICU hospitalization. There was a high prevalence rate of anxiety and depression in the family members of critically ill cancer patients. The prevalence rate for anxiety in this study was similar to most other studies done to date.[2,3] However the higher prevalence of depression in this study may be due to the time frame of evaluation for such symptoms in the caregiver.

This study confirms that there is a strong influence of religion, gender, ethnicity, socioeconomic status, and past experience that not only affects the patients but also families. Most of these studies have found that being a female was an independent risk factor for both anxiety and/or depression.[1] This study also confirms the results of a survey by the National Alliance of Caregivers and the Association for the Advancement of Retired Persons. Most of the caregivers were women, and one-third of them suffered from significant physical illness and/or emotional stress.[4]

When someone is critically ill, the burden of making complex decisions about their care usually falls on their family members. Previous advance directives or known wishes from patients are also known to decrease stress in family members.[5] This makes it essential to address the issue of advance directive much earlier in the course of the disease rather than when someone is critically ill in the ICU. In addition, the burden of making such complex decisions by family can also be alleviated by communicating with families honestly and truthfully, encouraging their questions, and responding to their questions within a reasonable time.

Culture and ethnicity may have a major influence on the family support system. Some studies in the United States have shown that involving pastoral care and palliative care medicine specialists during the family meetings for end-of-life discussions may help reduce the anxiety and depression among the family members.[6] In countries where pastoral care and palliative care medicine specialists are available, it might be worthwhile to involve them in the care of a cancer patient early on during the course of the disease rather than wait for the patient to be acutely ill in the ICU.

M. Mehta, MD

V. K. Rajput, MD

References

1. McAdam JL, Puntillo K. Symptoms experienced by family members of patients in intensive care units. *Am J Crit Care*. 2009;18:200-209.
2. Young E, Eddleston J, Ingleby S, et al. Returning home after intensive care: a comparison of symptoms of anxiety and depression in ICU and elective cardiac surgery patients and their relatives. *Intensive Care Med*. 2005;31:86-91.
3. Pochard F, Azoulay E, Chevret S, et al, French FAMIREA Group. Symptoms of anxiety and depression in family members of intensive care unit patients: ethical hypothesis regarding decision-making capacity. *Crit Care Med*. 2001;29: 1893-1897.
4. Jennings B, Ryndes T, D'Onofrio C, Baily MA. Access to hospice care. Expanding boundaries, overcoming barriers. *Hastings Cen Rep*. 2003;Suppl:S3-S21.

5. Tilden VP, Tolle SW, Nelson CA, Fields J. Family decision making to withdraw life-sustaining treatments from hospitalized patients. *Nurs Res.* 2001;50:105-115.
6. Gries CJ, Curtis JR, Wall RJ, Engelberg RA. Family member satisfaction with end-of-life decision making in the ICU. *Chest.* 2008;133:704-712.

Early exercise in critically ill patients enhances short-term functional recovery

Burtin C, Clerckx B, Robbeets C, et al (Katholieke Universiteit Leuven, Belgium; et al)

Crit Care Med 37:2499-2505, 2009

Objectives.—To investigate whether a daily exercise session, using a bedside cycle ergometer, is a safe and effective intervention in preventing or attenuating the decrease in functional exercise capacity, functional status, and quadriceps force that is associated with prolonged intensive care unit stay. A prolonged stay in the intensive care unit is associated with muscle dysfunction, which may contribute to an impaired functional status up to 1 yr after hospital discharge. No evidence is available concerning the effectiveness of an early exercise training intervention to prevent these detrimental complications.

Design.—Randomized controlled trial.

Setting.—Medical and surgical intensive care unit at University Hospital Gasthuisberg.

Patients.—Ninety critically ill patients were included as soon as their cardiorespiratory condition allowed bedside cycling exercise (starting from day 5), given they still had an expected prolonged intensive care unit stay of at least 7 more days.

Interventions.—Both groups received respiratory physiotherapy and a daily standardized passive or active motion session of upper and lower limbs. In addition, the treatment group performed a passive or active exercise training session for 20 mins/day, using a bedside ergometer.

Measurements and Main Results.—All outcome data are reflective for survivors. Quadriceps force and functional status were assessed at intensive care unit discharge and hospital discharge. Six-minute walking distance was measured at hospital discharge. No adverse events were identified during and immediately after the exercise training. At intensive care unit discharge, quadriceps force and functional status were not different between groups. At hospital discharge, 6-min walking distance, isometric quadriceps force, and the subjective feeling of functional well-being (as measured with "Physical Functioning" item of the Short Form 36 Health Survey questionnaire) were significantly higher in the treatment group ($p < .05$).

Conclusions.—Early exercise training in critically ill intensive care unit survivors enhanced recovery of functional exercise capacity, self-perceived functional status, and muscle force at hospital discharge.

▶ One of the new and exciting frontiers in critical care is the outcome success related to early mobility and aggressiveness of physical therapy during the early part of critical illness. Previous dogma was that during the intense front-end part of critical illness, particularly when mechanical ventilator support was required, attention should be toward disease process itself, delaying rehabilitation until after the initial recovery and ICU discharge. More and more data indicate that this is not true. In fact, ambulation with endotracheal tube in place while still receiving positive pressure ventilator support, as well as early aggressive physical therapy, improves intermediate and long-term outcome. This innovative study of bedside cycling continues to add to our understanding that more movement is better across the board.

R. P. Dellinger, MD

Critical Illness Outcomes in Specialty versus General Intensive Care Units
Lott JP, Iwashyna TJ, Christie JD, et al (Univ of Pennsylvania School of Medicine, Philadelphia; Univ of Michigan School of Medicine, Ann Arbor; et al)
Am J Respir Crit Care Med 179:676-683, 2009

Rationale.—General intensive care units (ICUs) provide care across a wide range of diagnoses, whereas specialty ICUs provide diagnosis-specific care. Risk-adjusted outcome differences across such units are unknown.

Objectives.—To determine the association between specialty ICU care and the outcome of critical illness.

Methods.—We conducted a retrospective cohort study design analyzing patients admitted to 124 ICUs participating in the Acute Physiology and Chronic Health Evaluation IV from January 2002 to December 2005. We examined 84,182 patients admitted to specialty and general ICUs with an admitting diagnosis or procedure of acute coronary syndrome, ischemic stroke, intracranial hemorrhage, pneumonia, abdominal surgery, or coronary-artery bypass graft surgery. ICU type was determined by a local data coordinator at each site. Patients were classified by admission to a general ICU, a diagnosis-appropriate ("ideal") specialty ICU, or a diagnosis-inappropriate ("non-ideal") specialty ICU. The primary outcomes were in-hospital mortality and ICU length of stay.

Measurements and Main Results.—After adjusting for important confounders, there were no significant differences in risk-adjusted mortality between general versus ideal specialty ICUs for all conditions other than pneumonia. Risk-adjusted mortality was significantly greater for patients admitted to non-ideal specialty ICUs. There was no consistent effect of specialization on length of stay for all patients or for ICU survivors.

Conclusions.—Ideal specialty ICU care appears to offer no survival benefit over general ICU care for select common diagnoses. Non-ideal specialty ICU care (i.e., "boarding") is associated with increased risk-adjusted mortality.

▶ Hospitals have been steadily dealing with overcrowding in emergency departments, reaching maximal capacity within the hospital, and are hard-pressed to find methods to improve workflow to reduce crowding. Reaching maximal capacity may prompt decisions to board critically ill patients in areas other than the specialized intensive care unit (ICU). These areas may include the recovery area, step/down intermediate care units with monitoring, and may also require boarding in the emergency department (ED). However, boarding ICU patients is not recommended by the American College of Emergency Physicians due to adverse effects and access to the ED.[1] In this situation to improve workflow, having to admit a patient to the "ideal" ICU may interfere with patient flow more so than admission to a general ICU.

Lott and colleagues conducted a retrospective cohort study of 84000 patients using the Acute Physiology and Chronic Health Evaluation (APACHE) IV database, in patients admitted with 1 of 6 specific diagnoses to 124 ICUs in the United States. The purpose of this study was to determine the association between specialty ICU and hospital mortality and ICU length of stay in diverse populations of critically ill. Boarding in a nonspecialized ICU had no statistically significant effect on length of stay. Similar findings have been reported in the trauma patient population supporting that the location or specialized ICU did not have an impact on mortality.[2] Limitations of this study include the retrospective design using APACHE IV with more than half of the patients in the initial dataset being excluded for a diagnosis not included in this study. Excluding a large diversity of diagnoses makes it difficult for the results to be generalizable, bearing the question, "What we do with this group?" A potential limitation not addressed in this study is the participant hospital within the APACHE IV database being a proprietary dataset, which may draw a specific type of hospital interested in research and risk-adjusted data analysis.

Conceivably, getting the critically ill patient to an ICU with close monitoring and attention is of utmost importance compared with being in an "ideal" specialized unit. In these tight economic times, improving efficiency in patient flow is of importance in most hospitals around the world.

C. A. Schorr, RN, MSN

References

1. American College of Emergency Physicians. Boarding of admitted and intensive care patients in the emergency department. *Ann Emerg Med.* 2008;52:188-189.
2. Duane TM, Rao IR, Aboutanos MB, Wolfe LG, Malhotra AK. Are trauma patients better off in a trauma ICU? *J Emerg Trauma Shock.* 2008;1:74-77.

End-of-life practices in 282 intensive care units: data from the SAPS 3 database
Azoulay É, on behalf of the SAPS 3 investigators (Hôpital Saint-Louis et Université Paris 7, France; et al)
Intensive Care Med 35:623-630, 2009

Objective.—To report incidence and characteristics of decisions to forgo life-sustaining therapies (DFLSTs) in the 282 ICUs who contributed to the SAPS3 database.

Methods.—We reviewed data on DFLSTs in 14,488 patients. Independent predictors of DFLSTs have been identified by stepwise logistic regression.

Results.—DFLSTs occurred in 1,239 (8.6%) patients [677 (54.6%) withholding and 562 (45.4%) withdrawal decisions]. Hospital mortality was 21% (3,050/14,488); 36.2% (1,105) deaths occurred after DFLSTs. Across the participating ICUs, hospital mortality in patients with DFLSTs ranged from 80.3 to 95.4% and time from admission to decisions ranged from 2 to 4 days. Independent predictors of decisions to forgo LSTs included 13 variables associated with increased incidence of DFLSTs and 7 variables associated with decrease incidence of DFLST. Among hospital and ICU-related variables, a higher number of nurses per bed was associated with increased incidence of DFLST, while availability of an emergency department in the same hospital, presence of a full time ICU-specialist and doctors presence during nights and week-ends were associated with a decreased incidence of DFLST.

Conclusion.—This large study identifies structural variables that are associated with substantial variations in the incidence and the characteristics of decisions to forgo life-sustaining therapies.

▶ The Simplified Acute Physiology Score III (SAPS 3) Outcomes Research Group is an organized front involved in laying down internationally recognized guidelines for betterment of ICU performances through observational studies. This study is a part of the same agenda and the investigators aimed to look at the incidence and presence of previously unidentified predictors and variables playing a role in decisions to forgo life-sustaining therapies (DFLSTs) at system and organizational level. It was seen that more deaths occurred once the DFLST was made, which has also been proven by past studies. The characteristics that decreased the likelihood of DFLSTs included factors such as a higher nurse-per-patient ratio, the presence of in-house intensivists during nights and week-ends, among others, while those that increased the likelihood of DFLSTs were hospitals without emergency departments, smaller ICUs, and large number of physicians per ICU bed. Studies done in the past, like the ETHICUS study[1] and others, have already demonstrated associations of chronic comorbid conditions, severity of disease, mechanical ventilator dependence, and patient's cultural and regional background with increased incidence of DFLSTs. This study, through its meticulous data collection and variation analysis, was successful in outlining many previously unknown factors that play a role in

DFLSTs. The number of nurses and physicians, observation of disparity between weekends and weekdays, and many other organizational and system-related factors seem intriguing for their statistical difference between the groups. The study again confirmed that physicians are more comfortable withholding treatment than withdrawing the treatment. Increased ICU mortality on withdrawing may be interpreted as futile care. However, another follow-up study would need to be planned to question why these characteristics would affect the decisions made in the ICU for these sick and vulnerable patients.

The big debate about DFLSTs has been regarding the ethical viewpoint. The popular thought, with which this reviewer concurs, is that modifying a health care setting to increase or decrease the possibility of an event such as DFLST would hardly be morally acceptable. In the United States many of the DFLST decisions are based on availability of advance directives and living wills and discussions with surrogate heath care proxy or family members with substitute judgments. The proactive role of ethics committees and socioethical and legal laws may have impact on this result and the difference between the United States and European countries. The decision to forgo treatment should always be individualized to the particular patient and should not be generalized on a population as a whole. In summary, though this study interestingly focuses on multitudinous factors influencing DFLSTs, tipping the scales one way or another by their implementation would add the unnecessary burden of costs to a health care setting and at the same time create ethical dilemmas for physicians.

V. Punjabi, MD

V. K. Rajput, MD

Reference

1. Sprung CL, Woodcock T, Sjokvist P, et al. Reasons, considerations, difficulties and documentation of end-of-life decisions in European intensive care units: the ETHI-CUS study. *Intensive Care Med.* 2008;34:271-277 [erratum in: *Intensive Care Med* 2008; 34:392-393].

Mandatory Ethics Consultation Policy
Romano ME, Wahlander SB, Lang BH, et al (Columbia Univ, NY; et al)
Mayo Clin Proc 84:581-585, 2009

Objective.—To describe ethics consultations at a single institution that has a mandatory ethics consultation policy.

Patients and Methods.—We retrospectively reviewed the medical records of all adult patients who were admitted to the Intensive care unit at Columbia University Medical Center and had an ethics consultation between August 1, 2006, and July 31, 2007. All mandatory and non-mandatory ethics consultations were reviewed. Patient diagnosis, prognosis, presence of do-not-resuscitate order, presence of written advance directives, reason for the ethics consultation, and survival data were collected. The number of ethics consultations hospital-wide from January 1, 2000, to December 31, 2007, was collected.

Results.—The total number of mandatory and nonmandatory ethics consultations requested was 168. Of these consultations, 108 (64%) were considered mandatory, and 60 (36%) were considered nonmandatory. Between January 1, 2000, and December 31, 2007, the total number of ethics consultations increased 84%.

Conclusion.—The increase in the total number of ethics consultations is interpreted as a positive outcome of the mandatory policy. The mandatory ethics consultation policy has possibly increased exposure to ethics consultant-physician interactions, increased learning for physicians, and raised awareness among physicians and nurses of potential ethics assistance.

▶ Although no one can absolutely determine the benefit or harm of an extra day or 2 days for a terminally ill patient in the intensive care unit, there should be a 1- to 2-day time period that is identifiable in most patients as a time when those involved in the care of the patient determine that continued medical intervention is not going to alter outcome of a patient. The main problem that arises is when the personal beliefs and values of physicians and other health care workers cloud their ability to make the right decision for that patient with or without an advance directive and health care proxy. There is constant tension between patient autonomy and beneficence. Ethics consultation is a tool to ensure its preservation and optimal balance. These consultations help ICU physicians and families cope with any dilemma that may arise. As noted in the article, ICU physicians must manage 2 important aspects of patient care: provide life-sustaining care and provide the patient and family the opportunity to discuss issues such as end-of-life care and life support considerations. To provide patients and families the chance to discuss their thoughts as well as physicians to ensure those under their care are provided ample time to express their concerns, Columbia University Medical Center began a policy for mandatory ethical consultations when dealing with certain patient situations, mainly withdrawal or withholding of life support.

In this study, the total number of ethics consults increased by 84% over 6 to 7 years. The study determined that this large increase in the number of consultations was a positive outcome of having a mandatory ethics consultation policy. However, the results would have appeared more promising if there was an increase in nonmandatory consultations as opposed to the total number of nonmandatory and mandatory consults. A large increase would have represented the valuable information and education physicians and other health care professionals received during mandatory consults and hence, their increased inclination to order nonmandatory consults. No other available study has been published that provides information about ethics consultations that are mandatory. An abundance of literature exists in favor of ethics consultations to be instituted as a standard and common method in the ICU and throughout the hospital. A 2003 study published in the *Journal of the American Medical Association* suggested that patient surrogates, physicians, and other health care workers found ethics consultations to be helpful and would request/order consultations in the future. The randomized control trial found that 80% of the 108 patient/patient surrogates interviewed a few weeks after an ethics consultation responded that they "agreed or strongly agreed that they would seek them [ethics consultations] again and recommend them to others."[1] The same study also found that there was no difference in mortality between those who received consults and those who didn't but that there was a "significant reduction in likely nonbeneficial treatments." Total hospital days, days spent in the ICU, and days receiving ventilation were also decreased. In another study, the same researchers found that there was a significant cost reduction of about $150000 for a 40-bed ICU for 50 enrolled patients.[2] Along with the satisfaction and cost decreases gained from ethics consultations, a study at the Mayo Clinic noted that frequent ethics consultations led to further education of health care employees and reported 70% of the ethical dilemmas were resolved by consultations, without the need to assemble a full multidisciplinary review team.[3] Correspondingly, the article under discussion similarly noted that ethics consultation "has possibly increased exposure to ethics consultant-physician interactions, increased learning for physicians, and raised awareness among physicians and nurses of potential ethics assistance." Knowledge gained by health care workers may prevent conflict and lead to swift resolution in patient care.

This study and many others are simply suggesting that patients, their families, physicians, and others should be given the opportunity to discuss the situation thoroughly and constantly in real time with the added perspective of an outside neutral facilitator in the form of an ethics consultation. All health care employees and their patients or patient surrogates have been found to think these consultations are beneficial. Although not mandatory in most places, ethics consultations are slowly becoming the standard in the hospital setting when ethical dilemmas arise.

R. Parekh, BA, BS

V. K. Rajput, MD

References

1. Schneiderman LJ, Gilmer T, Teetzel HD, et al. Effect of ethics consultations on nonbeneficial life-sustaining treatment in the intensive care unit: a randomized controlled trial. *JAMA*. 2003;290:1166-1172.
2. Gilmer T, Schneiderman LJ, Teetzel H, et al. The costs of nonbeneficial treatment in the intensive care setting. *Health Aff (Millwood)*. 2005;24:961-971.
3. Swetz K, Crowley ME, Hook C, Mueller P. Report of 255 clinical ethics consultations and review of the literature. *Mayo Clin Proc*. 2007;82:686-691.

Admission of incompetent patients to intensive care: Doctors' responsiveness to family wishes

Escher M, Perneger TV, Heidegger CP, et al (Geneva Univ Hosps, Switzerland)
Crit Care Med 37:528-532, 2009

Objective.—When a patient is incompetent, the family is often considered to be a natural surrogate. The doctors' responsiveness to family wishes may vary. We explored if doctors' personal characteristics were associated with responsiveness to the relatives' wishes when admission to the intensive care unit (ICU) is considered.

Methods.—In a mail survey, we asked all Swiss ICU doctors to decide on the admission of a hypothetical incompetent patient presenting with hemolytic uremic syndrome. Each participant was randomly allocated to a version of the scenario in which the family asked either that "everything be done" or that the patient be "spared useless suffering."

Main Results.—Overall, 232 (60.9%) questionnaires were returned. When the family asked that "everything be done," 60% of doctors chose to admit the hypothetical patient, but when the family asked that she be spared useless suffering, only 39% did so (odds ratio [OR] 2.6, confidence interval 1.5–4.6). This OR captures responsiveness to family wishes. It varied across subgroups of ICU doctors. Characteristics associated with greater responsiveness to family wishes were older age (OR 6.0 vs. 1.2, $p = 0.002$), nonuniversity work setting (OR 4.2 vs. 1.0, $p = 0.012$), less time devoted to intensive care practice (OR 4.0 vs. 1.5, $p = 0.036$), and greater self-confidence in ethical knowledge (OR 3.4 vs. 1.7, $p = 0.044$).

Conclusions.—Older doctors and those working in regional hospitals were more responsive to family wishes when assessing an incompetent patient for ICU admission. These findings emphasize the need for effective advance care planning.

▶ Medical care in any era and in any location is a function not only of the state of medical science, but also of the social, political, and economic system in which it exists. Ethical issues in hospital medicine have unique concerns because of their clinical setting. These include the need for rapid decision making that is often based on incomplete information and the difficulty in establishing trust when there is lack of a previous patient-physician relationship. When it comes to making medical decisions for incompetent patients, physicians often rely on the patient's family to guide their assessments. Overall, the study found that senior doctors, those who worked in a nonuniversity setting and those who spent 50% or less of their time in ICU practice, were more responsive to the family's wishes.

The authors wanted to explore the personal characteristics of physicians involved in decision making. It is difficult to believe that a dichotomous "yes" or "no" answer to a hypothetical case would reflect the reality of clinical reasoning a physician conducts when dealing with the complexities of a real patient with a myriad of complex clinical factors and emotional family input. Physicians are influenced by their own ethical and legal knowledge about medical decision making. For example, another international study similarly analyzed physician characteristics that influenced decision making across 7 countries, and found that United States physicians chose the more aggressive options when given a clinical vignette with an incompetent patient. They also found that, overall, older physicians were still more likely to choose less aggressive options.[1] This is interesting because in the United States, where shared decision making is increasingly valued and family relatives are frequently relied upon as next of kin when patients are incompetent, one might suspect that younger physicians trained in a new cultural era would be more likely to work with family wishes. Of course, this trend may be due to other factors, such as older physicians having increased years of medical experience, which often provides more confidence in personal medical decisions when choosing alternative, more conservative treatment options.

Mental capacity can change over time. Physicians should do what they can to catch the patient in a lucid state—even lightening up on the medication if necessary—to include him or her in the decision-making process. Physicians may find it difficult to perform an unbiased capacity assessment, particularly when the patient's choice goes against their recommendations, but it is important to remember that the purpose of capacity assessment is to evaluate the person's ability to understand relevant information and to appreciate the consequences of a decision. Medical decision making is a difficult area to tangibly investigate, and physicians everywhere are faced with the task of balancing medical opinions with ethical ones that often involve family wishes. Overall, this study does well by bringing out awareness of both objective factors and personal biases that influence our decisions.

D. Doshi, BA

V. K. Rajput, MD

Reference

1. Alemayehu E, Molly DW, Guyatt GH, et al. Variability in physician's decisions on caring for chronically ill elderly patients: an international study. *CMAJ.* 1991;144:1133-1138.

Miscellaneous

Hospital Teaching Intensity, Patient Race, and Surgical Outcomes

Silber JH, Rosenbaum PR, Romano PS, et al (The Children's Hosp of Philadelphia; Univ of Pennsylvania; Univ of California Davis School of Medicine, Sacramento; et al)
Arch Surg 144:113-120, 2009

Objectives.—To determine if the lower mortality often observed in teaching-intensive hospitals is because of lower complication rates or lower death rates after complications (failure to rescue) and whether the benefits at these hospitals accrue equally to white and black patients, since black patients receive a disproportionate share of their care at teaching-intensive hospitals.

Design.—A retrospective study of patient outcomes and teaching intensity using logistic regression models, with and without adjusting for hospital fixed and random effects.

Setting.—Three thousand two hundred seventy acute care hospitals in the United States.

Patients.—Medicare claims on general, orthopedic, and vascular surgery admissions in the United States for 2000-2005 (N = 4 658 954 unique patients).

Main Outcome Measures.—Thirty-day mortality, in-hospital complications, and failure to rescue (the probability of death following complications).

Results.—Combining all surgeries, compared with non-teaching hospitals, patients at very major teaching hospitals demonstrated a 15% lower odds of death (P < .001), no difference in complications, and a 15% lower odds of death after complications (failure to rescue) (P < .001). These relative benefits associated with higher resident-to-bed ratio were not experienced by black patients, for whom the odds of mortality and failure to rescue were similar at teaching and nonteaching hospitals, a pattern that is significantly different from that of white patients (P < 001).

Conclusions.—Survival after surgery is higher at hospitals with higher teaching intensity. Improved survival is because of lower mortality after complications (better failure to rescue) and generally not because of fewer complications. However, this better survival and failure to rescue at teaching-intensive hospitals is seen for white patients, not for black patients.

▶ Studies supported by the Agency for Healthcare Research and Quality (AHRQ) report racial disparities in patient care, including conditions such as heart disease, asthma, breast cancer, human immunodeficiency virus (HIV) infection, and nursing home care.[1] Eliminating racial and ethnic disparities in health care with a focus on access to high-quality care has continued to gain attention within the United States government. The questions that will need to be addressed are in part related to differences in access, hospital characteristics, insurance status, and strategies for improvement. Silber and colleagues set out to determine whether there were outcome differences in teaching versus nonteaching hospitals and whether or not there were any racial differences associated with these outcomes. In this 5-year retrospective study, including more than 4.5 million Medicare surgical patients admitted for general orthopedic and vascular surgery from more than 3200 acute care hospitals, the authors sought to measure outcomes of 30-day mortality, in-hospital complications, and failure to rescue, resulting in death. In this study, unadjusted outcomes by race and teaching intensity find higher mortality and complications in black patients compared with white patients. The authors report a significant finding of the lower mortality rate in surgical patients was mainly due to fewer deaths among patients having experienced a postoperative complication (ie, failure to rescue). However, white patients had lower mortality and failure to rescue rates at teaching-intensive hospitals than in black patients. As the authors indicate, other studies have found similar results of lower risk-adjusted mortality after major surgery in hospitals with higher teaching intensity (using the resident-to-bed ratio). The findings in this study do not fully explain why this racial disparity exists in this patient population. Unending effort in health care outcomes research will continue to be great interest and importance as we search for additional answers.

C. A. Schorr, RN, MSN

Reference

1. *Addressing Racial and Ethnic Disparities in Health Care Fact Sheet. AHRQ Publication No. 00-PO41.* Rockville, MD: Agency for Healthcare Research and Quality; February 2000. http://www.ahrq.gov/research/disparit.htm. Accessed September 30, 2009.

A 'shock room' for early management of the acutely ill

Piagnerelli M, Van Nuffelen M, Maetens Y, et al (Université Libre de Bruxelles, Brussels, Belgium)
Anaesth Intensive Care 37:426-431, 2009

Our 850-bed, academic, tertiary care hospital uses a four-bed dedicated 'shock room' situated between the Departments of Emergency Medicine and Intensive Care to stabilise all acutely ill patients from outside or inside the hospital before transfer to the intensive care unit or other department. Admitted patients stay a maximum of four hours in the shock room. In this article we describe our experiences using this shock room by detailing the demographic data, including time and source of admission, diagnosis and outcome, for the 2514 patients admitted to the shock room in 2006. The most common reasons for admission were cardiac (33%) and neurological (21%) diagnoses. After diagnosis and initial treatment, 54% of patients were transferred to an intensive care unit or a coronary care unit; 2.5% of patients died in the shock room. The shock room provides a useful area of collaboration between emergency department and intensive care unit staff and enables acutely ill patients to be assessed and treated rapidly to optimise outcomes.

▶ Aggressive resuscitation and appropriate antimicrobial administration have contributed to a systematic management approach of acutely ill septic shock patients. This early delivery of timely care has been demonstrated to improve outcomes.[1-3] Coordinating a unit capable of early patient identification, diagnosis, and initiation of effective treatment enables optimization of care for the critically ill patient. In this descriptive one-year study by Piagnerelli and colleagues, they report their experience of using a shock room as an environment for both the emergency department and intensive care unit staff to assess and treat patients requiring acute stabilization. This report found that the shock room provided the benefit of rapid diagnosis and management and facilitated appropriate admission to the ICU. Important but not so surprising findings of this program were decreased time to central line catheter placement, first antibiotic administration, fluid administration, and ICU admission. The authors present an interesting concept, but the value of such a system would require a study with a comparative group. Although the authors report that with this type of study it would be hard to demonstrate an outcome improvement, there is a cost for establishing such a program, and an association with improved outcomes may support institutions considering using a similar dedicated unit. The remaining question for the clinician may be, should we take our team to the patient or bring the patient to the team? Whether we determine that a rapid response team or a shock room is more effective, collaboration among the emergency department and ICU staff is essential. Efforts such as the shock room may unite these 2 groups in caring for the acutely ill patients and foster teamwork. The successful interaction may promote additional projects and joint protocols, leading to more efficient and effective treatment within the institution.

C. A. Schorr, RN, MSN

References

1. Rivers E, Nguyen B, Havstad S, et al, Early Goal-Directed Therapy Collaborative Group. Early goal-directed therapy in the treatment of severe sepsis and septic shock. *N Engl J Med.* 2001;345:1368-1377.
2. Kumar A, Ellis P, Arabi Y, et al. Initiation of inappropriate antimicrobial therapy results in a 5-fold reduction of survival in human septic shock. *Chest.* 20 August 2009; [Epub ahead of print].
3. Rivers EP, McIntyre L, Morro DC, Rivers KK. Early and innovative interventions for severe sepsis and septic shock: taking advantage of a window of opportunity. *CMAJ.* 2005;173:1054-1065.

Admission of incompetent patients to intensive care: Doctors' responsiveness to family wishes

Escher M, Perneger TV, Heidegger CP, et al (Geneva Univ Hosps, Switzerland)
Crit Care Med 37:528-532, 2009

Objective.—When a patient is incompetent, the family is often considered to be a natural surrogate. The doctors' responsiveness to family wishes may vary. We explored if doctors' personal characteristics were associated with responsiveness to the relatives' wishes when admission to the intensive care unit (ICU) is considered.

Methods.—In a mail survey, we asked all Swiss ICU doctors to decide on the admission of a hypothetical incompetent patient presenting with hemolytic uremic syndrome. Each participant was randomly allocated to a version of the scenario in which the family asked either that "everything be done" or that the patient be "spared useless suffering."

Main Results.—Overall, 232 (60.9%) questionnaires were returned. When the family asked that "everything be done," 60% of doctors chose to admit the hypothetical patient, but when the family asked that she be spared useless suffering, only 39% did so (odds ratio [OR] 2.6, confidence interval 1.5–4.6). This OR captures responsiveness to family wishes. It varied across subgroups of ICU doctors. Characteristics associated with greater responsiveness to family wishes were older age (OR 6.0 vs. 1.2, $p = 0.002$), nonuniversity work setting (OR 4.2 vs. 1.0, $p = 0.012$), less time devoted to intensive care practice (OR 4.0 vs. 1.5, $p = 0.036$), and greater self-confidence in ethical knowledge (OR 3.4 vs. 1.7, $p = 0.044$).

Conclusions.—Older doctors and those working in regional hospitals were more responsive to family wishes when assessing an incompetent patient for ICU admission. These findings emphasize the need for effective advance care planning.

▶ Do you hear what I hear? Listening is the first skill we learn as a child and is often ignored in genuine family communication encounters. Critically ill patients presenting to the ICU are often incapable of making decisions, due to therapies surrounding their severe illness, and rely on their relatives to make decisions on their behalf. When an incompetent critically ill patient presents to the ICU, do doctors really listen and follow the family's request to continue with aggressive care or maintain comfort for their loved one, or is it a dialog, with the doctor ultimately making the final decision? In this study by Escher, Swiss Society of Intensive Care Medicine doctors were sent an anonymous questionnaire using a hypothetical incompetent patient scenario. Each participant was given 1 of 8 randomly allocated versions of the questionnaire. The study was designed to have half of the physicians receive a version where the relatives wanted everything done and half asked that the patient be spared needless suffering. Despite a low return rate, the study has identified several characteristics worth discussion. The results of this study report that younger doctors were more likely to disregard the family wishes. In contrast, a doctor with confidence in his or her ethical knowledge was associated with a greater responsiveness to the relatives' request. This confidence may come with education and experience and may also come with age. In a study by Curtis et al, missed opportunities at the end of life were recognized as a failure to listen, respond, and provide emotional support to families.[1] Listening is an art in those who do it well, making every effort to hear something. Mastering active listening takes into account not only the words but also how they are said, including nonverbal cues. Perhaps doctors with confidence can educate those who have yet to master the skill of active listening, ensuring that our patients' voices are heard through the words of their loved ones.

C. A. Schorr, RN, MSN

Reference

1. Curtis JR, Engelberg RA, Wenrich MD, Shannon SE, Treece PD, Rubenfeld GD. Missed opportunities during family conferences about end-of-life care in the intensive care unit. *Am J Respir Crit Care Med.* 2005;171:844-849.

Survey of First-Year Medical Students to Assess Their Knowledge and Attitudes Toward Organ Transplantation and Donation

Mekahli D, Liutkus A, Fargue S, et al (Hôpital Edouard-Herriot and Université Lyon 1, France)
Transplant Proc 41:634-638, 2009

Background.—The important shortage of organ donors is still a fundamental public health problem in France. Improving the knowledge and attitudes of health care professionals could help to promote organ donation. The aim of this survey was to evaluate the level of knowledge of medical students and their gaps about organ donation prior to any medical course.

Materials and Methods.—A survey was conducted among 571 first-year medical students at a medical faculty in Lyon. Their knowledge, attitudes, personal views, and perceptions toward organ donation and transplantation were investigated prior to any medical course. A 31-item anonymous questionnaire including queries about personal views of organ donation, factual knowledge, and awareness of French law was distributed to the students.

Results.—To "willingness to donate a kidney to a relative," 97.7% of respondents consented, 0.9% objected, and 1.4% did not answer. Their attitudes toward cadaveric organ donation were different: 81.1% agreed, 13.5% refused, and 5.4% did not answer. Regarding their knowledge about which organs could be transplanted, 95% of the respondents were aware of the possibility to transplant a face and 14% thought that xenotransplantation was performed nowadays.

Conclusions.—First-year medical students have a good knowledge level regarding the organ donation and transplantation system prior to their medical course. Some gaps remain which could be improved. The results of this study supported a greater emphasis on providing information regarding transplantation in medical schools to improve the knowledge of future health care professionals. A follow-up survey of the participants at the end of their medical course will be interesting to assess the progress of their attitudes.

▶ When patients present with failing organs, transplantation from living or deceased donors offers the best possibility for survival and decreased future morbidity as well as enhanced cost-effectiveness for all parties involved. However, there remains an enormous difference between the supply of organs and the demand for organs despite various efforts to decrease the incongruity. Strategies varying from laws in place for presumed consent, which allows organs to be used if there are no previous written objections, to further education of medical personnel in the field of transplantation have been used to increase the donation rate. This study examined the knowledge and attitudes of medical students before any didactic training in different parts of transplantation. A study conducted in Italy in 2005 showed that there was no difference in organ donation and transplantation knowledge among 5 different fields:

medicine, agricultural, veterinary medicine, educational sciences, and psychology.[1]

Overall, the study found that the medical students had "relatively good knowledge about organ donation and transplantation" and therefore they could be used as future avenues of information for organ donors. However, the study could have been strengthened if it were to show if these students would gain more knowledge about transplantation as they progressed through medical school and if afterward they would still be more inclined to encourage their patients about donation as an Italian study showed in 2005.[2] There was a national campaign in 2006 to educate the French population about transplantation, and this may have influenced the selected students. In the United States, a survey administered to first- and second-year students showed significant gaps in knowledge regarding organ donation and transplantation and suggested further education should be instilled in medical school curriculums.[3] There were major knowledge gaps when physicians and nurses were surveyed in 2008 in Qatar, identifying definite areas where education may be useful.[4] More importantly, not all physicians were willing to donate organs themselves, which poses the question, is it fair for a physician to tell patients to donate organs when they themselves would not donate? It seems from these studies that having increased transplantation knowledge or being more educated in general does not necessarily translate into physicians suggesting and educating patients in the future.

Although informative, the study could be expanded to include a concomitant survey of fourth-year medical students from the same schools to view the knowledge gained after didactic and clinical teaching and assess if there are possible areas for improvement. Studies regarding physician attitudes and knowledge should also be assessed to observe current methods of practice. The ethical issues intertwined with organ transplantation are extensive. Informed versus presumed consent and personal physician attitudes versus practiced physician attitudes are 2 areas of consideration. These areas hold enormous potential in increasing the donation rates and increasing the amount of lives saved every year.

R. Parekh, BA, BS
V. K. Rajput, MD

References

1. Canova D, De Bona M, Rimunati R, Ermani M, Naccarato R, Burra P. Understanding of and attitudes to organ donation and transplantation: a survey among Italian university students. *Clin Transplant*. 2006;20:307-312.
2. Burra P, De Bona D, Canova M, et al. Changing attitude to organ donation and transplantation in university students during the years of medical school in Italy. *Transplant Proc*. 2005;37:547-550.
3. Essman C, Thorton J. Assessing medical student knowledge, attitudes and behaviors regarding organ donation. *Transplant Proc*. 2006;38:2745-2750.
4. Bener A, El-Shoubaki H, Al-Maslamani Y. Do we need to maximize the knowledge and attitude of physician and nurses toward organ donation and transplant? *Exp Clin Tranplant*. 2008;6:249-253.

Non–Heart-Beating Donors: An Inquiry to ICU Nurses in a Belgian University Hospital

Vincent J-L, Maetens Y, Vanderwallen C, et al (Université Libre de Bruxelles, Brussels, Belgium)
Transplant Proc 41:579-581, 2009

Demand for organs for transplantation continues to be greater than supply. Non–heart-beating donation (NHBD) has been reintroduced to reverse this trend. We describe the findings of a short questionnaire that determined the attitudes and feelings of nursing staff in a department of intensive care with an established NHBD program. Despite several educational sessions, only 3% of the nurses thought they were adequately informed about NHBD. Thirty-eight percent of nurses were less comfortable with NHBD than with brain death organ donation. NHBD is an ethically controversial area but one that can improve organ availability for transplantation. Adequate education, ongoing audit, and full transparency are needed in units that use NHBD.

▶ The study involved a survey of intensive-care nurses in a Belgian University hospital regarding their understanding of and ethical beliefs about non-heart-beating donation (NHBD) or donation after cardiac death (DCD). Most nurses felt that they are not well informed about this procedure. The study revealed large differences in opinions about NHBD, including 27% reporting having no problem with the procedure and 33% being uncomfortable or very uncomfortable.

This study is from a single western European country with an ethnically homogenous population of nurses. It would have shown more insight into this complex ethical-moral conflict if nurses and other health professionals from a multicultural population had given their opinion, a problem that has also hampered previous studies.[1] On the contrary, an ethnically heterogeneous nursing population from California showed majority approval for DCD before and after an educational intervention.[2]

The most critical question in NHBD or DCD is the time between the withdrawal of cardiopulmonary support and the declaration of death. This question was not well answered as almost half of the nurses did not describe a difference between brain death and NHBD organ donation. Interestingly, only 50% believe that complete cardiorespiratory death is necessary for the initiation of organ donation. This reveals a lack of understanding of this complex ethical dilemma, further shown by the 97% of respondents who claimed they were not adequately informed about NHBD. Previous studies have shown that nurses can have effective roles in NHBD and DCD discussions with family if properly educated on the subject.[3,4]

The need for education on NHBD limits our conclusions about the ethical or moral issues surrounding NHBD for the nurses in this study. A follow-up survey of the nurses after more adequate instruction on this topic, and a survey with a deeper exploration of ethical-moral conflict in NHBD, will help us to provide more meaningful education to all health care professionals.

N. Samras, BSE, MPH
V. K. Rajput, MD

References

1. Kent B, Owens RG. Conflicting attitudes to corneal and organ donation: a study of nurses' attitudes to organ donation. *Int J Nurs Stud.* 1995;32:484-492.
2. Mathur M, Taylor S, Tiras K, Wilson M, Abd-Allah S. Pediatric critical care nurses' perceptions, knowledge, and attitudes regarding organ donation after cardiac death. *Pediatr Crit Care Med.* 2008;3:261-269.
3. Pelletier ML. The needs of family members of organ and tissue donors. *Heart Lung.* 1993;22:151-157.
4. Hannah S. Increasing awareness of tissue donation: in the non-heart beating donor. *Intensive Crit Care Nurs.* 2004;20:292-298.

The Interface of Law and Medical Ethics in Medical Intensive Care
Kapp MB (Southern Illinois Univ Schools of Medicine and Law, Carbondale)
Chest 136:904-909, 2009

The delivery of medical care in the intensive care setting is subject to various legal principles and processes, as well as important ethical precepts. This article outlines the basic medicine-law interface, explaining the concepts of medical jurisprudence and forensic medicine. It then provides fundamental information about the current American medical malpractice system, including a brief discussion of the elements of a medical malpractice claim, the public policy rationales and goals purportedly undergirding the system, and potential alternatives to the existing medical malpractice system in the United States. Recognizing that the challenge, in the entire range of intensive care as in other medical settings, is adhering in practice to ethical principles while at the same time trying to minimize the providers' possible exposure to legal risks, the article identifies a number of components to the art of delivering care ethically and effectively within a pervasive legal environment, as follows: interfacing positively with the institutional legal counsel and risk management departments; utilizing (as appropriate) clinical practice guidelines or parameters; and pursuing continuing medical-legal education.

▶ Marshall Kapp describes the interface of lawyers, doctors, evidence-based medicine, and defensive medicine. Ethics at the bedside of the critically ill patient is complex. Both law and ethics provide rules of conduct to follow. Law stems from legislative statues, administrative agency rules, or court decisions that often vary in different locales and are enforceable only in those jurisdictions where they prevail. Ethics incorporates the broad values and beliefs of correct conduct. Good ethics often makes good law, whereas good law does not necessarily make good ethics. Significant overlap exists between legal and ethical decision making. A key difference between ethics and law is that ethics relies heavily on the individual person's values. Even without formal training health care professional or intensivists can and often should make ethically sound decisions—what is best for the patient under the current known circumstances. It can be argued that the law is the common ethos for a pluralistic society like the United States, and that law and lawyers are what hold a pluralistic society together. It can be further argued that resolving controversial medical ethical issues has been the domain of American law, not philosophy or medicine, in particular when professional liability is involved. Unfortunately, the best legal medical decision may not be the best ethical decision.

A good relationship between physicians and the legal team is certainly helpful, both to relieve the concerns of the physicians and to flesh out issues before they become larger. Unfortunately, under the current construct of tort liability, to protect their clients (the physicians or hospitals), lawyers generally will advise their clients against ethical medicine in favor of defensive medicine, despite the fact that it serves neither the client nor the patient from the perspective of cost or comfort.

One of the traditional rationales for our system of professional tort liability, as noted by Kapps has been to encourage physicians and others to provide quality care, to prevent digressions, and to improve quality of care in the future. Today, however, many other mechanisms have been developed to provide the deterrence function and to make health care quality much more transparent. Hospitals are required to report serious preventable incidents and numerous quality core measures to state and federal agencies. Much of this data is publicly available and, more importantly, easily available on the Internet. Further, governmental and private payors are increasingly requiring reporting of certain surgical events, such as wrong-site surgery and certain hospital-acquired conditions and refusing payment for treatment for such conditions.

Some lawyers have argued that all this reporting and public availability of such data relieves important privileges and could disadvantage physicians and hospitals in malpractice claims. Nevertheless, given the transparency demanded in so many professions and their representative organizations, it seems indisputable that transparency is the future. The question is how this might affect medical ethics and tort liability.

One might suggest that these quality and incident reporting mechanisms are at least as effective at providing the deterrence function as a single malpractice lawsuit. If that is the case, have we evolved to a point where we are able to look at professional tort liability differently, in a fashion that will provide for some level of compensation for patients who are subjected to a medical mistake, while recognizing that we now have a better method of deterrence: Can we achieve effective quality transparency while avoiding what many would perceive as inappropriately high jury verdict financial awards? If so, we can remove from tort liability the stick of deterrence, doctors can focus best practice congruent with the quality reporting measures, and the reliance on defensive medicine and potentially excessive testing and treatment can be reduced.

S. M. Dostmann, JD
V. K. Rajput, MD

13 Pharmacology/ Sedation-Analgesia

Randomized trial of light versus deep sedation on mental health after critical illness

Treggiari MM, Romand J-A, Yanez ND, et al (Univ of Washington, Seattle; Univ of Geneva, Switzerland)
Crit Care Med 37:2527-2534, 2009

Objectives.—To investigate if light sedation favorably affects subsequent patient mental health compared with deep sedation. Symptoms of posttraumatic stress disorder are common in patients after they have undergone prolonged mechanical ventilation and are associated with sedation depth.

Design.—Randomized, open-label, controlled trial.

Setting.—Single tertiary care center.

Patients.—Adult patients requiring mechanical ventilation.

Interventions.—Patients were randomized to receive either light (patient awake and cooperative) or deep sedation (patient asleep, awakening upon physical stimulation).

Measurements and Main Results.—Self-reported measures of posttraumatic stress disorder, anxiety, and depression were collected at intensive care unit discharge and 4 wks later. The primary outcomes were symptoms of posttraumatic stress disorder, anxiety, and depression 4 wks after intensive care unit discharge.

A total of 137 patients were assigned to either the light (n = 69) or the deep sedation (n = 68) group. Seven patients withdrew consent and one patient was randomized in error, leaving 129 patients (n = 65 in light sedation and n = 64 in deep sedation) available for analysis. At the 4-wk follow-up, patients in the deep sedation group tended to have more posttraumatic stress disorder symptoms ($p = .07$); the deep sedation group had more trouble remembering the event (37% vs. 14%; $p = .02$) and more disturbing memories of the intensive care unit (18% vs. 4%; $p = .05$). Patients in the light sedation group had an average one day less being ventilated and 1.5 fewer days in the intensive care unit. There were no differences between the two groups in the occurrence of anxiety and depression, and also no difference in mortality or in the incidence of adverse events.

Conclusions.—These data suggest that a strategy of light sedation affords benefits with regard to reduction of intensive care unit stay and duration of ventilation without negatively affecting subsequent patient mental health or patient safety.

▶ I can remember during my critical care training that deep sedation was the norm. This was before the days of "sedation vacations." It was unfortunately not unusual that some caregiver would, on a particular day, have the insight in an unresponsive patient to stop benzodiazepines and find that not only did it have no effect on the patient, but also the patient remained deeply sedated, and with the sedation off it was still days before the patient aroused. We have come a long way since then with "sedation vacations," but we are still learning that, as with many things in life, less is better. This article supports light sedation. On several recent occasions I have challenged my ICU fellow to see if by the end of our week's rotation he or she can have everybody off of benzodiazepines.

R. P. Dellinger, MD

Article Index

Chapter 1: Airways/Lungs

Chapter 2: Cardiovascular

Chapter 3: Hemodynamics and Monitoring

Chapter 4: Burns

Chapter 5: Infectious Disease

Chapter 6: Postoperative Management

Chapter 7: Sepsis/Septic Shock

Chapter 9: Renal

Chapter 10: Trauma and Overdose

Chapter 11: Neurologic: Traumatic and Non-traumatic

Chapter 12: Ethics/Socioeconomic/Administrative Issues

Chapter 13: Pharmacology/Sedation-Analgesia

Author Index